Transformational Tool Kit for Front Line Nurses

Editor

FRANCISCA CISNEROS FARRAR

NURSING CLINICS
OF NORTH AMERICA

www.nursing.theclinics.com

Consulting Editor
STEPHEN D. KRAU

March 2015 • Volume 50 • Number 1

ELSEVIER

1600 John F. Kennedy Boulevard • Suite 1800 • Philadelphia, Pennsylvania, 19103-2899

http://www.theclinics.com

NURSING CLINICS OF NORTH AMERICA Volume 50, Number 1
March 2015 ISSN 0029-6465, ISBN-13: 978-0-323-35660-2

Editor: Kerry Holland
Developmental Editor: Casey Jackson

Nursing Clinics of North America (ISSN 0029-6465) is published quarterly by Elsevier Inc., 360 Park Avenue South, New York, NY 10010-1710. Months of issue are March, June, September, and December. Periodicals postage paid at New York, NY and additional mailing offices. Subscription price per year is, $150.00 (US individuals), $400.00 (US institutions), $275.00 (international individuals), $488.00 (international institutions), $220.00 (Canadian individuals), $488.00 (Canadian institutions), $85.00 (US students), and $135.00 (international students). To receive student/resident rate, orders must be accompanied by name of affiliated institution, date of term, and the signature of program/residency coordinator on institution letterhead. Orders will be billed at individual rate until proof of status is received. Foreign air speed delivery is included in all *Clinics* subscription prices. All prices are subject to change without notice. **POSTMASTER:** Send address changes to *Nursing Clinics*, Elsevier Health Sciences Division, Subscription Customer Service, 3251 Riverport Lane, Maryland Heights, MO 63043. **Customer Service: Telephone: 1-800-654-2452** (U.S. and Canada); **1-314-447-8871 (outside U.S. and Canada). Fax: 1-314-447-8029. E-mail: journalscustomerservice-usa@elsevier.com** (for print support) and **journalsonlinesupport-usa@elsevier.com** (for online support).

Nursing Clinics of North America is covered in *EMBASE/Excerpta Medica, MEDLINE/PubMed (Index Medicus), Social Sciences Citation Index, Current Contents, ASCA, Cumulative Index to Nursing, RNdex Top 100,* and Allied Health Literature and International Nursing Index (INI).

Contributors

CONSULTING EDITOR

STEPHEN D. KRAU, PhD, RN, CNE
Associate Professor, Vanderbilt University Medical Center, School of Nursing, Nashville, Tennessee

EDITOR

FRANCISCA CISNEROS FARRAR, EdD, MSN
Professor, School of Nursing, Austin Peay State University, Clarksville, Tennessee

AUTHORS

LINDA K. DARNELL, MSN, RN
Assistant Professor, School of Nursing, Austin Peay State University, Clarksville, Tennessee

DORIS DAVENPORT, DSN, RN, PNP
Professor, School of Nursing, Austin Peay State University, Clarksville, Tennessee

DEBORAH ELLISON, PhD, RN
Associate Professor, School of Nursing, Austin Peay State University, Clarksville, Tennessee

FRANCISCA CISNEROS FARRAR, EdD, MSN
Professor, School of Nursing, Austin Peay State University, Clarksville, Tennessee

AMANDA J. FLAGG, PhD, MSN, EdM, RN, ACNS-BC, CNE
Assistant Professor, School of Nursing, Middle Tennessee State University, Murfreesboro, Tennessee

KEMPA S. FRENCH, RN, MSN, FNP-BC
Associate Professor, School of Nursing, Austin Peay State University, Clarksville, Tennessee; Doctoral Student, College of Nursing, Medical University of South Carolina, Charleston, South Carolina

BETH HALLMARK, PhD, RN, MSN
Director of Simulation, Belmont University College of Health Sciences and Nursing, Nashville, Tennessee

KRISTEN HERSHEY, PhD(c), MSN, RN, CNE
Associate Professor, Austin Peay State University, Clarksville, Tennessee

SHONDELL V. HICKSON, DNP, APN, ACNS-BC, FNP-BC
Assistant Professor, School of Nursing, Austin Peay State University, Clarksville, Tennessee

ROBERT W. KOCH, DNSc, RN
Director of Professional Development, The West Cancer Center, Memphis, Tennessee

JODI KUSHNER, MSN, RN
Assistant Professor, School of Nursing, Austin Peay State University, Clarksville, Tennessee

STEPHEN W. LOMAX, RN, MBA, MSN
Retired Army Colonel, Assistant Professor, School of Nursing, Austin Peay State University, Clarksville, Tennessee

PATRICIA MECHAN, PT, MPH
Director, Consulting, Education, & Clinical Services, Guldmann, Belmont, Massachusetts

PATTY ORR, EdD, MSN, RN
Director School of Nursing, Chair of Excellence, Associate Professor, Austin Peay State University, Clarksville, Tennessee

LAURA D. OWENS, PhD, RN
Assistant Professor, Loewenberg School of Nursing, University of Memphis, Memphis, Tennessee

MARIA A. REVELL, PhD, MSN, RN, COI
Associate Professor, Division of Nursing, Tennessee State University, Nashville, Tennessee

EVE RICE, MSN, PNP
Assistant Professor, School of Nursing, Austin Peay State University, Clarksville, Tennessee

TASHA RUFFIN, MSN, RN
Assistant Professor, School of Nursing, Austin Peay State University, Clarksville, Tennessee

LYNNE SHORES, PhD, RN
Professor of Nursing, Belmont University College of Health Sciences and Nursing, Nashville, Tennessee

SHERRI STEVENS, PhD, RN
Associate Professor, Nursing, Middle Tennessee State University, Murfreesboro, Tennessee

DANIELLE WHITE, RN, MSN
Associate Professor, School of Nursing, Austin Peay State University, Clarksville, Tennessee

JUDY WOODWARD, MSN, RN
State Director for Quality Improvement, Department of Health, Nashville, Tennessee

Contents

This article provides a theoretic framework for culturally diverse practice, provides a model for developing cultural competency, and provides best-practice guidelines for conducting a cultural assessment on patients to identify their diverse needs to integrate into a patient-centered plan of care. The role of ethics is discussed to empower mutual respect, equality, and trust building in patients to promote positive health care outcomes. Cultural diversity tool kits from the National League for Nursing and the American Association of Colleges of Nursing are reviewed to provide educational resources to the front line nurse.

Health care in the United States is changing rapidly under pressure from both political and professional stakeholders, and one area on the front line of required change is the discipline of case management. Historically, case management has worked to defragment the health care delivery system for clients and increase access to health care. Case management will have an expanded role resulting from Affordable Care Act initiatives to improve health care. This article includes definitions of case management, current issues related to case management, case management standards of practice, and a case study of the management of pediatric chronic disease.

Preventing 30-day readmissions to hospitals is a top priority in the era of health care reform. New regulations will be costly to health care facilities because of payment guidelines. The most frequently readmitted medical conditions are acute myocardial infarction, heart failure, and pneumonia. The transition from the hospital and into the home has been classified as a vulnerable time for many patients. During this time of transition patients may fail to fully understand their discharge instructions. Ineffective communication, low health literacy, and compliance issues contribute to readmissions. Telehealth and the use of technology may be used to prevent some readmissions.

In this article, the principles behind high-reliability organizations and a culture of safety are explored. Three areas in which health care has the greatest potential for improvement in safety culture are also discussed: a nonpunitive response to error, handoffs and transitions, and safe staffing. Tools for frontline nurses to help improve their organization's culture of safety in these areas are reviewed. Information is also given for nurses responding to error, including participating in root-cause analysis and supporting health care workers involved in adverse events.

NURSING CLINICS OF NORTH AMERICA

DOWNLOAD Free App!

Review Articles THE CLINICS

NOW AVAILABLE FOR YOUR iPhone and iPad

Foreword

"Good Care, Good Science": A Mantra as We Move Toward Success

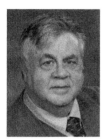

Stephen D. Krau, PhD, RN, CNE
Consulting Editor

The rate of major changes in the health care system has increased phenomenally in the last decade. Some changes seem here to stay, while others are deemed inadequate, useless, and to some extent, the award of political influence. For multiple reasons, the nursing professional is pivotal in the identification and support for outcomes related to these changes. Nurses traverse all dimensions of the health care system and various aspects of multiple patient populations. By number and expertise, nurses are integral to these changes and to the success of these changes.[1] While focusing on the care of patients and populations, and encountering new and deadly global challenges, it is easy to become diverted from the changes of health care delivery and the challenges they present. The complexity of nursing aligned with the uncertainty of the evolving health care system demands new thoughts, new models, and more and ongoing education.

Within this uncertainty, there are expectations that demand attention from leaders so that frontline nurses can deliver the quality of care that we have come to expect and deserve. To this end, it is clear that managers need to reevaluate their expectations of frontline nurses and are now tested not just to manage, but to lead. One element of this strategy demands that nurse managers need to work with frontline nurses to refine and narrow the scope of priorities,[2] as clearly articulated by Larkin and colleagues in "Good Care, Good Science."[2] The priorities must not only be clear and meaningful to frontline nurses but also should foster the ability of nurses at the bedside to prioritize evidence-based benchmarks and indicators, and implement evidence-based practices to produce quality outcomes.[2]

Although this may seem oversimplified, due to many factors, it is quite complex. Not only have priorities for many health care systems shifted, but also there has also been a change in science. As we discover new methods and new protocols, and with the

http://dx.doi.org/10.1016/j.cnur.2014.12.002
0029-6465/15/$ – see front matter
nursing.theclinics.com

discovery of new diseases, the context has morphed very much like an animal or plant. In addition, the rules, the foci, and the stakeholders seemed to have become unclear. This issue of *Nursing Clinics of North America* presents an array of articles to help the frontline nurse understand some of these changes and to help them find their roles, their duties, and their contributions to these ongoing shifts. In other words, to maintain quality, success, and "good care" by the use of "good science."

Stephen D. Krau, PhD, RN, CNE
Vanderbilt University Medical Center
School of Nursing
461 21st Avenue South
Nashville, TN 37240, USA

E-mail address:
steve.krau@vanderbilt.edu

REFERENCES

1. Carroll VS. Reimagining nursing quality in accountable care landscape. J Neurosci Nurs 2011;43:285.
2. Larkin JM, Lorenz H, Rack L, et al. Good care, good science: leveraging frontline staff for quality. Nurs Adm Q 2012;36:188–93.

Preface

Empowering Frontline Nurses for Success

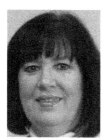

Francisca Cisneros Farrar, EdD, MSN
Editor

Health care reform and value-based care have transformed health care delivery models. Quality indicators and health care policies have been developed in response to value-based care to meet performance outcomes for full reimbursement. Frontline nurses are expected to meet benchmarks and develop plans of care to provide safe, quality, and accountable care. If benchmarks are not met, financial penalties can occur.[1] Most frontline nurses do not understand value-based care models and their role in promoting positive outcomes for reimbursement. They are not included in nurse executive meetings and are only told about changes in policies in unit meetings. Current challenging health care delivery models require clinical skills supported by evidence-based data. This issue of *Nursing Clinics of North America* serves as a best practice handbook for frontline nurses by providing resources to develop clinical skills needed for these new models of care.

The first series of articles provide a theoretical framework and resources to guide clinical practice. The article regarding embracing change discusses change to theories and charges to nurses from professional organizations that guide both transformational and incremental planned change. The article on evidence-based care demonstrates the role of research in providing a framework for useful protocols and guidelines to implement care activities. The article written about quality care indicators discusses key quality health organization and various measures of quality care as a framework for documenting quality patient care.

The second series of articles provide a tool kit and resources for clinical practice skills. The article written about communication skills points out that miscommunication is a major cause of errors. Shared governance models and interprofessional communication are practice models that offer ways of improving communication. The article on interprofessional collaborative care skills validates that frontline nurses must transition from working in a silo to working with an interprofessional team. The article provides a tool kit to develop interprofessional collaborative care skills. The article on

Nurs Clin N Am 50 (2015) xiii–xiv
http://dx.doi.org/10.1016/j.cnur.2014.12.001
0029-6465/15/$ – see front matter © 2015 Published by Elsevier Inc.

nursing.theclinics.com

the role of patient-centered care explores how this partnership is the key focus in providing quality health care and increasing patient satisfaction. The article concerning health literacy discusses using a universal approach as a tool for frontline nurses to assess patient concerns and preferences, comparing resources to identified needs, using teach-back to verify comprehension, and survey for other needs. The next article is about cultural competency prepares the frontline nurse for cultural care and provides a tool kit to develop cultural competency skills.

The article on case management empowers frontline nurses in the role of partnering with case management to provide quality and patient-centered care with the transition of the patient to the community. The following article about preventing 30-day readmission provides skills for discharge education and transitional care. The article on culture of safety explores the principles behind high-reliability organizations and culture of safety, focusing on three improvement areas for safety—a nonpunitive response to error, handoffs and transitions, and safe staffing. The article on ergonomics presents a tool kit to empower a culture of safety using the national standards for safe patient handling and mobility to prevent injury to frontline nurses and their patients. The article concerning healthy practice environment provides a tool kit to advocate for a healthy environment and lifestyle. The last article is about our growing aging population and provides a tool kit of gerontologic skills to meet the older adult's unique needs.

The cumulative articles in this issue can be used as a best practice handbook to meet the challenges of new health care delivery models. Theoretical frameworks are presented to provide the foundation for an evidence-based plan of care to meet quality indicator benchmarks. Frontline nurses can use the clinical skill tool kit as a supplement to develop clinical expertise needed to provide safe, quality, and accountable care.

Francisca Cisneros Farrar, EdD, MSN
Austin Peay State University School of Nursing
PO Box 4658
Clarksville, TN 37044, USA

E-mail address:
farrarf@apsu.edu

REFERENCE

1. Department of Health and Human Services Centers for Medicare and Medicaid Services. Hospital value-based purchasing from the Medicare learning network. Available at: http://www.cms.gov/Medicare. Accessed August 1, 2014.

Embracing Change

Patty Orr, EdD, MSN, RN, Doris Davenport, DSN, RN, PNP*

KEYWORDS

- Affordable care act • Care coordination • Change • Change theory • Employment
- Healthcare outcomes • Hospital readmissions • Institute of Medicine

KEY POINTS

- Nurses have an obligation to ensure that all care interventions are based on the latest evidence-based practice.
- All nurses need to learn how to develop leadership and innovation skills and to positively change nursing practice and contribute to cost-effective health care for populations.
- To ensure patients that the care given is evidence-based and current, nurses must be lifelong learners, and lifelong learning requires constant change and adaptation.
- Embracing change theory as a framework for effecting change at the bedside or at the organizational level will likely ensure success where failure is so often encountered.

INTRODUCTION

As a practicing nurse, there are many claims to how one spends professional work time and personal time, and the 2 options command strains in the decisions nurses make regarding professional and personal commitments of time and effort. The idea of being a change agent and thriving amidst change seems overwhelming at times. However, many changes are presently occurring in the United States that are affecting nurses' professional lives and require the nurse to be open to change. There are many driving forces presently in the evolving design and financing of health care that are impacting the need for change from nurses; these variables include a poor international ranking in quality of health care, professional education requirement goals issued by the Institute of Medicine (IOM), change in focus of care delivery models, the Affordable Care Act (ACA) implementation, quality assurance requirements and reporting responsibilities of quality metrics, and reimbursement for health care services. The time is now for nurses to be lifelong learners prepared for change and to serve as a change agent in any health care setting. All nurses need to learn

Disclosures: None.

School of Nursing, Austin Peay State University, 601 College Street, Clarksville, TN 37040, USA

* Corresponding author.

E-mail address: davenportd@apsu.edu

how to develop leadership and innovation skills and to positively change nursing practice and contribute to cost-effective health care for populations.

Nurses have an obligation to ensure that all care interventions are based on the latest evidence-based practice. To ensure patients that the care given is evidence-based and current, nurses must be lifelong learners, and lifelong learning requires constant change and adaptation. As the health care system is in a state of evolution, patients are expecting to be included in informed decision-making regarding their health care choices. Informed decision-making requires developing a relationship with patients so that the nurse can understand what is important and meaningful in each patient's life. Quality relationships with patients also assist patients to value their health status and to embrace behavior change that improves health status. This article describes the challenges and innovations that are presently emerging in the health care environment and prepares the nurse for thriving in the multiple settings where health care reform is occurring. The nurse is guided in using change theory to prepare professionally to meet the changing employment needs as a valued employee participating in the new care delivery models. Finally, the nurse is introduced to national efforts to improve quality and safety and is guided in instituting change processes that support the nurse in taking active involvement for contributing to the financial success of the enterprise where the nurse practices.

CHALLENGES THAT REQUIRE CHANGE BY NURSES

There are presently many challenges in health care in the United States that will demand nurses to embrace change as health care emerges into a more accountable system of care. A respected recent report ranks the United States last in quality when compared with 10 other western nations.[1] Although ranking last, the United States spent more than any of the other 10 nations. The United Kingdom spent $3405 per person on health care and the United States spent $8508; the United Kingdom ranked third in achieving certain health-related performance outcomes. The report stated that US providers have difficulty in sharing patient information and coordinating care dealing with administrative needs. Nurses can certainly contribute to coordinating care for patients and ensuring health-related information is shared between providers. Nursing must own the deficiencies in the US health care system and become a part of the solution.

The place of employment for nurses is gradually changing from the hospital as the central location to outpatient sites. Presently, approximately 60% of registered nurses (RNs) are employed in hospitals.[2] The Department of Labor expects the rate of employment in hospitals will slow, while increasing in outpatient settings.[3] More nursing services have increasingly transitioned to community, outpatient, and home settings. The Department of Labor projects RN employment to grow 19% from 2012 to 2022.[3] Uncertainty exists for nurses as hospitals face a shift from payment for number of admissions to payment for better quality and value.[4] According to Marilyn Tavenner, the Centers for Medicare and Medicaid Services (CMS) administrator, who is a nurse, both the outpatient and hospital areas of job opportunities for nurses will be related to ensuring improved quality, safety, and care coordination.[5] Nurses are critical for planning and executing effective discharge and transition from the hospital to alternate sites of care. To prevent readmissions, nursing skills in engaging patients and families in their health care before discharge and after discharge will be valued. Nurses also need to be looking at future trends in health care reform and plan for where jobs will grow based on the new incentives for providing preventive care interventions early in the care continuum.

Professional nurses often see change occurring in the setting where they work and practice nursing. The profession of nursing requires frequent change to be up-to-date in practicing evidence-based care interventions. In addition to providing evidence-based care, most nurses also face the need to change if they want to expand their careers and prepare to have the power to influence and transform the health care system. Expanding one's career opportunities often requires formal education and continuously learning and challenging oneself to grow and change to be viable in the emerging health care reform arena. Patients admitted to a hospital are there primarily for the interventions that nurses can provide. Independent of the setting, nurses are responsible in all settings for designing, leading, and asserting what needs to change so as to achieve measurable indicators of optimum quality care.

Nurses need to be prepared for and take advantage of the fundamental health care shift in who bears the risk for cost. Risk for cost is starting to shift to health providers and away from the insurers. Hospitals are needing to track and manage the patient's care to prevent readmissions, and to keep their patients healthy once discharged. Patients will need to be engaged with their providers, and the population will need evidence-based interventions that support the members to effectively execute their plan of care. Services will be required to be bundled, and revenues will likely be capped. Organizations will be rewarded for quality outcomes.[6] Under the CMS Hospital Valued-Based Purchasing Progam,[4] the hospital will lose revenue when demonstrating poor outcomes. Hospitals will more than ever need to actively manage their potential for profits and for losses. The changes should result in nurses asking: "What does this change in reimbursement for hospitals mean for me?" In simple terms it means that nurses will be valued when they are able to assist hospitals in achieving timely measurable health status improvement outcomes for patients. Nurses will have many opportunities to be a contributing part of a team that is incentivized to keep their population of patients healthy.

The Institute of Medicine Charge

In 2010, the IOM published a book entitled *The Future of Nursing: Leading Change, Advancing Health.*[7] The purpose of developing the book was to examine how the nursing profession could change from present status to building a better health care system. The report states that nurses must be prepared to "deliver patient-centered, equitable, safe, high-quality health care services; engage with physicians and other health care professionals to deliver efficient and effective care; and assume leadership roles in the redesign of the health care system."[7(xi)] The report proposes that the nursing profession must transform for nurses to assume roles that meet the health care needs of all of the US population. Nurses are at a challenging crossroad in their career where opportunities will increase for a nurse as a member of a health care team to be incentivized to keep large populations healthy and not needing as many costly disease management care interventions. To be effective in impacting better care delivery models, nurses must embrace change and take the crossroad that leads one to innovate in the delivery of care to patients. As included in the title of this landmark book, *The Future of Nursing: Leading Change, Advancing Health,*[7] the IOM is asking nurses to lead change.

Knowing the large numbers of nurses and their adaptive capacity for addressing change, the IOM recognizes nurses for their potential to transform the health care system. The IOM charges nurses to practice to the full extent of their education and training and asks nurses to achieve higher levels of education.[7] Nurses are being asked to contribute to improving the health of diverse US populations and to work as full partners with other health professionals to redesign health care in the United States. The IOM is asking nurses to embrace change, seeking further education to provide safe and quality health care, especially in public health, primary care, geriatrics, and in the community. Disease management and management of chronic disease are areas in which nurses are being asked to embrace so as to prevent exacerbations and disease progression, which are costly to the nation.

To achieve these changes and influence the transformation of health care, the nursing profession must produce leaders in all areas of nursing, including at the bedside. A nurse at the bedside or in the outpatient setting has the opportunity to shift some of the costs of inpatient care to more cost-effective outpatient care by helping people embrace wellness and self-care and lifestyle changes that promote health and prevent the development and/or slow the progression of chronic disease. Strong leadership, and care coordination competencies will result in nurses effectively addressing the varied needs of diverse populations, which will be needed to lead actions that improve access to care and promote effectiveness of care that drives improved patient outcomes. Leadership development achieved through education programs at all levels will be valued and sought in graduates that have furthered their nursing education. All nurses are asked to seek growth in their profession and develop partnerships inside and outside of the health care field.

Institute of Medicine and Transforming Practice

The key message by the IOM for transforming nursing practice is the challenge for nurses to "practice to the full extent of their education and training."[7(3–1)] However, there are many more messages under this message that gives nurses guidance on where they need to take action as they practice to the full extent possible. The IOM asks nurses to improve care by delivering more patient-centered care in the community and by providing primary care, rather than specialty care. This change in focus and setting will support prevention, quality improvement, and prevention of errors. The IOM believes nurses' versatility and skill set make them ready to address these changes of setting and focus of care.

As health care coverage improves with the ACA (2010), the nation will need to build a workforce with more primary care providers to meet the need for added access to care.[6] With population growth, an increase in people older than 65, and improved insurance coverage and access to care, it is projected that the United States will need 52,000 additional primary care physicians by 2025.[8] The American Medical Association states that there were only 246,090 primary care physicians in 2010 providing direct patient care.[8] Advance practice nurse practitioners will be part of the solution for providing access to primary care for many more Americans. Nurse practitioners play a critical role in providing primary care in the United States. In 2012 there were an estimated 154,000 licensed nurse practitioners and nearly half were practicing as a primary care provider.[9] A review of 26 studies published since 2000 found that the quality and outcomes of care from physician primary care providers and advance practice nurse practitioners to be similar.[10]

Research findings support that nursing care and leadership provided by RNs result in higher quality of care and improved safety.[11] Quality-improvement initiatives, such as interventions to prevent central line infections, which are led by nurses, result in reductions in infections. Having more RNs per patient, supportive leadership, and interprofessional relationships also lead to higher quality and safety in patient care delivery. Finally, RNs are successful in certain new models of care by providing chronic disease self-management instruction for patients and caregivers and by serving as care coordinators to help patients transition between care sites and providers.

The IOM in the *Future of Nursing*[7] gives nursing credit for improving the quality of care and safety for patients. Research has found that nurses are critical in leading the reduction of infection rates, preventing medication errors, and providing care interventions that prepare the patient for an effective transition to home and prevention of an unnecessary readmission.[7] The institution of many quality indicator programs has given nurses an opportunity to lead the achievement of improved patient outcomes by ensuring that systematic evidence-based processes that indicate optimum care are consistently defined, delivered, measured, evaluated, and reported. For health systems to achieve the highest quality of care, the providers need to embrace the nursing workforce as part of the solution for transforming health care.

Institute of Medicine and Transforming Nursing Education

Achieving higher levels of education was addressed in 2 of the IOM's *Future of Nursing* recommendations.[7] The first recommendation asks nursing to increase the number of nurses with a baccalaureate degree to 80% by 2020. The second recommendation is to double the number of nurses with a doctorate by 2020. The IOM makes the plea that "nursing education at all levels needs to provide better understanding of and experience in care management, quality-improvement methods, systems-level change management, and the reconceptualized roles of nurses in a reformed health care system".[7(4–1)] The case is made for nursing education to use formal education programs as the stage for seamless transition to achieving higher formal education goals and to learn to be a continual learner for life. The IOM report proclaims that entry-level nurses need to be ready to transition from their education program to many health care settings, with an increasing emphasis on students being prepared to function with competencies appropriate for community health facilities. The report emphasizes the need for entry-level nurses to have competencies in disease prevention, geriatrics, and health promotion in the outpatient setting, rather than primarily in providing care interventions in the acute care settings.

Bachelor of Science in Nursing (BSN) education was stressed as the necessary entry-level foundation for higher levels of evidence-based practice, teamwork, collaboration, and research. As nurses are being asked to have leadership skills for care coordination, the IOM report claimed that nurses need to have the competencies that are included in the American Association of Colleges of Nursing's *Essential of Baccalaureate Education for Professional Nursing Practice*.[12] More specifically, the report describes 3 prominent emerging expert skill sets that are needed from BSN graduates for achieving cost-effective high-quality care that drives optimum patient outcomes. The major 3 competency categories include (1) critical decision-making and use of technology to provide care interventions for complex and frail patients in the hospital setting; (2) ability to prevent acute care exacerbations and progression of disease by coordinating care and managing chronic disease in the outpatient setting; and (3) use of technology tools to provide effective quality care.

The IOM also recommended that all nurses engage in lifelong learning. For formal education to influence students to be lifelong learners, Orr and Ciampini[13] recommend that schools of nursing prepare BSN nurses to practice in evolving health care systems and community and public health settings during their BSN education. Formal nursing education can develop graduates that practice lifelong learning by providing students the opportunity to practice evidence-based care, execute research, and participate in interdisciplinary teamwork, collaboration, and care coordination while in school.[13]

Institute of Medicine Competency-Based Education

A discussion of competency-based education is included in the IOM report.[7] Traditional competencies and competencies needed for the reformed health care systems and changing environments of care delivery are outlined. This book discussed some of the traditional competencies, such as care management and coordination of care.[7] Added competencies include high-level decision-making, quality-improvement skills for achieving improved quality measurements and outcomes, systems thinking and development, and leadership skills for working in interprofessional teams.[7] The IOM encourages teaching that recognizes present competencies and ensures identified curriculum performance competencies are met. Education programs are encouraged to stress competencies that are clinically based and are essential for producing a graduate who has a skill set that is needed in the workforce. It is recommended that the focus be on high-level competencies, such as patient-centered decision-making skills that are applicable under many clinical scenarios in all care settings. In competency-based education, competencies are explicit to students, and students are required to demonstrate mastery in both theory and in simulation or at the clinical site of care.

Institute of Medicine Education for Advanced Practice Registered Nurses

The IOM report[7] describes the need for graduate-level advanced practice nurses who can practice as nurse practitioners and provide primary care, especially for underserved populations. With the US population needing more access to primary care, there is demand for building the primary care workforce, which includes nurse practitioners.[9] Job opportunities for nurse practitioners will grow as access to health care coverage increases with the ACA. According the Health Resources and Services Administration, there were 154,000 licensed nurse practitioners in 2012 and nearly half of nurse practitioners were working in primary care.[9] However, nurse practitioners certified in a primary care specialty included 76% of all nurse practitioners.[10] Nurse-managed health clinics using nurse practitioners offer career opportunities for nurses seeking change by advancing their education. Increased access to primary care is needed for individuals who in the past have not received access to care, especially care that focuses on wellness, prevention, and improved health status outcomes.

CHANGE IN REGISTERED NURSE EMPLOYMENT OPPORTUNITIES

The United States is presently experiencing a shift in the focus and location of health care for Medicare patients. The Medicare Payment Advisory Commission cites the goal of directing more resources to primary care.[14] The Commission explains that payment is being examined and promoted that will reward achieving population-based outcome measures that will result in improved prevention of hospital admissions for the population being managed. With the ACA's focus on prevention and population health, it is expected that the trend in movement from inpatient to outpatient and community services will increase.[14] Not only is the environment for nursing changing, the profession is poised for change. Each nurse must become tolerant of uncertainty, acknowledge the need for ongoing change, and realize that disruption can help a person move forward in his or her profession. When a person accepts disruption and change as a permanent part of life, one can embrace each new opportunity for growth.

Employment of RNs is projected to increase 19% from 2012 to 2022.[3] The projected increased growth in the need for RNs will occur for several reasons. The aging population with many more medical problems will increase, and this population will need more health services. RNs also will be needed to educate and support behavior change and self-care for patients with chronic conditions, such as diabetes, obesity, and heart disease. More health care initiatives will be focused on preventing and/or delaying progression of chronic disease as a result of federal health care reform. With the ACA, more individuals will have access to care and will need nursing care. With the Medicare Hospital Readmission Reduction Program, hospitals will need RNs to effectively provide discharge planning and follow-up care to prevent readmissions. These same patients will then seek care at outpatient centers, long-term care facilities and from home health services. The projected RN employment need represents a significant shift in employment opportunities from hospital to outpatient settings.

NATIONAL MOVEMENTS TO IMPACT HEALTH CARE OUTCOMES

Several national movements support and promote changes in the practice of nursing. In the hospital setting, the CMS Value-Based Purchasing Program defines quality indicators and outcomes that are expected with the Medicare population. The movement to assess, report, and improve indicators that represent the status of safety and quality of outcomes is prevalent in most health care delivery sites, including inpatient, outpatient, surgery centers, long-term care facilities, and hospice. Another national movement is the visionary actions being taken by the Institute for Healthcare Improvement (IHI). The IHI, founded by Dr Don Berwick, has a 3-decade history of commitment to redesigning health care. The IHI recognizes the need for a health system that focuses on the health interventions of a population, the individuals in that population, and the cost of providing care to that population.[15] The system is called the Triple Aim, which provides a framework for optimizing the outcomes for populations. IHI also addresses how Accountable Care Organizations (ACOs) will help achieve the Triple Aim.[16]

Centers for Medicare and Medicaid Services Hospital Value-Based Purchasing Program

The CMS Hospital Value-Based Purchasing (VBP) program is an initiative that provides incentives to acute care hospitals for their performance in achieving quality-of-care measurements for Medicare and Medicaid patients.[17] The VBP was developed with the goal to reimburse hospitals based on patient outcomes instead of the number of services provided. Hospitals are rewarded for following clinical best-practices and for how well patients evaluate their inpatient experience of care and does not incentivize only for volume of services a hospital provides. The VBP was established as part of the ACA of 2010 and began in 2013 applying payments according to certain quality measures and the improvement in performance compared with baseline. The VBP program affects CMS payment in 2985 hospitals.[17]

Measures include processes of care, experience of care, patient outcomes, and efficiency of delivery.[17] There are 13 specific clinical process measurements, such as discharge instructions, prophylactic antibiotic received within 1 hour before surgical incision, and cardiac surgery patients with controlled 6:00 AM postoperative serum glucose. Patient experience of care includes 8 measurements, such as nurse communication, doctor communication, and overall hospital rating. The 5 outcome measures are as follows: acute myocardial infarction 30-day mortality rate, heart failure 30-day mortality rate, pneumonia 30-day mortality rate, composite complication/patient safety for selected indicators, and central line–assisted bloodstream infection. The efficiency domain measure is Medicare spending per beneficiary. Many of these measures are nurse sensitive and/or influenced by nurse intervention. With this CMS pay-for-performance program, nurses' leadership and interventions will be critical to a hospital organization. The hospital is reimbursed based on the calculation of a total performance score that is based on the clinical process measures (weighted 70% of total score) and the patient experience measures (weighted 30% of total score). RNs are critical to achieving these outcomes in the VBP program.

Also of importance in identifying the value and need for nurses employed in hospital settings are 2 studies with Linda Aiken as an author. Aiken and colleagues[11] published research outcomes in *Lancet* that validated the importance of nurse staffing, particularly bachelor degree nurses, in decreasing rates of mortality in European hospital settings. Another similar research article with Aiken as the third author studied hospitals in the United States and demonstrated similar outcomes.[18] The first cited study found that adding 1 patient to a nurse's workload resulted in a 7% increase in the likelihood of an inpatient dying within 30 days of admission. The investigators also found that there was a 7% decrease in the likelihood of an inpatient dying within 30 days of admission for every 10% increase in bachelor degree nurses in the staffing mix.[18] More specifically, these findings from this retrospective observational study imply that when nurses care for an average of 6 patients and 60% of nurses have a bachelor's degree in nursing, there would be a 30% lower mortality rate compared with when only 30% of nurses have a bachelor degree and each nurse has an average of 8 patients.[18]

Quality and Safety Indicator Programs

Poor-quality health care not only impacts the health status of patients, but it is very costly. According to the IOM, 30% of health care spending in 2009 did not provide any value in improving patient outcomes.[19] Causes of the financial waste included administrative ineffectiveness, fraud, and poor-quality care that is not based on evidence-based practice. Poor quality also can be misuse, overuse, or underuse of care interventions. In addition, poor quality results in lost work for patients and poor reputations for the organization. Incentives that promote quality evidence-based care and positive outcomes is the most cost-effective care,[19] and the RN is the critical provider of many of the interventions that satisfy the quality indicator measurements.[20]

Besides the CMS VBP program, there are many other quality indicator measurement programs that are specific for many different health care delivery settings. These quality programs contribute to the increasing need for RNs delivering evidence-based care interventions. The National Nursing Database of Quality Indicators is a nationally recognized nurse sensitive quality indicator program.[21] The measured indicators all require nursing interventions or nurse staffing to achieve the goal of each indicator of quality. The Agency for Healthcare Research and Quality (AHRQ) also measures hospital quality and safety performance.[22] AHRQ provides hospitals a statistical software package to use with their data measurement. The National Committee for Quality Assurance has a quality indicator program called the Healthcare Effectiveness Data and Information Set (HEDIS) and is used by health plans to measure performance by providers in the outpatient setting.[23] HEDIS quality indicator measurements support the comparison of performance of health plans.

Hospital Readmission Reduction Program

With past rates of approximately 20% of Medicare patients being readmitted to the hospital within 30 days of hospital discharge, the Hospital Readmission Reduction Program was developed.[24] Recent rates for the final quarter of 2012 dropped to 17.8% and this decline is credited to the ACA.[25] The Hospital Readmission

Reduction Program was established by the ACA to reduce unnecessary readmissions. Hospitals with high numbers of readmissions for acute myocardial infarction, heart failure, and pneumonia that are above the national average receive a penalty and reduced payments.[24] Nurses are valuable when they focus on preparing the patient for discharge, home self-care, and follow-up by telephone with the patient after discharge. By preventing a readmission, the nurse is positively impacting their organization's profit margin.[20] To help others see the improvements in readmission rates, the nurse can lead the tracking of the change in readmissions on a unit by collecting readmission data and doing a run chart to determine the trend, whether positive or negative. Let the trend of results motivate the nursing staff for continued improvement or to increase interventions to prevent readmissions. Understanding and documenting the institution's cost saving is also motivating for continued improvement.

Institute for Healthcare Improvement Triple Aim for Populations

The goals of the Triple Aim are focused on improving the health of the population, enhancing the experience and outcomes of the patient, and reducing per capita cost of care.[26] Understanding and working to achieve the IHI Triple Aim initiative is pertinent for RNs. RNs have a proven history of not just focusing on the care interventions in acute care, but looking at the total patient and helping each patient optimize his or her ability to provide self-care for improving health status. For the RN to be effective in the Triple Aim, the nurse must look more acutely at the patients in their communities and ultimately at the population of the community. Knowing that a focus on prevention and high-quality care early in the disease process is the most cost-effective care, RNs will have opportunities to be a significant part of the solution as a health care team member to impact care interventions that lower costs for the population being served.

The first step in organizations achieving the Triple Aim is for the organization to identify or choose what population to work with for that population to be impacted by the 3 dimensions of the Triple Aim goal.[27] Actions to take for the identified population include deliver excellent high-quality care interventions, achieve optimum patient outcomes for the population, and lower the cost from previous baseline. Populations are defined as individuals in a health system, practice panel, or a specific health plan; employees of an organization; or patients in an identified ACO.[27] The population also can be a community defined by geography. This geographic community segment has similar needs or health problems to be solved and will likely receive care paid for from different payers.

A population is managed by a health team to have improved health and cost outcomes for that group of people. David Lawrence, the author of the *Chronic Care Model*, is often viewed as the first visionary of population management.[28] This model proposed proactive systems of health care delivery to meet the needs of populations instead of reacting to exacerbations of illness and acute care needs.[28] Population health and management is still in its early stages and will need new collaboration, skills to assess population needs, and innovative methods to impact large numbers of people for them to embrace behavior change that keeps them healthy and prevents disease. RNs will be essential in population management, and to be effective in this new model, they will need to embrace change in their practice to focus on population management. To be effective in achieving the Triple Aim, nurses will need to be high-performing team members who are skilled in improving quality of care, encouraging participants to make positive lifestyle choices that affect long-term health, reducing costs, and ensuring patient satisfaction with innovation in care delivery.

Health Care Reform

Key components of the ACA include protecting consumers from abuses of insurance companies, providing to consumers certain free preventive services, open enrollment for health insurance, and access to affordable health insurance and ACOs and medical homes. The ACA proposed patient-centered medical homes (PCMHs) and ACOs as provisions to decrease medical error and costs of care by promoting interprofessional collaboration and teamwork. The goal of the ACA entails providing improved access to primary care through insurance reform, the institution of evidence-based practice, collaboration, wellness promotion, and decreasing costs through fewer readmissions to hospitals. Care coordination and transition management are interventions needed in these models of care to achieve high quality and safety for at-risk patients with multiple chronic diseases. The ACA also provides incentives to increase the primary care workforce, which includes primary care physicians, nurse practitioners, and physician assistants. The incentives include scholarships and loan repayments for doctors and nurses, with added tax benefit if serving in underserved or health professional shortage areas. The ACA is a driving force in health care change from individual to population health, which gives nursing the opportunity to take specific actions in this new era. These actions for nurses to take include preventing underlying risk factors at the individual, family, and community levels and assisting patients to become active themselves in managing their underlying risk factors.[29]

PROJECTED CHANGES IN NURSING PRACTICE

The ACA changes in health care in the United States offer the visionary nurse a different view of where change in nursing practice may be going.[30] The value of what a nurse will need to offer to the organization will include quality clinical care, but the nurse will also want to engage in a practice that drives financial outcomes for the employer. Nurses need to understand health care reform and the financial incentives associated with the reform to improve outcomes for patients and to improve the financial outcomes for the organization that provides the structure to deliver the nursing care. Sharing responsibility for the financial outcomes of an organization requires a change in the practice of nurses. Change requires the nurse to see the need to measure nursing sensitive quality indicators and outcomes, measure the financial outcomes, and then to report the value of nursing actions.

Care Coordination

Knowing that 49% of health care spending in the United States is driven by 5% of the population, there is significant opportunity for better coordination of care for people with multiple chronic diseases and psychosocial needs.[31] Patients with multiple chronic diseases cost up to 7 times as much as people with 1 chronic disease.[31] The IHI proposes a Care Coordination Model to provide better care at a lower cost.[32] The model proposes how to assign resources to meet the needs of these complex and high-cost patients. This Care Coordination model provides an excellent opportunity for RNs to provide the solution for effectively driving improved health status outcomes for a decreased cost. New systems are needed to provide primary care and coordination of care for patients needing multiple services, such as physical therapy, medication instruction, and specialist referral. Care coordination and transition management are new job entities for RNs in outpatient settings, such as the PCMHs. Improved interprofessional collaboration, care coordination, and teamwork in ambulatory care settings will result in prevention and wellness promotion and decreased cost for complex patient populations with multiple chronic diseases.

The goal for transition management is to prevent and reduce hospital readmissions and have the patient experience high-quality, timely, and on-purpose care treatments. This model of care needs to create economic value by saving the cost of complications and hospitalizations over the cost of the nursing care and interventions. Given the need for ACOs to provide high-quality care that promotes improved health status and prevents exacerbations and complications, there is a need for care coordination and transition management models that effectively define the competencies of the care coordinators, the interventions they will take for a patient population, and the expected patient outcomes. In this new position in the care coordination model, the nurse will need to develop the skills to problem-solve with patients and professional team members to assist patients to navigate all referrals efficiently and effectively and to learn the self-care needed for optimal management of their chronic diseases.[30]

Ambulatory and Community Health Nursing

The ambulatory care nurse role is evolving to meet the needs of the Health Reform Act. With the new delivery models, PCMH and the ACO, ambulatory nurses will need to impact quality and safety indicators. The services that ambulatory nurses provide must be defined as critical processes that will impact improved patient outcomes and cost metrics, which in turn will maximize outpatient reimbursement and improved health status of the population being served. ACOs have incentives to reduce hospital and emergency room costs and maximize total care cost savings.[31] The ACA is designed to decrease health care needs and costs. The vision entails cost savings by using the electronic health record across health providers and settings and by promoting health and preventing disease before the patient develops chronic diseases that require complicated health services and possible hospitalization.

Cost-effective preventive care will need nurses to help patients stay healthy by promoting healthy lifestyles. If patients develop multiple chronic diseases, nurses will need to advocate for the patient to take actions for optimum evidence-based self-care and prevention of exacerbations. The provider will no longer be incentivized for fee-for-service care. Instead, the health team will be incentivized to keep the patient as healthy as possible by using telephonic and electronic care interventions to monitor and teach patients at home. In addition, the RN can use evidence-based algorithms for triage, education, and counseling the patient to prevent unnecessary ambulatory or emergency department visits and admission to the hospital.[31] To achieve optimum quality indicator evaluation, benchmarking, and improved patient outcomes, communication between interdisciplinary team members is essential to prevent errors and maximize quality. Nurses with leadership, administrative, and emotional intelligence can be excellent facilitators of quality team performance.

Nursing care is shifting from acute care health services to community-oriented services, such as prevention, disease prevention and management, and home care. Community health needs nurses with transformational leadership skills in this time of change to provide early preventive interventions, manage long-term conditions, and to prevent exacerbations and progression of disease processes.[32] Leadership skills are needed for the purpose of accomplishing goals and to realize a vision. Community nursing needs nurses with leadership skills to function in a team to achieve client and family welfare and improve health status outcomes for the clients. The community health nurse also needs leadership skills to develop effective relationships with patients and team members. Community nursing employment opportunities are increasing, and it is believed that leadership is essential in community nursing teams.[32]

EMBRACING CHANGE

Having a knowledge base in change theory will assist the nurse in embracing change and providing value in one's professional roles as health care reform gains traction. The nurse can provide emerging value as the focus of health care transitions from individual to population management and from fee-for-service to lowering per capita cost of care through improving a population's health status. More job opportunities will be in the outpatient arena to promote health and prevent disease progression. The nurse needs to learn to act as a change agent in defining and executing innovative solutions to the problems in health care.

Understanding change theory will give the nurse the knowledge and tools to be successful in leading the change needed for the next decade.

CHANGE THEORY AS FRAMEWORK FOR PRACTICE

Change is a process, whether it is transformational or incremental. Embracing change theory as a framework for effecting change at the bedside or at the organizational level will likely ensure success where failure is so often encountered. Nursing has been challenged to achieve the change that will be necessary to move practice to the next level. Success will depend largely on the ability to use a theoretic model of change.

Lewin's Theory of Change

Kurt Lewin (1952) studied change extensively and published multiple theories related to planned change.[33] Field theory, group dynamics, action research, and a 3-step process for change are the structural components of Lewin's Theory of Change. Field theory consists of the idea that a situation is the totality of the influences that formed it. The influences are described as forces that may affect both the structure of the group and the individual within that group. According to Lewin, group behavior consists of interactions and forces that are often symbolic. This relationship is known as the field, in which change in any aspect results in a change in group behavior or the behavior of the individual within the group. Lewin's early work with group dynamics provided the basis for determining that the behavior of a group was not due to the individuals who made up the group, but rather that the group had a dynamic independent of the individual members. Therefore, to effect change within a group, the level of intervention required is at the level of the group. Action research is composed of planning, action, and reflecting about the results of the action. Lewin's 3-step model of change is the fourth component of his Theory of Planned Change (**Table 1**).[33]

Table 1 Lewin's 3-step model of change	
Step 1. Unfreezing	Recognition that change is needed. According to field theory, the group (or individual) equilibrium must be destabilized. Entrenched behaviors can be only discarded if they are challenged.
Step 2. Moving (transitioning)	Unfreezing creates the conditions to learn new behaviors. Change is accomplished through action research at both the individual and group levels. Moving does not ensure that change will be sustained.
Step 3. Refreezing	The process of reestablishment of equilibrium.

Adapted from Lewin K. Field theory in social science: selected theoretical papers. New York: Harper & Row; 1951. p. 1052.

Rogers' Diffusion of Innovations Theory

Rogers expanded on Lewin's 3-step model for change.[34] Rogers' diffusion of innovations theory explains change within a given social system. Rogers contends if an innovation has relative advantage, compatibility, complexity, divisibility, and communicability that it is more likely to be adopted. Relative advantage is the perception that the innovation has advantages for current practice. Compatibility is consistency with the potential adopter's values, past experiences, and needs at either the group or individual level. Complexity has to do with the sustainability of the change, more complex ideas are likely to endure even though innovation that is easy to understand may be more quickly implemented. Divisibility means that the innovation may be introduced on a small scale. Communicability means that the innovation will produce observable results that are easily described and communicated to encourage diffusion (**Table 2**).[34]

Two other theories are frequently used in nursing: Lippitt's Change Theory and Reddin's Change Theory.[35] Both of the theories have commonalities with Lewin and Rogers. Lippitt, Reddin, and Rogers all expanded on Lewin's work, developing steps or phases that incorporate concepts of Lewin's force fields, active research, and group dynamics.[33,35,36] Additionally, Lippitt and Reddin have composed the language in their theories to be readily identifiable with that of the nursing process, which makes them easily adaptable to the nursing practice environment (**Table 3**).

Kotter's 8-Step Process for Leading Change

A fifth theory that bears consideration, especially for transformational change, is Kotter's 8-Step Process for Leading Change.[37] This theory provides broader guidelines for the leaders that will be charged with implementing change. Utilization of this theory in effecting change in large organizations has been successful in the implementation of electronic medical records within contemporary maternity services, health care management projects, and respiratory care departments.[38–40] Lacina[41] used Kotter's 8-step process as a framework to assist in the transformation of the Department of Defense military health system in establishing medical stability operations (**Table 4**).

Kotter's 8-Step Process for Leading Change seems to be a viable option for both incremental and transformational change. **Table 5** provides specific activities that may be engaged to operationalize the steps in the theory and avoid some of the pitfalls leading to failure, which were originally identified by Kotter.[37]

Table 2 Roger's diffusion of innovations theory	
Phase 1. Awareness	Awareness and knowledge of the innovation.
Phase 2. Interest	If there is enough interest in the innovation, the change process progresses.
Phase 3. Evaluation	Adopters of change evaluate the merits of the innovation when faced with a decision about adoption or rejection.
Phase 4. Trial	Trialability means that the innovation can be implemented in part or in whole, and may be evaluated at intervals.
Phase 5. Adoption	Adoption is the final phase in which the innovation is either rejected or adopted. If rejected, it may be considered at a later time.

Adapted from Rogers EM. Diffusion of Innovation, 4th edition. New York: The Free Press; 1996.

Table 3
Comparison of Reddin and Lippitt theories of change

Reddin	Lippitt
Diagnosis	Diagnosis
Mutual objective setting	Assessing motivation and capacity for change
Group emphasis	Assessing change agents, motivation, and resources
Maximum information	Selecting progressive change objective
Discussion of implementation	Choosing the appropriate role of the change agent
Use of ceremony and ritual	Maintaining change
Resistance interpretation	Terminating the helping relationship

Data from Roussel L. Management and leadership for nurse administrators, 6th edition. Burlington (MA): Jones and Barlett; 2013; and Mitchell G. Selecting the best theory to implement planned change. Nurs Manag (Harrow) 2013;20(1):32–7.

Table 4
Kotter's 8-step process for leading change

1. Establishing a sense of urgency	Others must see the need for change and feel that it is important enough that action must be taken: convince stakeholder that the status quo is more dangerous than change.
2. Creating a guiding coalition	The coalition should have key members with enough power that progress will not be threatened. The members of the coalition should be credible, able to make informed decisions, and be able to drive the change.
3. Developing a change vision.	The coalition should work to create a vision and establish strategies to achieve that vision.
4. Communicating the vision for buy-in.	All stakeholders should have a clear understanding of the vision and consider it achievable.
5. Empowering broad-based action.	Institutional and/or organizational barriers should be eliminated or reduced as much as possible. Encourage risk taking and new ideas.
6. Generating short-term wins.	Recognize and celebrate success as it occurs. Design and implement goals that are observable.
7. Never letting up: continuing to build on the change.	Keep the momentum positive by encouraging new ideas, bringing in new people, and continuing to reduce barriers.
8. Embed the new way of working.	Communicate the relationship of the change to institutional (any unit) success.

From Kotter JP. Leading change. Boston: Harvard Business Press, 1996. Used with permission from Kotter International, Cambridge, MA. Available at: http://iiiserver.lib.apsu.edu/search~S1?/aKotter%2C+John+P.%2C+1947-/akotter+john+p+1947/-3%2C-1%2C0%2CZ/l856&FF=akotter+john+p+1947&7%2C%2C11%2C1%2C0. Accessed August 19, 2014.

Table 5
Suggestions for activities and dangers: Kotter's 8-step process for leading change

Components	Activities Leading to Success	Dangers Leading to Failure
Step 1	Assess the environment in which the change will occur. What are the challenges and opportunities? Create a *sense of urgency* about the needed change, convincing the stakeholders that the status quo will result in a negative outcome. Appeal to the emotions surrounding the issue rather than the analytical approach.	Allowing too much complacency. Underestimating resistance to change. Relying only on the analytical approach, appealing to the cognitive domain only.
Step 2	Assemble a leadership *coalition* that has shared commitment. Ensure that the coalition has the power to effect the change or decrease the barriers to change. Encourage activities of team building for the coalition.	Lack of power in leadership choices. Members of the coalition have no experience in teamwork.
Step 3	The coalition should develop a *vision* that is understandable in terms of goals and values embedded in the change. The team must ask the hard question related to the future the change will create, what will it look like?	Over communication of the vision. The vision is too complicated. Not understanding the importance of vision in the change process.
Step 4	*Communication* must be clear, persistent, and use a variety of delivery systems. The communication should answer questions related to how the change will affect all stakeholders. The coalition should begin to exhibit behaviors they are attempting to achieve.	Over communication of the vision. Ineffective role modeling by the leadership team.
Step 5	Encourage new ideas and risk taking. *Empower* others to act on the vision. Remove barriers that are obstructing the vision.	Failure to recognize, remediate, or remove individuals with power who resist the change. Permitting barriers to change to persist.
Step 6	Celebrate *short-term wins* in the change process. Early in the process, design observable short-term, achievable goals that contribute to the long-term goal.	Not creating or recognizing short-term wins.
Step 7	Look for examples that the change is working. This is a time to assess and possibly make changes in the leadership coalition to get a fresh look at how the change is evolving. Build on the change, *never let up.*	Declaring victory or success too soon.
Step 8	Make sure that the change is *embedded* in the social norms and values of the institution/organization. Design activities that demonstrate that the change has implications for organizational success.	Failing to embed the change in the culture of the institution/organization.

From Kotter JP. Leading change. Boston: Harvard Business Press, 1996. Used with permission from Kotter International, Cambridge, MA. Available at: http://iiiserver.lib.apsu.edu/search~S1?/aKotter%2C+Joh n+P.%2C+1947-/akotter+john+p+1947-/3%2C-1%2C0%2CZ/I856&FF=akotter+john+p+1947&7%2C%2C11%2C1%2C0. Accessed August 19, 2014.

SUMMARY

Without question, nursing education and practice have many challenges to meet the demands of an evolving health care system. The ability to drive better patient outcomes and effectively manage chronic disease will determine nursing's place in the health care hierarchy. We must seek a national identity that is recognized for our ability to meet the challenges of today's health care needs by having a solid grasp on how to achieve successful change. A sense of urgency has already been created by the challenges and charges that confront nurses at all levels of practice. As a discipline, we must be able to translate that sense of urgency into change that will preserve our professional values as we move into an uncertain future. Kotter's[37] 8 steps for leading change is not a step-by-step process: one step may be used to enhance another step and much of the success is dependent on the leadership skill sets. There will be continued challenges and there will be unanticipated setbacks, but using a theoretic framework as described in this article will enhance the chance of success.

REFERENCES

1. Bernstein L. Once again, U.S. has most expensive, least effective health care system in survey. Washington Post 2014.
2. US Bureau of Labor Statistics. Occupational Outlook Handbook: registered nurses work environment. Available at: http://www.bls.gov/ooh/Healthcare/Registered-nurses.htm. Accessed June 18, 2014.
3. US Bureau of Labor Statistics. Occupational Outlook Handbook: job outlook. Available at: http://www.bls.gov/ooh/Healthcare/Registered-nurses.htm. Accessed June 18, 2014.
4. Department of Health and Human Services Centers for Medicare and Medicaid Services. Hospital value-based purchasing from the Medicare learning network. Available at: http://www.cms.gov/Medicare. Accessed August 1, 2014.
5. The American Nurse. ANA, CMS officials meet to discuss health care reform, nurses' roles. The American Nurse, March/April 2014.
6. Department of Health and Human Services. Key Features of the Affordable Care Act by year. Available at: http://www.HHS.gov/healthcare/facts/timeline/timeline-text.html. Accessed June 30, 2014.
7. Institute of Medicine. The future of nursing: leading change, advancing health. Washington, DC: The National Academies Press; 2010.
8. Petterson SM, Liaw WR, Phillips RP, et al. Projecting US primary care physician workforce needs: 2010-2025. Ann Fam Med 2012;10:503–9.
9. Department of Health and Human Services. HRSA health workforce nations sample survey of nurse practitioners. Available at: http://bhpr.hrsa.gov/healthworkforce/supplydeman/nursing/nursepractitionersurvey. Accessed July 9, 2014.
10. Robert Wood Johnson. Health Affairs Health Policy Briefs. Nurse practitioners and primary care. Available at: http://www.healthaffairs.org/healthpolicybriefs/brief.php?brief_id=79. Accessed August 3, 2014.
11. Aiken L, Sloane D, Bruyneel L. Nurse staffing and education and hospital mortality in nine European countries: a retrospective observational study. Lancet 2014; 383:1824–30.
12. American Association of Colleges of Nursing. AACN essential of baccalaureate education. Available at: http://www.aacn.nche.edu. Accessed November 4, 2013.

13. Orr P, Ciampini L. A BSN action guide for responding to the 2011 Institute of Medicine recommendations. In: Caputi L, editor. Innovations in Nursing Education Building the Future of Nursing. Baltimore (MD): Lippincott, Williams and Wilkins; 2014. p. 161–8.
14. Medicare Payment Advisory Commission, Report to the Congress. Medicare and the health care delivery system. Available at: http://www.medpac.gov. Accessed July 5, 2014.
15. Institute for Healthcare Improvement. ACOs: about us vision, mission, and values. Available at: http://ihi.org/about/pages/ihivisionand values.aspx. Accessed May 30, 2014.
16. Institute for Healthcare Improvement. A step in the right direction. Available at: www.ihi.org. Accessed July 10, 2014.
17. Department of Health and Human Services Centers for Medicare and Medicaid Services. Hospital value-based purchasing. ICN 907664, March 2013.
18. Kelly LA, Mc Hugh MD, Aiken LH. Nurse outcomes in magnet and non-magnet hospitals. J Nurs Adm 2011;41:428–33.
19. National Academy of Sciences, National Academy of Engineering, Institute of Medicine, and National Research Council. Transformation of health systems needed to improve care and reduce costs. Available at: http://www8.nationalacademies.org/onpinews/newsitem.aspx?RecordID=13444. Accessed July 15, 2014.
20. Ewoldt LL. Healthcare reform; resolve to increase your knowledge in 2014. American Nurse Today 2004;9:8–11.
21. Montalvo, I. National database of nursing quality indicators. The Online Journal of Issues in Nursing. Available at: http://www.nursingworld.org/Main MenuCategories/ANAMarketplace/ANAPeriodicals/OJIN. Accessed August 4, 2014.
22. Agency for Healthcare Research and Quality. Inpatient quality indicators overview. Available at: http://www.qualityindicators.ahrq.gov/Modules/iqi_resources.aspx. Accessed August 4, 2014.
23. National Commission for Quality Assurance. HEDIS and performance measurement. Available at: http://www.ncqa.org/HEDISQuality Measurement.aspx. Accessed August 4, 2014.
24. Centers for Medicare and Medicaid Services. Readmissions reduction program. Available at: http://www.cms.gov/Medicare/Medicare-Fee-for-Service-Payment/Acute Inpatient PPs. Accessed July 15, 2014.
25. AMN Healthcare. CMS: Hospital readmissions declined in late 2012, ACA credited. Available at: http://amnhealthcare.com/latest-healthcare news/cms-hospital readmissions-declined. Accessed August 8, 2014.
26. Institute for Healthcare Improvement. Triple aim for populations. Available at: http://www.ihi.org/Topics/TripleAim/Pages/default.aspx?utm_campaign=tw&utm_source=hs_email. Accessed June 9, 2014.
27. Institute for Healthcare Improvement. Populations, population health, and the evolution of population management: making sense of the terminology in US health care today. Available at: http://www.ihi.org/communities/blogs/_layouts/ihi/community/blog/itemview.aspx?List. Accessed June 9, 2014.
28. Lawrence D. From chaos to care the promise of team-based medicine. Cambridge (MA): Perseus Publishing; 2002.
29. U.S. Department of Health and Human Services. Key factors of the Affordable Care Act by year. Available at: http://www.hhs.gov/healthcare/facts/timeline/timeline-text.html. Accessed August 9, 2014.

30. Haas SA, Swan BA. Developing the value proposition for the role of the registered nurse in care coordination and transition in management in ambulatory care settings. Nurs Econ 2014;32:70–9.

31. Agency for Healthcare Research and Quality. High concentration of US health care expenditures. Available at: http://www.ahrq.gov/research/findings/factsheets/costs/expriach/index.html. Accessed August 9, 2014.

32. Institute for Healthcare Improvement. Care coordination model: better care at lower cost for people with multiple health and social issues. Available at: http://www.ihi.org/resources/Pages/IHIWhitePapers/IHICareCoordinationModelWhitePaper.aspx. Accessed July 18, 2014.

33. Lewin K. Field theory on social science. London: Routledge and Kegan Paul; 1952.

34. Rogers EM. Diffusion of innovation. 4th edition. New York: The Free Press; 1996.

35. Roussel L. Management and leadership for nurse administrators. 6th edition. Burlington (MA): Jones and Bartlett; 2013.

36. Mitchell G. Selecting the best theory to implement planned change. Nurs Manag (Harrow) 2013;20(1):32–7.

37. Kotter JP. Leading change. 1947 [electronic]. Available at: http://iiiserver.lib.apsu.edu/search~S1?/aKotter%2C+John+P.%2C+1947-/akotter+john+p+1947/-3%2C-1%2C0%2CZ/l856&FF=akotter+john+p+1947&7%2C%2C11%2C1%2C0. Accessed August 19 2014.

38. Barnfather T. Critical evaluation and refection on the role of the supervisor of midwives within the maternity services. Br J Midwifery 2013;21(7):503–9.

39. Campbell RJ. Change management in health care. Health Care Manag (Frederick) 2008;27(1):23–39.

40. Stoller JK. Implementing change in respiratory care. Respir Care 2010;55(6): 749–57.

41. Lacina D. Medical stability operations: one approach to transforming the Department of Defense military health system. Mil Med 2012;177(10):1119–24.

Role of Research in Best Practices

Maria A. Revell, PhD, MSN, RN, COI

KEYWORDS

- Evidence-based practice • Research • Nursing education • Outcomes
- Certification

KEY POINTS

- Evidence-based care is imperative to the promotion of best practices.
- Research is available that promotes care activities for key activities and interventions that should be used for promotion of care activities related to catheter-associated urinary tract infections (CAUTIs), ventilator-associated pneumonia (VAP)/infection, family presence during cardiopulmonary resuscitation, and other patient care problems.
- Obtaining certification and active involvement in professional organizations can serve as a foundation to individually maintaining nursing knowledge and promoting expertise.
- Using research evidence, obtaining certification, and active involvement in professional organizations can bridge the gap between paper and practice, promoting the use of patient management protocols and guidelines that are objective and scientific.

INTRODUCTION

Nursing knowledge has been transformed from decades of factual mouth-to-mouth information to current-day synthesized research evidence. This new knowledge is being converted into clinically useful protocols and guidelines. These allow interdisciplinary care management that blends expertise for the best patient outcome. This outcome can be measured and validated to re-energize research as it moves across all involved disciplines. How has this evolution occurred? Not without changes to the very core of nursing's educational and health care elements, which form the foundation of patient management. The need for a research base is articulated in the Institute of Medicine's *The Future of Nursing*[1] report (2010),where health care is identified as more complicated and requiring research and evidence-based practice (EBP) for the delivery of high-quality patient care. This report also notes how nursing's future will include new functions or roles for nurses. Nursing research is systematic inquiry into ways of knowing for the profession. It serves to answer questions and "develop, refine and expand knowledge."[2]

Disclosure: None.
Division of Nursing, Tennessee State University, 214 Jon Paul Court, Murfreesboro, TN 37128, USA
E-mail address: oshum.mr@gmail.com

PROBLEM

Research has evolved as a guiding standard for nursing practice. The profession is expected to base its care on evidence discovered through analyses. Although barriers to research utilization (RU) remain, nurses are more and more accepting of the need to use research as the foundation for their clinical nursing actions. Barriers to RU have been conceptualized by several investigators.[3] Five domains have been suggested for barriers, which include (1) quality of research, (2) access to research, (3) process of RU, (4) attitude and knowledge of nurses, (5) and organization.[3] Three core elements of RU have been conceptualized, consisting of (1) level and nature of the evidence, which include poor quality and inconsistent research results and failure; (2) context or environment for RU, which includes organizations that are task driven and little to no continuing education for nurses; and (3) method for implementation, which includes inflexible style and inappropriate characteristics.[4]

General research barrier domains have been conceptualized.[5] These include (1) physician related (which can include other health care professionals), (2) patient related, and (3) health system related. Physician-related barriers include lack of knowledge due to the multitude of research, some of which may give differing results, and time constraints to read and review this research. Patient-related barriers include time and financial constraints, polypharmacy, and failure to change behaviors that pose hazards to a healthy lifestyle. Health system–related barriers include concerns about high health care cost, large numbers of uninsured and underinsured individuals entering the health care system, and failure of systems to have systematic approaches to management of the chronically ill. Barriers to RU have been identified by other researchers, which can be categorized into these conceptual elements and domains.[5] Research has been gathered around nurses' perceptions of barriers to the utilization of research.[5,6] Findings are clustered around problems in interpreting and using research, perceived lack of organizational support for research, lack of clinical credibility for research studies, failure of a clear clinical direction from research findings, and lack of skills and motivation to use research. Nurses in a study on barriers to research utilization had a desire for research to be delivered by another resource and no desire to become directly involved in research themselves.[6]

Barriers to RU in the clinical setting have been investigated. The greatest barriers are constraints in time, lack of awareness of research literature available for specific problems, insufficient authority related to needed changes, inadequate critical appraisal skills, and lack of organizational support for implementation.[7] Time has been identified as the most frequent barrier to implementation of research.[8] Cost of implementation was the second most frequently identified barrier, with others including no or limited knowledge regarding research by nurses in the organization and no interest in research implementation by organizational leaders. Research also identified that several nurses indicated that they were not aware of EBP or what it meant.[8]

The United States is not alone in its quest to overcome research barriers. Barriers in Australian nurses not only are similar to those in the United States but also mirrored those of nurses in the United Kingdom and Northern Ireland.[7]

STRATEGIES TO OVERCOME RESEARCH BARRIERS

Overcoming the many barriers is an important step in moving research from paper to practice. Using evidence to verify patient interventions promotes the best possible outcomes. EBP is an integration of individual clinical expertise and the best available evidence retrieved from research.[9] This form of practice improves health care outcomes. Transitioning this evidence from paper to practice is the culmination of RU.

RU incorporates the use of groundbreaking research to move from identification of clinical problems to evidence affirmation and utilization. Use of an algorithm can help nurses move research from paper to actual utilization (**Fig. 1**). RU begins with identification of a clinical problem and culminates in 1 of 2 decisions. If there is sufficient information to validate use of an intervention, a nurse can proceed with implementation. If, after literature search and critique, there is insufficient or ambiguous information, there should be reinitiation of a literature search to identify evidence for alternate interventions. Use of databases not previously investigated may facilitate retrieval of appropriate information to validate care intervention.

MANAGEMENT OF PATIENT CARE PROBLEMS/INTERVENTIONS

Hospital-acquired infection prevention is one of the 20 "priority areas" identified in the Institute of Medicine's 2003 report, *Transforming Health Care Quality*.[10]

The IOM publication further focused attention of the public, policy makers, and health care community on opportunities to improve patient safety that were previously reported in the Institute of Medicine's 2000 report, *To Err Is Human: Building a Safer Health System*.[11]

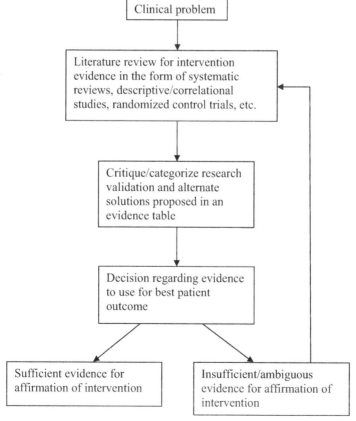

Fig. 1. RU algorithm.

Nurses face numerous issues in patient care management. Some of these include catheter-associated infections, VAP, family presence during cardiopulmonary resuscitation, failure to maintain adherence to proper hand hygiene, early mobilization/early exercise, central venous catheter blood stream infection, and communication failure between health care providers. Research has been done that addresses each of these issues, which can be used by nurses to manage patients based on the best research evidence (**Table 1**).

Catheter-Associated Urinary Tract Infection

CAUTIs have been the most common hospital-acquired infections until the past few years, when research has focused on reduction. Catheters have been commonly used in most acute care institutions and have been the source of many urinary tract infections.[46] CAUTIs are common and costly. Interest in reduction of hospital-acquired CAUTIs has been prompted through mandated public reporting,[47] the 2008 Association for Professionals in Infection Control and Epidemiology (APIC) Targeting Zero Campaign,[48] and removal of reimbursement on October 1, 2008, by Medicare. Since this time, there have been several research-initiated, catheter-associated interventions for prevention of urinary tract infections (see **Table 1**). APIC developed a comprehensive guide in 2008 that can be used by critical care nurses to address CAUTIs.[48] Research has demonstrated not only how bundle approaches can be implemented to reduce infections but also how removal of silver alloy catheters, which are more costly, did not significantly affect CAUTI rates.[12]

Ventilator-Associated Pneumonia/Infection

Nurses are the first line of defense to the prevention of many infections, which includes prevention of bacterial colonization of the respiratory tract. Interventions to prevent infections must begin no later than the time of intubation. Identification of risk factors that may lead to increased susceptibility must be considered during care management. Risks have been divided into 3 categories: (1) host related, (2) device related, and (3) personnel related.[49] Host-related risks for infection may include underlying medical conditions (chronic obstructive pulmonary disease, immunosuppression, and so forth), body position, level of consciousness, and medications. Device-related categories include the endotracheal tube itself along with ventilator circuit and use of an orogastric or nasogastric tube. Personnel-related categories include improper and infrequent hand washing and failure to use or properly use protective equipment between infected patients. Evidence-based clinical practice guidelines have been developed in an effort to prevent and reduce the incidence of VAP[50] along with strategies related to circuit management (see **Table 1**).

Family Presence During Cardiopulmonary Resuscitation

Family can be foundational to a patient's psychological health. They can serve as a psychological comfort during procedures that are painful or uncomfortable. This is recognized through visitation practices in acute care organizations that allow and actively promote visitation by family and friends through flexible visitation hours that extend throughout the day and evening. This family presence has expanded to include end-of-life activities, for instance cardiopulmonary resuscitation. In a public opinion poll, 50% to 96% of individuals believed that family should have the option of being present during not only resuscitation but also during invasive procedures.[50] Despite feelings that this increases caregiver stress and that family members will be in the way, research has validated the opposite.[24,51] Researchers have identified many benefits to family members' presence during cardiopulmonary

Table 1
Select research based findings for patient care issues

Management of Patient Care Issues	Select Research-Based Findings
CAUTIs	• Use of guidelines, nurse-driven interventions, system-wide product changes, and patient and family involvement[12] • Use of guidelines to judge appropriateness of catheter use[13] • Use of a reminder system for removal[14] • Catheter removal as soon as clinically possible[15] • Bladder prevention bundles, which may include daily assessment, minimizing urethral trauma, hand washing, frequent drainage bag emptying, electronic reminders or stop orders, and removal when feasible[16] • Use of a collaborative model for transformational change[15]
VAP	• Orotracheal intubation can reduce incidence of infection and sinusitis[17] • Semirecumbent positioning at 45° from horizontal to reduce potential[18,19] • Use of heated humidifiers rather than heat and moisture exchangers[20] • Chlorhexidine use in oral care[21–23]
Family presence during cardiopulmonary resuscitation	• Does not increase emotional stress in health professionals[24] • Does not interfere with health care patient efforts[24] • Does not result in medicolegal claim initiative by family of patient[24] • Conflicts may result from differences of opinion between health care providers[25] • Critical care professionals do not support current ECC and CPR 2000 guidelines[26]
Failure to maintain adherence to proper hand hygiene	• A multifaceted approach of education, reminders, performance feedback, facilities and products, use of role models, active ward management, and setting norms and targets is beneficial.[27] • Using education can improve compliance[28,29] • Doubling the amount of alcohol gel hand disinfectant used can result in improved surface area and lower bacterial count on caregiver hands[30]
Early mobilization/early exercise	• Ambulation of mechanically ventilated patients to reduce length of stay[31] • Individually tailored exercise training can improve muscle force at discharge[32] • Whole-body rehabilitation can decrease delirium duration and result in better functional outcomes[33]
Central venous catheter blood stream infection	• Insertion and maintenance bundles, which include training (operator and assistant), removal as soon as feasible, hand hygiene, daily dressing inspection with changes occurring when soiled, and discouragement of catheter changes over guide wires and blood sampling[34] • Sequential infection control education and performance feedback[35,36] • Use of maximal barrier protection[37–39] • Use of sutureless securement device[40] • Evaluate new innovations prior to use; mechanical valves may increase infection rate[40–42]

(continued on next page)

Table 1 *(continued)*	
Management of Patient Care Issues	**Select Research-Based Findings**
Communication failure between health care providers	• Efforts should be engaged to increase and improve effective communication among health care workers in order to improve care delivery[43] • Utilization of a daily goals form may assist in collaborative communication[44] • Implementation of an educational program using techniques inclusive of video and PowerPoint presentations, practice scenarios, SBAR practice, visual reminders, champions and Web-based training can serve to improve interdisciplinary communication[45]

Abbreviations: CPR, cardiopulmonary resuscitation; ECC, emergency cardiovascular care.

resuscitation (see **Table 1**). One foundational finding is that family presence removes doubt and validates severity of a patient's condition while insuring that all was done in an attempt to preserve life.[52]

Failure to Maintain Adherence to Hand Washing Practices

Infection control is an essential component of safe patient care. Hand hygiene is a foundational component of the infection control bundle in any patient care area. The need to improve and sustain proper hand hygiene has been recognized by the World Health Organization in their Clean Care is Safer Care initiative.[53] Poor hand hygiene may be linked to hospital-acquired infections.

Barriers to proper hand hygiene can be broken into 2 main categories: professional and organizational (**Fig. 2**). Work culture can significantly affect how nurses view the importance of hand hygiene as well as their perception of the time needed to address hygiene between and among patients. Education can affect nurse attitude development related to the importance of hand hygiene in the health care setting. Mentors and other health care workers can affect actions resulting from interrelated attitudes.[54,55]

The organizational focus can portray how important hand hygiene is in the overall scheme of patient care management. Failure to develop policies, protocols, and monitoring practices with sufficient sanctions for noncompliance does little to encourage compliance. Product availability and the type of products can affect use because they may have detrimental effects on the skin, which may reduce use by nurses (see **Fig. 2**).

Addressing barriers involves awareness of placing the issue of hand washing at the forefront for persons and organizations. Education can be a foundational initiative in addressing hand hygiene from a professional and organizational focus.[56] Working to

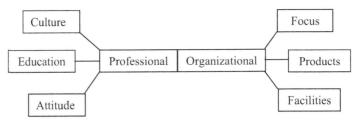

Fig. 2. Barriers to proper hand hygiene.

address issues of skin alterations can promote use and improve compliance (see **Table 1**).

Early Mobilization/Early Exercise

Until recent years, patients in ICUs were kept immobilized with safety restraints to maintain the integrity of life-saving equipment. Some postsurgery patients were also kept immobilized or on bed restriction. These restrictions led to patients with increased weakness and decreased activity tolerance. The resulting ICU-acquired paresis affected both muscles and nerves and is referred to as critical illness polyneuropathy or critical illness myopathy.

Prolonged bed rest and inactivity are commonly identified factors that hasten a switch in the muscle fibers from slow-contracting fatigue-resistant myosin isoforms (type I) to fast-twitching isoforms (type II). These promote the effects of prolonged forced bed rest, which include muscle atrophy, reduced total muscle mass, decreased exercise capacity, contractures, foot drop, decreased bone density, pressure ulcers, reduced lung volumes, and pneumonia.[57] In consideration of these prolonged immobility consequences, it is important for nurses to initiate activities to reduce the potential for muscle atrophy and other deleterious effects. Research has been ongoing that validates early mobilization and/or early exercise for patients despite needed interventional equipment (see **Table 1**). These activities can improve patient outcomes.

Central Venous Catheter Blood Stream Infection

Central venous catheters are used in ICUs and surgical and medical surgical units to have access for circulating body fluid measurement and intravenous fluid administration of various viscosities. Despite their life-saving qualities, these catheters can predispose patients to serious blood stream infections. According to the Joint Commission, blood stream infections comprise 14% of all hospital-acquired infections.[58] Patients who acquire blood stream infections have prolonged hospitalizations as well as an increased costs of health care. These infections can also cause adverse consequences that lead to deterioration of a patient's current condition, leading to increased morbidity and mortality.[34] Research has identified methods that can be used to reduce infection, which include hand hygiene, aseptic technique with barrier precautions used during insertion, insertion operator and assistant training, avoidance of femoral sites, and port cleaning with alcohol prior to use (see **Table 1**).

Communication Failure Between Health Care Providers

Interdiciplinary communication is imperative to the promotion of patient care. In order to respond in a timely manner and appropriately, communication is the foundation for relay of necessary information. With the current emphasis on length of stay, reduction of adverse events, and postdischarge follow-up to prevent readmission, communication is foundational to these goals. Poor communication and miscommunication between members of the health care team can result in poor quality of patient care. This failure to communicate can also result in medical errors and patient harm.[59] There are several barriers to effective communication in health care. These include

- Complexity of health care that can involve numerous providers of various roles
- The unpredictable nature of care response and patient changing condition
- Structure of acute care facilities, clinics, and care provider offices that may promote a hierarchical structure for communication
- Educational preparation that focuses on individual roles

Nurses should actively solicit and engage in activities that can improve communication in their designated care setting. Systematic approaches to improving communication include educational courses in various formats (Web based, PowerPoint, and so forth) and activities, such as use of Situation, Background, Assessment, Recommendation (SBAR) and daily goals forms for standardization of communication formats (see **Table 1**).

CERTIFICATION IN A SPECIALTY AREA

Certification is voluntary evidence of expertise in a specific area of nursing practice. It validates high-quality, competent patient management by individuals who are successful in achieving this recognition.[60] Certification gives formal acknowledgment of cognitive knowledge, skills, and clinical experience in a specialty area. There are approximately 115 various nursing specialty certifications through 45 nursing and interdisciplinary organizations.[61,62]

Certification has been linked to empowerment in nursing[63] and to higher salaries and/or benefits.[64] Nurses also report that certification promotes an increased sense of practice control and autonomy as well as enhanced collaboration and communication.[65]

Investigation has occurred into the difference in perceptions of empowerment between nurses with and without national nursing certifications.[66] Statistical analysis demonstrated that certified nurses had higher perceptions of formal power than noncertified nurses in this acute care facility ($P<.038$) and informal power ($P<.000$). Certified nurses also indicated a higher perception of access to information ($P<.0100$), which may be an organizational benefit because certification is often linked to membership. This research suggested a positive benefit to certification for nurses.[66]

Other researchers have also identified better outcomes for patients based on nurse certification.[67,68] Findings identified that units with fewer certified nurses had an increased probability of more patient falls. This inverse relationship supports nurse certification as a worthwhile investment for organizations in an effort to improve patient safety outcomes related to falls.

ACTIVE INVOLVEMENT IN PROFESSIONAL ORGANIZATIONS

Professional organizations provide nurses with tools and access to knowledge that promote a high level of excellence. These organizations provide numerous opportunities that may provide nurses with[69]

- Guidelines for clinical practice
- Evidence-based protocols
- Patient safety initiatives
- Algorithms for patient management
- Networking opportunities
- Continuing education opportunities
- Resources for career development
- Scholarships and grants

Active involvement in professional organizations allows nurses to be engaged in shared governance and decision making processes that affect practice standards and issues of concern to the profession in general and affect specific areas of nursing care management in particular.[70] Nurses have the opportunity to engage in review of standards and offer suggestions and opinions. They further engage in activities that affect governing of the organization through elections and voting.

Involvement in professional organizations can promote career development.[71] Professional organizations often provide clinical practice guidelines and evidence-based protocols that have been through review and validation. These can improve patient outcomes and reduce adverse events. Using these guidelines and protocols can ease nurse entry into the profession and serve to refresh professional excitement for nurses who are currently involved in care activities.

RESOURCES TO PROMOTE CONTINUED USE OF EVIDENCE IN PATIENT CARE

There are many resources to assist in using research for evidence-based care in nursing. Research-based protocols can be key to this process for nurses who are already time and energy deficient. Having key links for easy identification can be beneficial and several of these are listed with a brief description for easy reviewing:

- The American Association of Critical-Care Nurses has evidence-based resources, which include practice alerts, tool kits, protocols, and Thunder studies, among other key topics, located at http://www.aacn.org/wd/practice/content/ebp.pcms?menu=practice.
- The Academy of Medical-Surgical Nurses has EBP resources that include foundational information about EBP and specifics regarding patient care (nutrition, end of life, care of older adults, and so forth), located at https://www.amsn.org/practice-resources/evidence-based-practice.
- The American Nurses Association Web site has information from the International Council of Nurses Evidence-Based Practice Resource, which includes steps on how to acquire and actually use research in nursing practice and opportunities for research funding, located at http://www.nursingworld.org/Research-Toolkit/ICN-Evidence-Based-Practice-Resource.
- The Agency for Healthcare Research and Quality, Evidence-based Practice Centers Program, has research findings and report summaries of scientific literature and numerous topics that include blood disorders, endocrine conditions, obstetric and gynecologic conditions, cancer, and many more at http://www.ahrq.gov/research/findings/evidence-based-reports/index.html.
- The National Institute of Nursing Research has numerous internal links to further refine inquiries for specific research topics (eg, preventing infection or end of life) through selection of "Research Highlights" or "Quick Links" at http://www.ninr.nih.gov/.
- Sigma Theta Tau International, an honor society of nursing, has resources that promote utilization and transformation of research findings into nursing practice, with links to the Virginia Henderson Global Nursing e-Repository, a full-text repository, located at http://www.nursinglibrary.org/vhl/.
- The Cochrane Collaboration promotes retrieval of information from full-text reviews to protocols in formats that include podcasts on blood disorders, cancer, child health, complementary and alternative medicine, neurology, urology, wounds, and so forth at http://www.cochrane.org/.
- Nursing evidence-based information can also be obtained from research databases, such as the Cumulative Index to Nursing and Allied Health Literature (CINAHL), Medical Literature Analysis and Retrieval System Online (MEDLINE), or the Nursing Reference Center from the Elton B. Stevens Company (EBSCO) host. Some of these can be accessed free of charge through hospital or university sites that subscribe to these databases for their employees or students. In some instances, individual subscriptions are available.

These are but a few of the many resources available to nurses promoting evidence as a foundation for patient care management. It is important to individually locate those resources that are foundational to an area of nursing expertise and maintain contact though intermittent review of this information to stay current. It is only through the utilization of research that nursing will grow as a profession and deliver the best possible patient care.

SUMMARY

Although it is easy to become overwhelmed with changes in health care, it is imperative that nurses continue to engage in activities that promote the best patient outcomes. Use of evidence-based interventions, obtaining certification, and active involvement in professional organizations can serve as a foundation to individually maintaining nursing knowledge and promoting expertise. Using this professional triad can bridge the gap between paper and practice, promoting the use of patient management protocols and guidelines that are objective and scientific.

REFERENCES

1. Institute of Medicine. The future of nursing: leading change, advancing health. Washington, DC: National Academies Press; 2010 [prepared by Robert Wood Johnson Foundation Committee Initiative on the Future of Nursing].
2. Polit DF, Beck CT. Nursing research: generating and assessing evidence for nursing practice. 9th edition. Philadelphia: Wolters Kluwer Health/Lippincott Williams & Wilkins; 2012. p. 3.
3. Hunt J. Towards evidence based practice. Nurs Manag (Harrow) 1997;4:14–7. Available at: http://www.plosone.org/article/info%3Adoi%2F10.1371%2Fjournal. pone.0081908#B8.
4. Kitson A, Harvey G, McCormack B. Enabling the implementation of evidence based practice: a conceptual framework. Qual Health Care 1998;7:149–58. http://dx.doi. org/10.1136/qshc.7.3.149.
5. Rich MW. From clinical trials to clinical practice: bridging the GAP. JAMA 2002; 287:1321–3.
6. McCaughan D, Thompson C, Cullum N, et al. Acute care nurses perceptions of barriers to using research information in clinical decision-making. J Adv Nurs 2002;39(1):46–60.
7. Hutchinson AM, Johnston L. Bridging the divide: a survey of nurses' opinions regarding barriers to, and facilitators of, research utilization in the practice setting. J Clin Nurs 2004;13(3):304–15.
8. Koehn ML, Lehman K. Nurses' perceptions of evidence-based nursing practice. J Adv Nurs 2008;62(2):209–15. http://dx.doi.org/10.1111/j.1365-2648.2007.04589.x.
9. Drisko J. Evidence based practice. 2008. Available at: http://sophia.smith.edu/ ~jdrisko/evidence_based_practice.htm. Published March 11, 2004. Updated September 24, 2012. Accessed July 26, 2014.
10. Adams K, Corrigan J. Institute of Medicine Committee on identifying priority areas for quality improvement. Priority areas for national action: transforming health care quality. Washington, DC: National Academies Press; 2003. Available at: http://www.nap.edu/openbook.php?isbn=0309085438. Accessed July 28, 2014.
11. Kohn LT, Corrigan JM, Donaldson MS. Institute of Medicine Committee on Quality of Healthcare in America. To err is human: building a safer health system. Washington, DC: National Academy Press; 2000. Available at: http://www.nap. edu/openbook.php?record_id=9728&page=1. Accessed July 28, 2014.

12. Oman KS, Makic MB, Fink R, et al. Nurse-directed interventions to reduce catheter-associated urinary tract infections. Am J Infect Control 2012. http://dx.doi.org/10.1016/j.ajic.2011.07.018.

13. Elpern EH, Killeen K, Ketchem A, et al. Reducing use of indwelling urinary catheters and associated urinary tract infections. Am J Crit Care 2009;18(6):535–42. http://dx.doi.org/10.4037/ajcc2009938.

14. Saint S, Olmsted RN, Fakih MG, et al. Translating health care-associated urinary tract infection prevention research into practice via bladder bundle. Jt Comm J Qual Patient Saf 2009;35(9):449–55. Available at: http://www.ncbi.nlm.nih.gov/pmc/articles/PMC2791398/. Accessed June 3, 2014.

15. Saint S, Kaufman SR, Rogers MA, et al. A reminder reduces urinary catheterization in hospitalized patients. Jt Comm J Qual Patient Saf 2005;31(8):455–62.

16. Meddings J, Rogers MA, Krein SL, et al. Reducing unnecessary urinary catheter use and other strategies to prevent catheter-associated urinary tract infection: an integrative review. BMJ Qual Saf 2013. http://dx.doi.org/10.1136/bmjqs-2012-001774.

17. Holzapfel I, Chevret S, Madinier G, et al. Influence of long term oro- or nasotracheal intubation on nosocomial maxillary sinusitis and pneumonia: results of a prospective, randomized, clinical trial. Crit Care Med 1993;21(8):1132–8.

18. Dodek P, Keenan S, Cook D, et al. Evidence-based clinical practice guideline for the prevention of ventilator-associated pneumonia. Ann Intern Med 2004;141(4):305–14.

19. Krein SL, Kowalski CP, Damschroder L, et al. Ventilator-associated pnwumonia in the United States: a multicenter mixed-methods study. Infect Control Hosp Epidemiol 2008;29(10):933–40. http://dx.doi.org/10.1086/591455.

20. Lorente L, Lecuona M, Jiménez M, et al. Tracheal suction by closed system without daily change versus open system. Intensive Care Med 2006;32(4):538–44.

21. Koeman M, vanderVen AJ, Hak E, et al. Oral decontamination with chlorhexidine reduces the indicence of ventilator-associated pneumonia. Am J Respir Crit Care Med 2006;173(12):1348–55. Available at: http://www.ncbi.nlm.nih.gov/pubmed/16603609. Accessed June 3, 2014.

22. Labeau S, Van de Vyker K, Brusselaers N, et al. Prevention of ventilator-associated pneumonia with oral antiseptics: a systematic review and meta-analysis. Lancet Infect Dis 2011;11(11):845–54.

23. Tantipong H, Morkchareonpong C, Jaiyindee S, et al. Randomized controlled trial and meta-analysis of oral decontamination with 2% chlorhexidine solution for the prevention of ventilator-associated pneumonia. Infect Control Hosp Epidemiol 2008;29(2):131–6.

24. Jabre P, Belpomme V, Azoulay F, et al. Family presence during cardiopulmonary resuscitation. N Engl J Med 2013;368(11):1008–18. http://dx.doi.org/10.1056/NEJMoa1203366. Available at: http://www.nejm.org/doi/full/10.1056/NEJMoa1203366. Accessed June 4, 2014.

25. Helmer SD, Smith RS, Dort JM, et al. Family presence during trauma resuscitation: a survey of AAST and ENA members. American Association for the Surgery Trauma. Emergency Nurses Association. J Trauma 2000;48(6):1015–22 [discussion: 1023–4].

26. McClenathan BM, Torrington KG, Uyehara CF. Family member presence during cardiopulmonary resuscitation: a survey of US and international critical care professionals. Chest 2002;122(6):2204–11.

27. Tromp M, Huis A, de Guchteneire I, et al. The short-term and long-term effectiveness of a multidisciplinary hand hygiene improvement program. Am J Infect Control 2012;40(8):732–6.

28. Huang J, Jiang D, Wang X, et al. Changing knowledge, behavior and practice related to universal precautions among hospital nurses in China. J Contin Educ Nurs 2002;33(5):217–24.

29. Macdonald DJ, McKillop EC, Trotter S, et al. Improving hand-washing performance – a crossover study of hand-washing in the orthopaedic department. Ann R Coll Surg Engl 2006;88(3):289–91. http://dx.doi.org/10.1308/003588406X98577. Available at: http://www.ncbi.nlm.nih.gov/pmc/articles/PMC1963687/#__ffn_sectitle. Accessed June 4, 2014.

30. Mcdonald D, Mckillip E, Trotter S, et al. One plunge or two? – hand disinfection with alcohol gel. Int J Qual Health Care 2006;18(2):120–2. http://dx.doi.org/10.1093/intqhc/mzi109. Available at: http://intqhc.oxfordjournals.org/content/18/2/120.full. Accessed June 4, 2014.

31. Kress JP. Clinical trials of early mobilization of critically ill patients. Crit Care Med 2009;37(10 Suppl):S442–7. http://dx.doi.org/10.1097/CCM.0b013e3181b6f9c0.

32. Burtin C, Clerckx B, Robbeets C, et al. Early exercise in critically ill patients enhances short-term functional recovery. Crit Care Med 2009;37(9):1–7.

33. Schweickert WD, Pohlman MC, Pohlman AS, et al. Early physical and occupational therapy in mechanically ventilated, critically ill patients: a randomised controlled trial. Lancet 2009;373:1874–82.

34. Longmate A, Ellis K, Boyle L, et al. Elimination of central-venous-catheter-related bloodstream infections from the intensive care unit. BMJ Qual Saf 2011;20(2):174–80. http://dx.doi.org/10.1136/bmjqs.2009.037200.

35. Rosenthal VD, Guzman S, Pezzotto SM, et al. Effect of an infection control program using education and performance feedback on rates of intravascular device-associated bloodstream infections in intensive care units in Argentina. Am J Infect Control 2003;31(7):405–9.

36. Yilmaz G, Caylan R, Aydin K, et al. Effect of education on the rate of and the understanding of risk factors for intravascular catheter–related infections. Infect Control Hosp Epidemiol 2007;28(6):689–94.

37. Raad II, Hohn DC, Gilbreath BJ, et al. Prevention of central venous catheter-related infections by using maximal sterile barrier precautions during insertion. Infect Control Hosp Epidemiol 1994;15(4 Pt 1):231–8.

38. Hu KK, Lipsky BA, Veenstra DL, et al. Using maximal sterile barriers to prevent central venous catheter-related infection: a systematic evidence-based review. Am J Infect Control 2004;32(3):142–6.

39. Hu KK, Veenstra DL, Lipsky BA, et al. Use of maximal sterile barriers during central vanous catheter insertion: clinical and economic outcomes. Clin Infect Dis 2004;39(10):1441–5. Available at: http://cid.oxfordjournals.org/content/39/10/1441.full. Accessed August 12, 2014.

40. Maragakis LL, Bradley KL, Song X, et al. Increased catheter-related bloodstream infection rates after introduction of a new mechanical valve intravenous access port. Infect Control Hosp Epidemiol 2006;27:67–70.

41. Jarvis WR, Murphy C, Hall KK, et al. Health care-associatd bloodstream infections associated with negative or positive-pressure of displacement mechanical valve needless connectors. Clin Infect Dis 2009;49:1821–7.

42. Chernecky C, Waller J. Comparative evaluation of five needleless intravenous connectors. J Adv Nurs 2011;67:1601–13.

43. Evanoff B, Potter P, Wolf L, et al. Can we talk? Priorities for patient care differed among health care providers Advances in Patient Safety. vol. 1. 2005. p. 5–14. Available at: http://www.ncbi.nlm.nih.gov/books/NBK20468/pdf/ch2.pdf. Accessed June 4, 2014.

44. Pronovost P, Berenholtz S, Dorman T, et al. Improving communication in the ICU using daily goals. J Crit Care 2003;18(2):71–5.
45. Dingley C, Daugherty K, Derieg MK, et al. Improving Patient Safety Through Provider Communication Strategy Enhancements. In: Henriksen K, Battles JB, Keyes MA, et al, editors. Advances in Patient Safety: New Directions and Alternative Approaches, (Vol. 3: Performance and Tools). Rockville (MD): Agency for Healthcare Research and Quality (US); 2008.
46. Warye KL, Murphy DM. Targeting zero health care-associated infections. Am J Infect Control 2008;36(10):683–4.
47. Brown J, Doloresco F III, Mylotte JM. "Never events": not every hospital-acquired infection is preventable. Clin Infect Dis 2009;49(5):743–6.
48. Association for Professionals in Infection Control and Epidemiology. Guide to the elimination of catheter-associated urinary tract infections (CAUTIs): developing and applying facility-based prevention in acute and long-term care settings. 2008. Available at: http://www.apic.org/resource_/eliminationguideform/c0790db8-2aca-4179-a7ae-676c27592de2/file/apic-cauti-guide.pdf. Accessed June 4, 2014.
49. Augustyn B. Ventilator-associated pneumonia: risk factors and prevention. Crit Care Nurse 2007;27(4):32–9. Available at: http://ccn.aacnjournals.org/content/27/4/32.full#T2. Accessed June 18, 2014.
50. Mazer MA, Cox LA, Capon A. The public's attitude and perception concerning witnessed cardiopulmonary resuscitation. Crit Care Med 2006;34(12):2925–8.
51. Sachetti A, Paston C, Carraccio C. Family members do not disrupt care when present during invasive procedures. Acad Emerg Med 2005;12(5):463–6.
52. Meyers TA, Eichhorn DJ, Guzzetta CE, et al. Family presence during invasive procedures and resuscitation: the experiences of family members, nurses, and physicians. Am J Nurs 2000;100(2):32–42.
53. World Health Organization. 'The first global patient safety challenge: clean care is safer care'. 2013. Available at: http://www.who.int/gpsc/en/. Published 2014. Accessed August 8, 2014.
54. Fishbein M, Ajzen I. Predicting and changing behavior: the reasoned action approach. New York: Psychology Press (Taylor & Fancis); 2010.
55. Aiello AE, Malinis M, Knapp JK, et al. The influence of knowledge, perceptions, and beliefs, on hand hygiene practices in nursing homes. Am J Infect Control 2009;37(2):164–7. http://dx.doi.org/10.1016/j.ajic.2008.04.258.
56. Al-Besides, Habib. Healthcare workers and hand hygiene practice: a literature review. The public 6.1. Available at: http://atp.uclan.ac.uk/buddypress/diffusion/?p=1515. Accessed June 18, 2014
57. Truong AD, Fan E, Brower RG, et al. Bench-to-bedside review: mobilizing patients in the intensive care unit-from pathophysiology to clinical trials. Crit Care 2009;13:216–23.
58. The Joint Commission. Preventing central line–associated bloodstream infections: a global challenge, a global perspective. Oak Brook (IL): Joint Commission Resources; 2012. Available at: http://www.PreventingCLABSIs.pdf. Accessed June 8, 2014.
59. Leonard M, Graham S, Bonacum D. The human factor: the critical importance of effective teamwork and communication in providing safe care. Qual Saf Health Care 2004;13:85–90.
60. Krapohl G, Manojlovich M, Redman R, et al. Nursing specialty certification and nursing-sensitive patient outcomes in the intensive care unit. Am J Crit Care 2010;19(6):490–9. http://dx.doi.org/10.4037/ajcc2010406.

61. Guide to nursing certification organizations: specialty certification organizations 2008. Dimens Crit Care Nurs 2008;27(4):171–2.
62. Your guide to certification: here's what you need to know to pursue recognition of your expertise. Am J Nurs [serial online] 2007;107(1 Suppl):26–38.
63. American Nurses Credentialing Center. ANCC Certification-opening a world of opportunities. 2014. Published 2014. Available at: http://www.nursecredentialing.org/Mission-Statement. Accessed June 4, 2014.
64. Stierle LJ, Mezey M, Schumann MJ, et al. Professional development: the nurse competence in aging initiative: encouraging expertise in the care of older adults. Am J Nurs 2006;106(9):93–6.
65. Cary AH. Certified registered nurses: results of the study of the certified workforce. Am J Nurs 2001;101:44–52.
66. Piazza IM, Donahue M, Dykes P, et al. Differences in perceptions of empowerment among nationally certified and noncertified nurses. J Nurs Adm 2006; 36(5):277–83.
67. Boltz M, Capezuti E, Wagner L, et al. Patient safety in medical-surgical units: can nurse certification make a difference? Medsurg Nurs 2013;22(1):26–37.
68. Schroeter K, Byrne MM, Klink K, et al. The impact of certification on certified perioperative nurses: a qualitative descriptive survey. ORNAC J 2012;30(3):35–45.
69. Sullivan D, Stevenson D. Promoting professional organization involvement. AORN J 2009;90(4):575–9. http://dx.doi.org/10.1016/j.aorn.2009.09.007.
70. Holleman G, Eliens A, vanVliet M, et al. Promotion of evidence-based practice by professional nursing associations: literature review. J Adv Nurs 2006;53(6):702–9. http://dx.doi.org/10.1111/j.1365-2648.2006.03776.x.
71. Martin A. Fostering career development through involvement in professional organizations. Am J Health Syst Pharm 2007;64(14):1472–3. http://dx.doi.org/10.2146/ajhp070096.

Understanding Quality Patient Care and the Role of the Practicing Nurse

 CrossMark

Laura D. Owens, PhD, RN[a], Robert W. Koch, DNSc, RN[b],*

KEYWORDS

- Health care quality • Affordable Care Act
- Center for Medicare and Medicaid Services (CMS)
- Institute of Healthcare Improvement (IHI)
- The Agency for Healthcare Research and Quality (AHRQ)
- National Database of Nursing Quality Indicators (NDNQI)

KEY POINTS

- Understanding the history of the quality initiative in health care is important in understanding the directions for the future.
- Health care quality is closely monitored by both private and public agencies charged with ensuring safe and efficient delivery of health services.
- Measuring quality in health care is the key to determining if desired outcomes are achieved.

INTRODUCTION

Nursing today requires more than caring for patients. Nurses must provide, manage, and document quality patient care measured within the patient care setting. This article discusses the history of the quality movement, key quality health care organizations, various measures of quality care, and the financial and professional practice implications for quality patient care.

HISTORY OF QUALITY MOVEMENT

Quality management in the United States can be traced to the 1920s and the work of Edward Deming, Walter A. Shewhart, and Joseph Juran.[1] All 3 laid the groundwork for current quality health care initiatives with their work that began in American industry.

Disclosure: The authors of this publication have not received any support (financial or otherwise) in the preparation of this article.
[a] Loewenberg School of Nursing, University of Memphis, Memphis, TN 38152, USA; [b] The West Cancer Center, Memphis, TN 38120, USA
* Corresponding author.
E-mail address: rkoch@WESTCLINIC.com

Deming's work in Japan during their postwar reconstruction led to significant industrial gains and business success in that country. Later, as the United States recognized his work, it became the turning point for quality control in the United States.[2] By the time of Deming's death in 1993, he had seen quality management efforts move from manufacturing to service industries, and finally, to health care.[3,4]

Dr Avedis Donabebian also contributed to the quality movement in the 1960s with his research on quality and outcomes research in medicine. His model used the aspects of structure, process, and outcomes to examine health care quality. Structure indicates the context in which the care is given, such as a hospital; process is the interaction between patients and providers, and outcomes are the effects of health care on patients and the population. The Donabedian model continues to influence health care quality evaluation today.[5,6]

In 1966, Medicare was signed into law under Title XVIII of the Social Security Act to provide health insurance to people 65 years of age and older and for those with certain disabilities and chronic diseases. Medicaid was signed into law as Title XIX of the Social Security Act to provide medical assistance for certain individuals with low income and resources. Both programs have undergone changes and expansion over their years of existence.[7] Measures to address quality in these services were established at the onset and have also changed over the course of time. Initially, in 1965, a set of conditions called "conditions of participation" were developed that addressed matters such as nursing services, staff credentials, and utilization review. Utilization review committees were established to identify whether hospitals and providers were meeting the conditions for participation. These committees were not considered successful partly because of a lack of means to identify ways to improve care.

In 1972, "Experimental Medical Care Review Organizations" were established by Congress and given the responsibility of reviewing both quality and appropriateness of care being delivered. These organizations were able to develop improvement strategies based on the findings of a quality review. The Experimental Review Organizations were more successful than the utilization review committees and led to the development of Medicare's Professional Standards Review Organizations (PSROs), which were charged with ensuring that hospitals and providers met Medicare guidelines for quality care. In 1983, the PSROs were replaced with Peer Review Organizations (PROs), which led to success in achieving goals of cost containment and quality improvement (QI). PROs continue to function as a Quality Improvement Organization under the current Centers for Medicare and Medicaid Services (CMS).[8]

Quality assurance (QA) models were the models initially used by hospitals as a method to maintain quality in the institution. In the 1980s, the approach of QI or quality management was added and used alongside QA models to improve the process of identifying root causes of poorer quality care and prevent future problems. Koch and Fairly[9] described some differences in QA and QI models of quality. QA activities tend to be inspection oriented to detect problems, whereas QI models are planning-oriented and focus on prevention. QA models tend to have a narrow focus, be reactive, and correct special problems, whereas QI models tend to have a cross-functional focus, are proactive, and attempt to correct the common causes of quality concerns. QA "models seek to ensure that current quality exists, whereas QI models assume that the process if ongoing and quality can always be improved."[10]

In the 1980s, the Healthcare Quality Improvement Initiative, developed by the Health Care Finance Administration (HCFA) and implemented as an effort to maintain QI in Medicare, allowed PSROs to apply a patient algorithm to data sets and claims history to identify how well care conformed to guidelines.[11] In the late 1980s, the Institute of Medicine (IOM) conducted a study commissioned by Congress to evaluate QA for

Medicare. The study found that many health services were inadequate and, following the IOM's report, the Health Care Finance Administration developed and implemented several QI initiatives that commenced in the early 1990s. Two publications by the IOM[12,13] focused national attention on quality issues in health care and the need for improvement. *To err is human: Building a safer health system*[12] identified safety gaps in health care and found that as many as 98,000 people died yearly because of preventable medical errors. *Crossing the quality chasm: A new health system for the 21st century*[13] placed blame on the health care system for failing to provide high-quality medical care to all people. With blame placed on the system rather than individuals, recommendations were made to make the system safer. Six dimensions were identified in the report as critical to improving health care quality and continue to remain as a framework for improving quality of care in the United States. Using these 6 dimensions, care should be safe, effective, patient-centered, timely, efficient, and equitable.[13]

In 2001, the Voluntary Hospital Association and the Institute for Healthcare Improvement (IHI) collaborated on an initiative called Idealized Design of the Intensive Care Unit and examined the structure and assumptions that were used to deliver care in intensive care units. The goal of the initiative was to determine how to achieve high levels of reliability in critical care and good outcomes, all while using concepts of enhanced teamwork and communication. The result of this initiative was the development of care bundles.[14] A care bundle is defined by the IHI as a small set of evidence-based interventions for a defined patient population and care setting. Originally, 2 bundles were developed out of the initiative research: the IHI ventilator bundle and the IHI central line bundle. Since the inception of this concept, more bundles have been developed, and the IHI reports that use of the bundles has significantly improved patient outcomes and care quality.[15]

In 2010, President Barack Obama signed The Patient Protection and Affordable Care Act into law. This law included an objective related to improving overall quality, while lowering costs and increasing access to health care. One of the law's quality-related provisions was the development of the Patient-Centered Outcomes Research Institute, a nonprofit institute that conducts clinical effectiveness research.[16]

KEY HEALTH CARE QUALITY ORGANIZATIONS
Joint Commission

In 1951, the Joint Commission for Accreditation of Healthcare was established as an independent, not-for-profit agency with the purpose of providing voluntary accreditation to hospitals for meeting quality-related guidelines. The name was changed to The Joint Commission for Healthcare Organizations in 1987 to reflect an expanded focus with more emphasis on organizational performance and is now known as the Joint Commission (JC). The JC has had a tremendous impact on quality planning and control in hospitals and currently accredits more than 20,500 hospitals. In the 1980s, JC developed requirements that hospitals have QA programs in place that not only reviewed care provided by hospitals but also included specific plans to remedy identified or suspected problems. In 1982, quarterly evaluations of nursing care were mandated (History of the Joint Commission, 2014). The year 1996 saw the establishment of the Sentinel Event Policy for the evaluation of sentinel events in relationship to the organization's accreditation status. The JC maintains a large database of reported sentinel events and their causes.[17]

As the JC shifted its focus of accreditation from organizational structure to organizational outcomes, the Agenda for Change initiative was launched. In 1997, ORYX was implemented to integrate outcome and other performance measures into the accreditation process, and information about accredited organizations was made available on a JC Web site known as Quality Check (www.qualitycheck.org). Organizations that were accredited by JC were required to collect data-specific clinical performance measures.[18] In 2002, JC implemented its core measures program as part of the ORYX initiative and targeted 4 areas: acute myocardial infarction, pneumonia, heart failure, and the surgical care improvement project. Since the implementation of the core measures program, many other core measures have been added, and the required number of core measures that hospitals are required to implement has increased. In 2012, core measures were reclassified as accountability measures, which are described as quality measures that meet 4 specific criteria and produce the greatest positive impact on patient outcomes when hospitals demonstrate improvement on them. The criteria are research, proximity, accuracy, and adverse effects.[19]

Also in 2002, the JC established its first annual National Patient Safety Goals for improving the safety of patient care in health care organizations. These goals were to become effective in 2003. Some of the current patient safety goals include improved communication between staff, correct patient identification, safe medication administration, and infection prevention. In the same year, the JC and the CMS launched Speak Up, a national campaign that urged patients to take a role in preventing health care errors and encouraged them to become active and involved, and informed participants of the health care team. In 2004, the World Health Organization launched its World Alliance for Patient Safety, and the JC was invited to be involved in several of the Alliance's initiatives. Throughout the decade, JC continued to expand its efforts related to improving quality in it accredited hospitals.

Center for Medicare and Medicaid Services

The CMS, formerly known as the HCFA and a department of the United States Department of Health and Human Services, plays an active role in quality measurement and setting quality standards in health care.[8] The Hospital Quality Initiative launched in 2001 made data related to health care quality available to the public. The purpose of this initiative was to enable the health care consumer to make well-informed decisions on hospital care, create incentives for hospitals to improve care, and create public accountability.[20] "Never events," identified in 2001 by the National Quality Foundation as sentinel events or medical errors that are serious and preventable and should simply never happen, are reported by the JC. CMS in 2007 began restricting payments in never events. Examples of these events include surgical events, product or device events, patient protection events, care management events, environmental events, radiologic events, or criminal events. One specific example of a never event is wrong site surgery.[21,22] CMS established the Quality Reporting and Hospital Value-Based Purchasing program in 2011 under the Affordable Care Act. Under this program, hospitals earn incentive payments based on their performance on clinical process measures and patient experience measures. The program was designed to improve quality of care while reducing inappropriate care and promoting better health outcomes thus leading to high-value care.[20] Providing high-value care is considered providing the highest quality care at the lowest cost. Value can be improved by either increasing quality or decreasing costs and includes both clinical outcomes and the patient's experience. Costs include monetary costs and harm to patient and/or the system.[23]

The Institute for Healthcare Improvement

The IHI was established in 1991 as an independent not-for-profit organization working to promote improvement in health care systems in the United States. IHI describes its mission as improving health and health care worldwide with a vision that all people have the best health and health care possible. IHI connects people and organizations with similar visions that are committed to health care reform and quality, provides educational opportunities for health care students and professionals, along with conducting and promoting research related to quality.[24]

The Agency for Healthcare Research and Quality

The Agency for Healthcare Research and Quality (AHRQ), supported by the Federal government, supports research to provide evidence-based information on health care outcomes, quality, cost, use, and access, ensuring that the evidence is understood by the consumer and the professional. AHRQ's research is designed to help consumers make more informed decisions, improve the quality of health care services, and inform policy.[25]

National Association for Healthcare Quality

The National Association for Healthcare Quality is dedicated to improving the quality of health care and supporting professionals involved in health care quality by providing educational and development opportunities. Professionals from hospitals and other health care organizations that are involved in all aspects of quality, such as QA, QI, core measures, and risk management, find professional education and support through NAHQ.[25]

The Institute for Safe Medication Practices

The ISMP, founded in 1979, is a not-for-profit organization with a goal of educating health care professionals and consumers about medication safety. ISMP works closely with health care providers, institutions, regulatory agencies, professional organizations, and the pharmaceutical industry to prevent medication errors. The organization provides an independent review of medication errors that have been voluntarily submitted by practitioners to a national Medical Error Reporting Program (MERP). All information derived from the MERP is shared with the US Food and Drug Administration and pharmaceutical companies whose products are mentioned in the reports. ISMP offers education for health care professionals and consumers through teleconferences, error reports, and consultations services.[26]

American Society for Quality

The American Society for Quality (ASQ) was founded in the 1940s and identifies itself as a global group of people passionate about quality. ASQ began its quality initiatives in manufacturing and industry and later expanded in the health care arena. The organization provides ongoing development, advancement, and promotion of quality concepts, principles, and techniques by offering education and professional certification to all those involved in the quality industry. Participation in standards development and research related to quality is also an integral component of ASQ's work.[25]

Hospital Compare

Hospital Compare[27] is a Web site developed by the CMS and the Hospital Quality Alliance that provides consumers with quality information about specific hospitals and allows them to compare with other hospitals and therefore make informed decisions. The Web site contains information about timely and effective care for certain conditions, such as heart attack or heart failure, readmission rates, complications and death rates, use of medical imaging, survey of patients' experiences, and Medicare payment rates. In 2013, information was added about the hospital value-based purchasing program.[27]

MEASURES OF QUALITY CARE

Few dispute the importance of nurses and nurse staffing on quality patient care. Nurses provide continuous care and must assess patient care needs, interact with the patient and family/caregivers, provide education as well as medications and treatments, and plan for community care after discharge to the appropriate setting, all at reasonable cost. However, how do nurses and the health care organizations that employ them measure quality care? Can quality nursing care impact an organization's financial goal to lower costs through decreased hospital readmissions, lengths of stay, and legal liability? Several groups have developed quality indicators to measure the outcomes of care in health care systems to address the economics of care delivery and minimize overall human suffering during illness.

Agency for Healthcare Research and Quality and Quality Indicators

One organization central to quality measurements initiative is the AHRQ. The AHRQ provides many tools for health care decision-making and research, including Quality Indicators (QIs), health care measurements determined through available hospital inpatient administrative data. These QIs can help define potential quality issues, pinpoint areas deserving further study, and evaluate and track changes over time. AHRQ currently offers QI modules on Prevention Quality Indicators (PQIs), Inpatient Quality Indicators, Patient Safety Quality Indicators, and Pediatric Quality Indicators. They offer free software to assist hospitals in determining quality of care and highlighting needs for further study (AHRQ; http://www.qualityindicators.ahrq.gov/). The AHRQ QI indicators are currently available for hospital use only and not other settings, such as long-term care, home care, or specific populations, such as rehabilitation, mental health or substance abuse, or nursing quality. To learn more about these AHRQ quality indicators, visit the AHRQ Web site.[28]

National Database of Nursing Quality Indicators

In March 1994, the American Nurses Association (ANA) began a multifaceted investigation of the impact of health care restructuring that resulted from increased cost-cutting measures in health care facilities, such as the use of unlicensed personal in patient care. Nursing's Safety and Quality Initiative worked with nurses and the public to inform nurses, consumers, and legislators about the important contribution of nurses to safe quality health care.[29]

In 1998, the National Center for Nursing Quality began advocating research and measurement for quality nursing care, such as studying the relationship between nurse staffing and quality patient care. The ANA funded an initiative to develop a national database on nursing-sensitive quality indicators, housed at the University of Kansas School of Nursing. The goal was to establish a standardized approach to uniform data collection that could be submitted by hospitals to impact quality patient care through nursing. ANA knew that nurses can and do make a difference in safe, quality patient care that is cost-effective. The 10 nursing-sensitive quality indicators determined for acute care settings are listed in **Box 1**.[29]

The nursing-sensitive quality indicators reflect the structure, process, and outcomes of nursing care, capturing data on care and/or outcomes most impacted by nursing. An example of a structure indicator is the education or certification of the nursing staff. Process indicators might include nursing assessment or nurse job satisfaction. An outcome of nursing care could be patient falls or pressure ulcers. Adverse patient outcomes may be related to institutional policies or medical decisions, so

---

Box 1
Nursing-sensitive quality indicators determined by American Nurses Association for acute care settings

Mix of RNs, LPNs, and unlicensed staff caring for patients in acute settings

Total nursing care hours provided per patient day

Pressure ulcers

Patient falls

Patient satisfaction with pain management

Patient satisfaction with educational information

Patient satisfaction with overall care

Patient satisfaction with nursing care

Nosocomial infection rate

Nurse staff satisfaction

---

these are not considered nursing-sensitive outcomes. To learn more about nursing-sensitive quality indicators, visit the ANA Web site.[30]

National Database of Nursing Quality Indicators (NDNQI) has worked to further define QI indicators with the National Quality Forum (NQF). Collaborating with the JC through a grant from the Robert Woods Johnson Foundation, the ANA developed microspecifications of NQF-endorsed nursing measures. The indicators under review are shown in **Box 2**.[30]

The project also collects information on the patient population (adult/pediatric), hospital category (teaching, nonteaching), type of unit (Critical Care, Step Down, Medical, Surgical, Combined Med-Surg, Rehab, and Psychiatric), and the number of staffed

---

Box 2
Additional nurse-sensitive quality indicators currently being reviewed

- Nursing hours per patient day (RN, LPN/LVN, and unlicensed assistive [UAP] hours per patient day)
- Nursing turnover
- Nosocomial infections
- Patient falls
- Patient falls with injury (injury levels)
- Pressure ulcer rate (community-acquired, hospital-acquired, and unit-acquired)
- Pediatric pain assessment, intervention, reassessment cycle
- Pediatric peripheral intravenous infiltration
- Psychiatric physical/sexual assault
- RN education/certification
- RN survey (job satisfaction scales, practice environment scales)
- Restraints
- Staff mix (RN, LPN/LVP, UAP, percentage agency staff)

beds designated by the hospital. Benefits for participating hospitals in NDNQI include support in QI efforts, staff education, RN retention and recruitment, research, patient recruitment, and helping satisfy regulatory or magnet status requirements.[30]

In 2014, Press Ganey, a company known for working collaboratively with health care providers to improve the patient experience through customer satisfaction, clinical safety, and financial measurement, acquired the NDNQI. As a proprietary database, Press Ganey will enhance the ability to work with nurses and nurse leaders to improve the patient care experience.

IMPLICATIONS FOR NURSING PRACTICE

As hospitals continue to face demands for participation in QI activities, the roles of nurses are increasing and becoming integral to QI initiatives. Nurses have a long history of evaluating the quality of nursing practice, beginning with the practice of Florence Nightingale and her role in measuring patient outcomes related to environmental conditions.[31] Over the years, the quality movement has grown and continues to evolve to meet the demands of an ever-changing health care system.

Draper and colleagues[32] assert that nurses play a pivotal role in helping hospitals meet QI guidelines and, by identifying the challenges nurses face in meeting those guidelines, hospitals can more effectively use the expert role that nurses play. Researchers collected information from 8 hospitals in 4 communities that were participating in the Robert Wood Johnson Foundation's Aligning Forces for Quality Program by conducting semistructured phone interviews with hospital leadership. Some critical approaches to help foster QI were identified by the hospital leaders, including a supporting hospital leadership that was actively engaged in quality work; setting expectations for all staff and not just nurses, emphasizing that quality is a shared responsibility; holding staff accountable as individuals; using physicians and nurses as champions to promote quality efforts; and providing ongoing useful feedback to engage staff effectively. Draper and colleagues also identified several challenges to nursing staff when implementing quality efforts. These challenges include adequacy of nursing staff if resources are scarce, engaging nurses at all levels from bedside to management, increasing numbers of QI activities, high level of administrative burden often associated with QI activities, and meeting the lack of preparation in traditional nursing education for the nurse's role in quality efforts.

Kovner and colleagues[33] found the almost 39% of new graduates thought they were poorly prepared to implement QI measures or to use QI techniques despite having received the content in the prelicensure program. Quality and Safety Education for Nurses was developed using funding by the Robert Wood Johnson Foundation to evaluate and enhance curricula related to quality and safety.[34] This project led to the establishment of prelicensure nursing competencies for knowledge, skills, and attitudes needed to improve the quality of health care systems. In 2008, The Essentials of Baccalaureate Education for Professional Nursing[35] was revised and required that students participate in the process of retrieval, appraisal, and synthesis of evidence to improve patient outcomes. This requirement also includes collaboration in the process with other members of the health care team. Kovner and colleagues recommend that hospitals and nurse educators' partner to provide more comprehensive QI education that enables all students to participate in QI projects before graduation.

Nursing as a profession has an obligation to continue to evaluate and improve nursing practice, as noted in 2 of the profession's guidelines for practice. In the ANA *Code of Ethics*, the "nurse promotes, advocates for, and strives to protect the health, safety, and rights of the patient."[36(p12)] The *Nursing: Scope & Standards of*

Box 3
Web sites for major quality organizations

- American Society for Quality: http://asq.org/index.aspx
- Centers for Medicare and Medicaid Services: http://cms.hhs.gov/
- Institute for Healthcare Improvement: http://www.ihi.org/Pages/default.aspx
- National Association for Healthcare Quality: http://www.nahq.org/
- National Center for Nursing Quality: http://www.nursingworld.org/ncnq
- National Quality Forum: http://www.qualityforum.org/Home.aspx
- Patient-Centered Outcomes Research Institute: http://www.pcori.org/
- The Agency for Healthcare Research and Quality: http://www.ahrq.gov/
- The Deming Institute: https://www.deming.org/
- The Joint Commission: http://www.jointcommission.org/
- The Institute for Safe Medication Practices: http://www.ismp.org/
- Quality and Safety Education for Nurses: http://qsen.org/

Practice, Standard 7, states "the registered nurse systematically enhances the quality and effectiveness of nursing practice."[37(p33)] To this end, the NDNQI was established by ANA in 1998 to allow ANA to collect data and improve nursing's knowledge of factors relating to quality of nursing care. Information from the database is available to member hospitals and can be used to improve patient care, improve quality outcomes, guide staffing decisions, assist in progression to Magnet status, and allow hospitals and nursing units to compare themselves to similar entities (**Box 3**).[38,39]

REFERENCES

1. Neave HR. The Deming dimension. Knoxville (TN): Statistic Press Control (SPC Press); 1990. Available at: http://www.spcpress.com/book_deming_dimension.php.
2. Deming the man. The W. Edwards Deming Institute; 2012. Available at: https://www.deming.org/theman/timeline.
3. Tritus M. (1988). Deming's way. Mechanical Engineering, 28, 38–45.
4. Staskson FC, Kopera A, Wilson RC. Taking the IOM quality challenge: providers can do a lot to meet the Institute of Medicine's call for improving the quality of healthcare (Institute of Medicine's quality control measures to improve the performance of healthcare services). Behav Healthc 2007;24:27–35.
5. Donabedian A. The quality of care: how can it be assessed? JAMA 1988;121(11):1145–50.
6. Marjoua Y, Bozic KJ. Brief history of quality movement in US healthcare. Curr Rev Musculoskelet Med 2012;5(4):265–73. http://dx.doi.org/10.1007/s12178-012-9137-8.
7. About us. The Institute for Healthcare Improvement; 2014. Available at: http://www.ihi.org/about/pages/ihivisionandvalues.aspx. Accessed August 2, 2014.
8. History. Centers for Medicare and Medicaid Services; 2014. Available at: http://cms.gov/About-CMS/Agency-Information/History/index.html.
9. Koch MW, Fairley TM. Integrated quality management: the key to improving nursing care quality. St Louis (MO): Mosby; 1993.

10. Marquis BL, Huston CJ. Leadership roles and management functions in nursing. 8th edition. Philadelphia: Wolters Kluwer Health Lippincott Williams and Wilkins; 2015.
11. Luce JM, Bindman AB, Lee PR. A brief history of health care quality assessment and improvement in the United Stated. West J Med 1994;160:263–8.
12. Institute of Medicine. To err is human: building a safer health system. Washington, DC: The National Academies Press; 2000.
13. Institute of Medicine. Crossing the quality chasm: a new health system for the 21st century. Washington, DC: The National Academies Press; 2001.
14. Resar R, Griffin FA, Haraden C, et al. Using care bundles to improve health care quality. IHI innovation series white paper. Cambridge (MA): Institute for Healthcare Improvement; 2012. Available at: www.IHI.org.
15. What is a bundle? Available at: http://www.ihi.org/resources/Pages/Improvement Stories/WhatIsaBundle.aspx. Accessed August 10, 2014.
16. About the law. US Department of Health and Human Services. Available at: http://www.hhs.gov/healthcare/rights/index.html.
17. Sentinel event data summary. Available at: http://www.jointcommission.org/sentinel_event.aspx.
18. Facts about ORYX for hospitals: National Hospital Quality Measures. 2013. Available at: http://www.jointcommission.org/facts_about_oryx_for_hospitals/.
19. What are accountability measures? Available at: http://www.jointcommission.org/about/JointCommissionFaqs.aspx?CategoryId=31#174.
20. Hospital quality initiative overview. Centers for Medicare & Medicaid Services; 2008. Available at: http://www.cms.hhs.gov/HospitalQualityInits/Downloads/Hospitaloverview.pdf. Accessed August 1, 2014.
21. US Department of Health and Human Services. Spotlight on...never event. 2012. Available at: http://oig.hhs.gov/newsroom/spotlight/2012/adverse.asp.
22. US Department of Health & Human Services, Agency for Healthcare Research and Quality. 2012. Patient safety primers: never events. Available at: http://www.psnet.ahrq.gov/primer.aspx?primerID53.
23. Porter M. What is value in health care? N Engl J Med 2010;363:2477–81.
24. About AHRQ. Agency for Healthcare Research and Quality; 2014. Available at: http://www.ahrq.gov/cpi/about/index.html. Accessed August 4, 2014.
25. Who we are. National Association for Healthcare Quality; 2014. Available at: http://www.nahq.org/about/whoweare/whoweare.html. Accessed August 10, 2014.
26. About ISMP. Institute for Safe Medicine Practices; 2014. Available at: http://www.ismp.org/about/default.asp.
27. Hospital Compare. 2014. Available at: http://www.cms.gov/Medicare/Quality-Initiatives-Patient-Assessment-Instruments/HospitalQualityInits/HospitalCompare.html.
28. Agency for Healthcare Research and Quality. Available at: http://www.qualityindicators.ahrq.gov/FAQs_Support/FAQ_QI_Overview.aspx.
29. ANA Indicator History. Available at: http://www.nursingworld.org/MainMenu Categories/ThePracticeofProfessionalNursing/PatientSafetyQuality/Research-Measurement/The-National-Database/Nursing-Sensitive-Indicators_1/ANA-Indicator-History.
30. Nursing-Sensitive Indicators. Available at: http://www.nursingworld.org/MainMenu Categories/ThePracticeofProfessionalNursing/PatientSafetyQuality/Research-Measurement/The-National-Database/Nursing-Sensitive-Indicators_1.

31. Dossey BM, Selanders LC, Beck DM, et al. Florence Nightingale today: healing, leadership, global action. Silver Spring (MD): Nursesbooks.org; 2005. Available at: www.nursingworld.org/books/pdescr.cfm?cnum=29#04FNT.

32. Draper DA, Felland LE, Liebhaber A, et al. The role of nurses in hospital quality improvement, vol. 3. Washington, DC: Center for Studying Healthcare System Change; 2008. Available at: www.hschange.com/CONTENT/972/972.pdf.

33. Kovner CK, Brewer CS, Yingrengreung S, et al. New nurses' views of quality improvement education. Jt Comm J Qual Patient Saf 2010;36(1):29–35. Available at: www.ncbi.nlm.nih.gov/pubmed/?term=new+nurses+views+of+quality+improvement+e ucation%5BTitle%5D.

34. Quality and Safety Education for Nursing Institute. The evolution of the quality and safety education for nurses (QSEN) initiative. 2012. Available at: http://qsen.org/about qsen/project-overview/.

35. American Association of Colleges of Nursing. The essentials of baccalaureate education for professional nursing practice. 2008. Available at: www.aacn.nche.edu/education resources/baccessentials08.pdf.

36. American Nurses Association. Code of ethics for nurses with interpretative statements. Washington, DC: American Nurses Publishing; 2001. p. 12.

37. American Nurse Association. Nursing: scope & standards of practice. Silver Spring (MD): Nursesbooks.org; 2004.

38. Montalvo I. The National Database of Nursing Quality Indicators. Online J Issues Nurs 2007;12(3). Available at: http://www.nursingworld.org/MainMenuCategories/ANAMarketplace/ANAPeriodicals/.

39. Press Ganey Associates, Inc. NDNQI. 2014. Available at: http://www.nursingquality.org/.

Communication Skills

Deborah Ellison, PhD, RN

KEYWORDS

- Miscommunication • Interprofessional communication • Shared governance

KEY POINTS

- Hospital medical errors are now considered the third leading cause of death in the United States.
- The US Joint Commission identified miscommunication as the main cause of serious, unexpected patient injuries and improving the effectiveness of communication among health care providers as a national patient safety goal.
- The IOM recommended looking at system improvements, rather than individual failures, when addressing medical and medication error.
- The implementation of interprofessional learning experiences is essential for nursing, given the nature of professional nursing practice and with around-the-clock coordination of care provided.
- Shared governance can provide safety initiatives; employees must have partnership, equity, and accountability.
- For shared governance to be beneficial ownership must occur at the point of service and occur with at least 90% of the decisions being made by those providing the point of care service.

INTRODUCTION

The quality of hospital nursing care has a direct impact on the quality and safety of patient care. Too often, inefficient workplace policies and practices prevent hospital nurses from focusing fully on the needs of their patients, and patient care and nurse job satisfaction suffer as a result. Communication involves a two-way process of expressive and receptive communication so that the message and responsibilities of the patient and health care provider are understood.[1] Communication should be timely, accurate, and useful to the sender and the receiver of the message.[2]

The US Joint Commission, a nonprofit health care accreditation organization, identified miscommunication as the main cause of serious, unexpected patient injuries and improving the effectiveness of communication among health care providers as a national patient safety goal.[1,3,4] The Joint Commission determined that miscommunication was the second common cause of sentinel events reported in the first 6 months

School of Nursing, Austin Peay State University, PO Box 4658, Clarksville, TN 37044, USA
E-mail address: ellisond@apsu.edu

Nurs Clin N Am 50 (2015) 45–57
http://dx.doi.org/10.1016/j.cnur.2014.10.004
0029-6465/15/$ – see front matter © 2015 Elsevier Inc. All rights reserved.

nursing.theclinics.com

of 2013.[5] The sentinel events relating to communication involved staff, physicians, administration, and patients' families.[5]

Each year medical errors contribute to the escalating costs of health care and can lead to life-altering, life-threatening, or fatal consequences for patients and their families. Paradis and coworkers[6] in a voluntary patient safety event study of three hospitals found medical errors increased costs by 17% and length of stay by 22%. In 2010, it was thought that bad hospital care contributed to the deaths of 180,000 patients (the Office of Inspector General for the Department of Health and Human Services).[7] As recently as 2013, it is thought that number is much higher and between 210,000 and 440,000.[8] Hospital medical errors are now considered the third leading cause of death in the United States.[8,9] The complexity and cost of health care impacts the way in which nurses and other health care professionals are expected to be educated, practice, and communicate.

HISTORICAL IMPLICATIONS

Many countries are concerned with the number of documented medical errors and are working to improve patient safety while decreasing cost. Reports have indicated 2.3% to 16.6% of patients were harmed by human error while hospitalized. Reports of medical errors have produced many resolutions and plans from the United Kingdom, United States, and Australia to improve interprofessional communication with the goal to improve patient outcomes.[10,11] Communication as a part of patient safety has been discussed for years, although it was not until the Institute of Medicine (IOM) published *To Err is Human: Building a Safer Health System* in 1999 that a serious look was taken at how interprofessional education (IPE) could impact patient safety.[12] This IOM publication reported that approximately 98,000 deaths occurred from medical errors annually in the United States. The IOM recommended looking at system improvements, rather than individual failures, when addressing medical and medication error. This publication was also the first in a series of IOM publications examining the quality and safety of the health care system.[13–16] Immediately after the first IOM publication, a national theme emerged calling for the transformation of health care to improve its quality and safety. *Crossing the Quality Chasm: A New Health System for the 21st Century*[13] proposed six aims for improving health care that include safe, effective, patient-centered, timely, efficient, and equitable care. *Health Professionals Education: A Bridge to Quality*[14] examined how health professionals are educated and recommended that all health professionals be prepared to deliver patient-centered care that is evidence-based and integrates informatics and quality improvement strategies within interdisciplinary models of care. The IOM reports examined the complexity of the health care system and recognized that health professionals needed to master new competencies in communication and teamwork to maintain and enhance the quality and safety of patient care.

NURSES' DAILY RESPONSIBILITY TO COMMUNICATION

The front-line nurse has the responsibility to provide direct patient care, patient satisfaction, care coordination, policy, safety, and communication; and that is just a few of the many responsibilities the professional nurse provides during a 12-hour shift. Every nurse has the opportunity to make a positive impact on patient outcomes through day-to-day advocacy for patients, nurses, and the nursing profession. Communication is a means of advocacy that can provide the avenue to which a positive impact is made. Levine, a nursing theorist,[17] has emphasized that nursing language must be crystal clear for understanding by all practitioners—a necessary skill in communication in professional practice models that emphasize transdisciplinary communication. Effective communication for the front-line nurse is a professional responsibility. For effective communication, the communication must have clarity and precision of message that relies on verification and collaborative problem solving, calm and supportive demeanor under stress, maintenance of mutual respect, and an authentic understanding of the unique role.[18]

Patient Satisfaction Scores

The need to improve quality in health care delivery is increasing. The Centers for Medicare and Medicaid Services (CMS), hospitals, and insurance providers alike are striving to better define and measure quality of health care. A major component of quality of health care is patient satisfaction. Furthermore, patient satisfaction is critical to how well patients do; research has identified a clear link between patient outcomes and patient satisfaction scores.[19]

Patient satisfaction is a key determinant of quality of care and an important component of pay-for-performance metrics. Under the CMS Hospital Inpatient Value-Based Purchasing program, Medicare reimbursements are linked to patient satisfaction and surveys completed by patients. Beginning in 2013, CMS makes value-based incentive payments to acute care hospitals based, in part, on the results of patient satisfaction surveys completed by patients.[19]

Patient satisfaction scores regarding care are indicators used in monitoring organizational effectiveness.[2] The survey results regarding patient experiences within a hospital environment are based on numerous encounters with a wide variety of individuals and locations. Nevertheless, organizations have implemented several programs to increase patient satisfaction scores over the last few years and continue those in many facilities today. **Table 1** outlines some of the most frequently used strategies to assist in increasing patient satisfaction scores that are nursing based. Nurses play an integral role in communications with patients and families and therefore impact patient satisfaction scores.

Professional Responsibility

The American Nurses Association Standards of Professional Nursing Practice provides standards for communication for professional nurses. "Standard 11. Communication" includes the following[24]:

- Assesses communication format preferences of health care consumers, families, and colleagues.
- Assesses his or her own communication skills in encounters with health care consumers, families, and colleagues.
- Seeks continuous improvement of communication and conflict resolution skills
- Conveys information to health care consumers, families, the interprofessional team, and others in communication formats that promote accuracy.
- Questions the rationale supporting care processes and decisions when they do not appear to be in the best interest of the patient.
- Discloses observations or concerns related to hazards and errors in care or the practice environment to the appropriate level.
- Maintains communication with other providers to minimize risks associated with transfers and transition in care delivery.
- Contributes to his or her own professional perspective in discussions with the interprofessional team.

Table 1 Nursing-based strategies to assist in increasing patient satisfaction scores		
Study	**Implementation**	**Outcomes**
Effects of rounding on patient satisfaction and patient safety on a medical surgical unit	Charge nurses made rounds on all patients on their floor every 2 h assessing the "Four P's": pain, potty, position, and presence	• Decrease in patient falls • Decrease in call light frequency • Increase in patient satisfaction scores[20]
The Studer Group's May 2007 study	Hourly patient rounding	Call lights decreased by 50% • Patients falls reduced by 33% • Hospital-acquired pressure ulcers reduced by 56% • Overall patient satisfaction increased by 71%[21]
Effects of nursing rounds on patients' call light use, satisfaction, and safety	Nurses rounding either 1- or 2-h intervals	Specific nursing actions performed at set intervals (more specifically, round either every hour or every 2 h) were associated with statistically significant reduced patient use of call lights and a reduction in patient falls and increased patient satisfaction[22]
Proactive patient rounding to increase customer service and satisfaction on the orthopedic unit	The "I Care" rounding model is a proactive and purposeful model that enables staff to anticipate patient needs before they occur	After implementation of the model, the nursing staff was able to see an increase in staff response times, improved patient satisfaction, and an improvement in staff anticipation of patient needs[23]

Data from Refs.[19–22]

CHALLENGES TO IMPROVING COMMUNICATION SKILLS

Barriers to effective communication include such factors as lack of time, hierarchies, defensiveness, varying communication styles, distraction, fatigue, and workload.[25] Nevertheless, there are challenges that go beyond barriers but are deeply rooted in organizations and professions. These include the culture of the organization, professional jargon, hierarchies, and organizational structure.

Culture and Climate

Health care systems across America have struggled with quality and safety issues and changing the culture of their organizations to meet the growing needs of society and changes in health care. These changes are difficult for many. Nevertheless, when change encompasses an organizational cultural change it can be complicated and overwhelming. This is because the culture of an organization is the sum of the organization's beliefs, norms, values, mission, philosophies, traditions, and sacred cows.[2] Organization culture can be further broken down into artifacts, perspectives, values, assumptions, symbols, language, and behaviors that have either been effective or accepted over time.[2] Culture is a social subsystem of the total organization and can be modified with managerial effort and skill.

Organizational culture and organizational climate are not interchangeable. The organizational climate is the emotional state, perceptions, and feelings shared by members or individuals of the system. It can be formal, relaxed, defensive, cautious, accepting, trusting, and so on.[2] It is essentially the employees' subjective impression or perception of their organization's policies, practices, and procedures, both formal and informal. Practicing nurses create or at the very least contribute to the creation of the climate perceived by patients and other staff.[2] If nurses contribute to the culture and climate of an organization, nurses have a professional responsibility to assist in change and not just be a part of the problem.

Nurses want a climate of administrative support that includes adequate staffing, effective communication, professional accountability, and trust. Organization climate can be changed. The front-line nurse can be a catalyst to changing the climate of their workplace and an impetus to others (**Box 1**).

Professional Jargon

Barriers, such as the use of jargon or professional hierarchy, which lay a foundation for other barriers to develop, include disciplines working and training in silos and having little practical understanding of each other's curricula and educational models, with the history of hierarchy of medical practice.[26,27] These lead to common barriers to interprofessional communication and collaboration practice. The more common barriers include personality differences; gender; culture and ethnicity; generational differences; historical interprofessional rivalries; complexity of care; and differences in accountability, payment, and rewards.[28]

Communication among members of the health care teams can be challenging for many reasons. Ineffective communication can make someone feel inferior, create dependence on electronic systems, and create linguistic and cultural barriers.[29]

One of the major reasons for ineffective communication is the use of professional jargon.[27,30] Professional jargon is exacerbated because past and current health professionals are not educated with students in other health care disciplines, and disciplines have created their own specific language.[27,30]

Box 1
Practice example: 1

In a small rural county hospital the new administration would like to change the culture and climate of the hospital. They arrived to find low staff moral throughout the hospital, although the hospital was doing well. Some of the nursing units were covering themselves when staffing was low, whereas others were being required to cover other units. When surveying the nursing staff several themes became apparent about the culture of the hospital.

1. Nursing staff reported they do not believe the administration is listening to them.

2. Nursing staff that have been at the hospital do not like that travel nurses are making more money than they are.

3. Some nursing units are not working as a team.

4. Communication between all parties seems to be suffering.

5. Decisions are being made without nursing input.

These are common themes in hospitals today. How does the front-line nurse go about changing the culture and climate in a clinical setting? How does this impact patient care, safety, and satisfaction?

Hierarchies

Hierarchies within health professionals are created by isolated education practices that are perpetuated in the professional workforce. Hierarchies are common within health care and can create dysfunctional communication patterns working against effective interprofessional teamwork.[27] These can create barriers to effective communication, teamwork, and effective patient-centered care.

Organizational Structure

Many facilities have an organizational structure that is management led with little to no voice of employees for changes being implemented. This top-down approach can create a barrier to effective communication. Professional nurses are trained to understand the "why" of practice. This top-down approach often lacks the communication to answer that question of why and the impact on patient care for the implementation of change (**Box 2**).

This type of top-down approach can lead to feelings of powerlessness over personal professional practice. The accountability to implement policies may not be accepted by staff nurses when lack of empowerment to effect the change that is needed can lead to burn out and disillusion for clinical practice.[31] The lack of control over professional practice from a top-down approach can lead to unnecessary hypercomplexity of the nursing work environment.[32] Ineffective communication, whether accurate or perceived, in a top-down approach can contribute to stress and leads to direct economic losses through low productivity, grievances, absenteeism, and turnover, which can all effect patient outcomes.[2]

PROFESSIONAL PRACTICE MODELS TO IMPROVE COMMUNICATION

The 2014 Affordable Care Act brought health care coverage to an estimated 32 to 51 million previously uninsured Americans, many of whom are expected to come with a plethora of untreated health issues.[33,34] The current health care system will be severely challenged to meet this need. Additional changes are set to take place to assist and ease the burden to health care institutions including financial incentives. These incentives include such items as rewards for care coordination, chronic disease management, improvement of care transition, and reduction of hospital readmissions all in hopes of improving patient outcome.[33,34] Because of an aging and diverse population living longer with chronic conditions, such as diabetes, heart disease, or cancer, that require coordinated care from a team of professionals it is not certain how this will be accomplished. Teams of providers (physicians, nurses, and other health care professionals) bring their collective knowledge and experiences to the table, providing a foundation of care and decision-making that no single provider can contribute.

Box 2
Practice example: 2

Your unit has been full for the last month and even though your unit is staffed, you have had a difficult time pulling a meeting together to discuss new evidence-based practice in postsurgical patients, about which you have been reading. This morning you received an email regarding a new policy for surgical patients that does not encompass all of the new evidence-base practice that has been published. You send an email to the director, and include the articles and information providing the evidence-based practice guidelines. After several days you receive an email explaining the policy has been evaluated and does encompass all necessary guidelines. What can you do now?

Interprofessional Communication

Health care and social service professionals are being called to engage IPE and inter-professional collaboration to provide efficient and effective care to clients and patients.[35] IPE is defined as "when students from two or more professions learn about, from and with each other to enable effective collaboration and improves health outcomes."[11] Despite the inherent benefit to patient outcomes, IPE remains relatively underdeveloped and undervalued in formal and continuing education for health care professionals.[36]

In 2011, an expert interprofessional panel identified four core interprofessional competencies and has called on all health professional educators to implement these competencies into their programs. The Interprofessional Education Collaborative Panel (IPEC) is composed of the following associations: the American Association of Colleges of Nursing, American Association of Colleges of Osteopathic Medicine, the American Association of Colleges of Pharmacy, the American Dental Education Association, the Association of American Medical Colleges, and the Association of Schools of Public Health.[30] The core competencies for IPE include: Domain 1, Values/Ethics for Interprofessional Practice; Domain 2, Roles/Responsibilities; Domain 3, Interprofessional Communication; and Domain 4, Teams and Teamwork.[30] The panel's intent was to build on each profession's expected competencies while defining interprofessional collaborative competencies.[30]

To assist with the transition within health care educational systems the IPEC was formed. The IPEC working group initially included experts from six disciplines collaborating to develop IPE core competencies that would be relevant across all six disciplines. The work of the panel identified and published IPE core competencies in 2011 to address the essential preparation of clinicians for interprofessional collaborative practice. The IPEC identified four core competency domains: (1) values and ethics, (2) roles and responsibilities, (3) interprofessional communication, and (4) team and teamwork.

Competency Domain 3: Interprofessional Communication

Health care administrators, professionals, and faculty are making an effort to implement effective communication procedures among all health care professionals. Communicating refers to aspects of openness, style, and expression of feelings and thoughts.[37] Such procedures include using read-back and call-out techniques for medical orders or using the technique known as SBAR, which requires the health professional who is communicating information about a patient to clearly relay the situation, background, action, and response to clinical situations. Although such techniques do offer assistance in effective communication, they do little to incorporate interprofessional concepts. Effective interprofessional communication competency is an essential professional skill that should be conceptualized and developed in all undergraduate health professional educational programs.[38] Although the literature supports the critical importance of effective communication for quality health care,[11,14,35,39] the fact remains that preparing and assessing communication competency in health care staff and licensed professionals is challenging. Communication skills move nurses in the direction of meeting the core competencies, which will assist them to engage in a collaborative practice.[30]

The IPEC provides a general competency statement for communication: "communicate with patients, families, communities, and other health professionals in a responsive and responsible manner that supports a team approach to the maintenance of health and the treatment of disease."[30] This statement is inclusive, but is not so restrictive that it cannot be used in all health care facilities. Competency development in the domain of interprofessional communication stressed using respectful language; organizing and communicating information with patients, families, and health team members in an understandable form; choosing effective communication tools and techniques; and communicating effectively in difficult situations.[30] Using the specific competency statements for communication the IPEC has developed should assist with reducing the communication challenges created by the use of jargon and hierarchies. Mastering the communication patterns and/or skills within an interprofessional team framework directly impacts all members of the health care team and future function of the team, but more importantly could impact patient outcomes (**Table 2**).

IPE is a prerequisite for enhanced communication among members of the health care team, improved quality of care, and better outcomes for patients.[35,39] Interprofessional communication and collaboration are promoted by policymakers as fundamental building blocks for improving patient care and meeting the demands of increasingly complex care.[27] The implementation of interprofessional learning

Table 2
IPEC competency domain 3

IPEC Competency Domain	Specific Interprofessional Competencies
Competency domain 3: interprofessional communication	1. Choose effective communication tools and techniques, including information systems and communication technologies, to facilitate discussions and interactions that enhance team function
	2. Organize and communicate information with patients, families, and health care team members in a form that is understandable, avoiding discipline-specific terminology when possible
	3. Express one's knowledge and opinions to team members involved in patient care with confidence, clarity, and respect, working to ensure common understanding of information and treatment and care decisions
	4. Listen actively, and encourage ideas and opinions of other team members
	5. Give timely, sensitive, instructive feedback to others about their performance on the team, responding respectfully as a team member to feedback from others
	6. Use respectful language appropriate for a given difficult situation, crucial conversation, or interprofessional conflict
	7. Recognize how one's own uniqueness, including experience level, expertise, culture, power, and hierarchy within the health care team, contributes to effective communication, conflict resolution, and positive interprofessional working relationships
	8. Communicate consistently the importance of teamwork in patient-centered and community-focused care

From Interprofessional Education Collaborative Expert Panel. Core competencies for interprofessional collaborative practice: Report of an expert panel. Washington, D.C. Interprofessional Education Collaborative; 2011.

Table 3
Shared governance principles

Core Concept	Purpose	Definition	Clarification
Principles of partnership	Links health care providers and patients along all points in the system	A collaborative relationship among all stakeholders and nursing required for professional empowerment	Is essential to building relationships, involves all staff members in decisions and processes, implies that each member has a key role in fulfilling the mission and purpose of the organization, and is critical to the health care system's effectiveness
Accountability	Is the core of shared governance	A willingness to invest in decision-making and express ownership in those decisions	It is often used interchanged with responsibility. Accountability has different characteristics, supports partnership, and is secured as staff produce positive outcomes. Accountability characteristics: • Defined by outcomes • Self-described • Embedded in roles • Dependent on partnerships • Shares valuation • Contributions-driven value
Equity	The best method for integrating staff roles and relationships into structures and processes to achieve positive patient outcomes	Maintains a focus on services, patients, and staff; is the foundation and measure of value; and says that no role is more important than any other	Although equity does not equal equality in terms of scope of practice, knowledge, authority, or responsibility, it does mean that each team member is essential to providing safe and effective care.
Ownership	To enable all team members to participate, ownership designates where work is done and by whom	Recognition and acceptance of the importance of everyone's work and of the fact that an organization's success is bound to how well individual staff members perform their jobs	Ownership requires all staff members to participate in devising purposes for the work. Activities may include participation in scheduling, joint staffing decisions, and shared unit responsibilities (eg, all nurses trained as a charge nurse).

Data from Refs.[42–45]

experiences is essential for nursing, given the nature of professional nursing practice and with around-the-clock coordination of care provided.

Shared Governance

Never before has the voice of the front-line nurse been so critical to patient outcomes, the nursing profession, health care facilities, and health care in general as it is today. Front-line nurses often believe they do not have the ability or the voice to make a change in their workplace. Judy Woodward stated "I do understand how that feels, having worked most of my life in facilities where nurses had little or no administrative support, were not respected and were powerless to make any changes" (Judy Woodward, MSN, RN, personal communication, 2014). This statement has been expressed by many professional nurses over the years. Now nurses have avenues to pursue that help advance the impact of nurses and drive health care changes using the concepts and strategies of Magnet.[40] One strategy that can be implemented is shared governance.

Shared governance is a model developed by Tim Porter-O'Grady. The intention is to provide direction for the professional practice of nursing. This model directs nurses to participate in the decision making that allows them to demonstrate accountability, the principles of partnership, equity, and ownership for their practice as a front-line nurse (Table 3).[41]

An increasing number of facilities have or are developing some level of shared governance structures to ensure that nurses at the point of care have a voice in decisions related to patient care and the work environment. The impact of registered nurses on patient outcomes is increasingly evident; and nursing input into organizational decision-making related to safety and quality initiatives is invaluable. Nurses are increasingly positioned to advocate more effectively than ever before not only for patients, but also for themselves and the nursing profession.[46]

If shared governance is to allow for cost-effective, safe service delivery and nurse empowerment, decision-making must be shared at the point of service. This means that the management structure must be decentralized. To make this happen, employee partnership equity, accountability, and ownership must occur at the point of service and occur with at least 90% of the decisions being made by those providing the point-of-care service.[42,46,47] Shared governance as a process demands new views and visions, and a willingness to risk the yet unknown results of shared decisions.[42,46]

SUMMARY

Front-line nurses today have a great responsibility not only in caring for their patients but also effectively communicating to everyone in the goal of safe patient care. The methods of communication used in the past are not sufficient for the changes in health care of today. Understanding the options front-line nurses have and must implement for effective communication paves the way for new graduates in the future. Implementing shared governance models and IPE together benefits all involved. Shared governance models can be simple or complex in health care organizations. Even starting on a small scale can improve empowerment and accountability within nursing units. Interprofessional teamwork and communication is not a fad and has begun to trickle into all aspects of education of disciplines and hospitals. Professional nurses have a responsibility to continuing education and patient safety. Therefore, moving to shared governance and IPE (specifically communication) must happen.

REFERENCES

1. The Joint Commission. Advancing effective communication, cultural competence, and patient- and family-centered care: a roadmap for hospitals. 2010. Available at: http://www.jointcommission.org/assets/1/6/ARoadmapforHospitalsfinalversion727.pdf. Accessed August 1, 2014.
2. Roussel LA. Management and leadership for nurse administrators. 6th edition. Burlington (MA): Jones & Bartlett Learning; 2013. Print.
3. The Joint Commission. Accreditation program: Ambulatory health care national patient safety goals. 2010. Available at: www.jointcommission.org. Accessed August 1, 2014.
4. The Joint Commission. R^3 Report requirement, rational, reference: a complimentary publication of the Joint Commission. 2011. Available at: http://www.jointcommission.org/assets/1/18/r3%20report%20issue%201%2020111.pdf. Accessed August 1, 2014.
5. Rodak S. 10 most identified sentinel event root causes. 2013. Available at: http://www.beckershospitalreview.com/quality/10-most-identified-sentinel-event-root-causes.html. Accessed August 2, 2014.
6. Paradis AR, Stewart VT, Bayley KB, et al. Excess cost and length of stay associated with voluntary patient safety events reports in hospitals. Am J Med Qual 2009;24:53–60.
7. Department of Health and Human Services, Office of the Inspector General. Adverse Events in Hospitals: National Incidence among Medicare Beneficiaries. Washington, DC; 2010. Available at: http://oig.hhs.gov/oei/reports/OEI-06-09-00090.pdf.
8. Allen M. How many die from medial mistakes in U.S. hospitals? 2013. Available at: http://www.npr.org/blogs/health/2013/09/20/224507654/how-many-die-from-medical-mistakes-in-u-s-hospitals. Accessed August 1, 2014.
9. McDonald I. Hospital medical errors now the third leading cause of death in the U.S. 2013. Available at: http://www.fiercehealthcare.com/story/hospital-medical-errors-third-leading-cause-death-dispute-to-err-is-human-report/2013-09-20. Accessed August 1, 2014.
10. Mitchell M, Groves M, Mitchell C, et al. Innovation in learning - An interprofessional approach to improving communication. Nurse Educ Pract 2010;10:379–84.
11. WHO. Framework for action on interprofessional education & collaborative practice. Geneva (Switzerland): World Health Organization; 2010. Available at: http://whqlibdoc.who.int/hq/2010/WHO_HRH_HPN_10.3_eng.pdf. Accessed July 15, 2014.
12. Institute of Medicine (IOM). To err is human: building a safer health system. Washington, DC: National Academies Press; 1999.
13. Institute of Medicine. Crossing the quality chasm: a new health system for the 21st century. Washington, DC: National Academies Press; 2001.
14. Institute of Medicine. Health professions education: a bridge to quality. Washington, DC: National Academies Press; 2003.
15. Institute of Medicine. Patient safety: achieving a new standard for care. Washington, DC: National Academies Press; 2004.
16. Institute of Medicine. Keeping patients safe: transforming the work environment of nurses. Washington, DC: National Academies Press; 2004.
17. Levine M. Antecedents from adjunctive disciplines: creation of nursing theory. Nurs Sci Q 1988;1(1):16–21.

18. Robinson FP, Borman G, Slimmer LW, et al. Perceptions of effective and ineffective nurse-physician communication in hospitals. Nurs Forum 2010;45:3.
19. Morris BJ, Jahangir AA, Sethi MK. Patient satisfaction: an emerging health policy issue: what the orthopaedic surgeon needs to know. Available at: http://www.aaos.org/news/aaosnow/jun13/advocacy5.asp. Accessed July 15, 2014.
20. Meade C, Bursell A, Ketelsen L. Effects of nursing rounds on patients' call light use, satisfaction, and safety. Am J Nurs 2006;106(9):58–70.
21. Studer Group. Hourly rounding supplement. Best practice: Sacred Heart Hospital. Pensacola (FL): Studer Group; 2007. Available at: http://www.studergroup.com/Hourly_rounding/hourly_rounding_supplement_sample_gs_1-5. Accessed June 9, 2009.
22. Woodard J. Effects of rounding on patient satisfaction and patient safety on a medical-surgical unit. Clin Nurse Spec 2009;23(4):200–6.
23. Tea C, Ellison M, Feghali F. Proactive patient rounding to increase customer service and satisfaction on an orthopedic unit. Orthop Nurs 2008;27(4):233–40.
24. American Nurses Association (ANA). School of nursing: scope and standards of practice. 2nd edition. Silver Spring (MD): American Nurses Association; 2001.
25. The American College of Obstetricians and Gynecologists. Committee opinion: Committee on patient safety and quality improvement. 2012. Available at: http://www.acog.org/Resources-And-Publications/Committee-Opinions/Committee-on-Patient-Safety-and-Quality-Improvement/Communication-Strategies-for-Patient-Handoffs. Accessed July 15, 2014.
26. Egan-Lee E, Baker L, Tobin S, et al. Neophyte facilitator experiences of interprofessional education: implications for faculty development. J Interprof Care 2011;25(5):333–8. Available at: http://dx.doi.org.library.capella.edu/10.3109/13561820.2011.562331.
27. Rice K, Zwarenstein M, Conn L, et al. An intervention to improve interprofessional collaboration and communications: a comparative qualitative study. J Interprof Care 2010;24(4):350–61.
28. Wood JA, Jackson DJ, Ziglar S, et al. Interprofessional communication. Drug Top 2011;155(8):42–53.
29. Liaw SY, Zhou WT, Lau TC, et al. An interprofessional communication training using simulation to enhance safe care for a deteriorating patient. Nurse Educ Today 2014;34:259–64.
30. Interprofessional Education Collaborative Expert Panel. Core competencies for interprofessional collaborative practice: report of an expert panel. Washington, DC: Interprofessional Education Collaborative; 2011. Available at: http://www.aacn.nche.edu/education-resources/ipecreport.pdf.
31. Linnen D, Rowley A. Encouraging clinical nurse empowerment. Nurs Manage 2014;43(11):45–8.
32. Castner J, Ceravolo D, Folt-Ramos K, et al. Nursing control over practice and teamwork. Online J Issues Nurs 2013;18(2):3.
33. Carrier E, Yee T, Garfield RL. The uninsured and their health care needs: how have they changed since the recession? The Henry J. Kaiser Family Foundation: Kaiser Commission on Medicaid and the Uninsured; 2011.
34. Wakefield M. Proceedings from team-based competencies: building a shared foundation for education and clinical practice. Washington, DC: 2011.
35. Thannhauser J, Russell-Mayhew S, Scott C. Measures of interprofessional education and collaboration. J Interprof Care 2010;24(4):336–49.
36. Benner P, Sutphen M, Leonard V, et al. Educating nurses: a call for radical transformation. San Francisco (CA): Jossey-Bass; 2010.

37. Essens PJ, Vogelaar AL, Mylle JJ, et al. Team effectiveness in complex settings: a framework. In: Salas E, Goodwin GF, Burke CS, editors. Team effectiveness in complex organizations. New York: Psychology Press; 2009. p. 293–320.

38. Boschma G, Einboden R, Groening M, et al. Strengthening communication education in an undergraduate nursing curriculum. Int J Nurs Educ Scholarsh 2010; 7(1):1–17.

39. Casimiro L, MacDonald CJ, Thompson T, et al. Grounding theories of W(e)Learn: a framework for online interprofessional education. J Interprof Care 2009;23(4): 390–400.

40. American Nurses Association. Fundamentals of magnet course. 2014. Available at: http://www.nursecredentialing.org/Magnet-Academy. Accessed August 1, 2014.

41. Swihart D, Porter-O'Grady T. Shared governance: a practical approach to reshaping professional nursing practice. Marblehead (MA): HCPro, Inc; 2006.

42. Porter-O'Grady T, Malloch K. Innovation leadership: creating the landscape of healthcare. Sudbury (MA): Jones and Bartlett Publishers; 2009.

43. Baston V. Shared governance in an integrated health care network. AORN J 2004;80(3):493–6, 498, 501–504, 506, 509–512.

44. Koloroutis M. Relationship-based care: a model for transforming practice. Minneapolis (MN): Creative Health Care Management; 2004.

45. Page A. Keeping patients safe: transforming the work environment of nurses. Washington, DC: The National Academies; 2004.

46. Tomajan K. Advocating for nurses and nursing. Online J Issues Nurs 2012;17(1): 4, 10913734.

47. Donohue-Porter P. Creating a culture of shared governance begins with developing the nurse as a scholar. Creat Nurs 2012;18(5):160–7.

Interprofessional Collaborative Care Skills for the Frontline Nurse

Stephen W. Lomax, RN, MBA, MSN*, Danielle White, RN, MSN

KEYWORDS

- Interprofessional collaborative care • Teamwork • Team building
- Phases of group formation • Interprofessional communication • Values and ethics
- Interprofessional team models of care • TeamSTEPPS

KEY POINTS

- Frontline nurses must transition from working in a silo to working with interprofessional teams. This transition is needed to provide high-quality, safe, and accountable care to empower positive patient outcomes.
- Frontline nurses need to respond to the charge from the Quality and Safety Education for Nurses, Joint Commission, and the Institute of Medicine to transform their delivery of care for complex and acute inpatients to interprofessional collaborative care.
- Frontline nurses need to understand the essential components (interprofessional teamwork, collaboration, and communication) of patient-centered care.
- Frontline nurses need education about teams and group process for the formation of interprofessional collaborative care skills.
- Frontline nurses can apply best practice care models such as nurse care coordination teams, the hospice team, and rapid response teams to develop their collaborative model of care.
- Resources such as Situation, Background, Assessment, Recommendation, and Interprofessional Education Collaborative Panel, and TeamSTEPPS, can be used to develop a toolkit for interprofessional collaborative care skills.

INTRODUCTION

Frontline nurses must embrace interprofessional collaborative care because health care reform has transformed health care delivery models that require nurses to work in an interprofessional world while caring for patients.[1] Many nurses work in silos providing care to their patients without consideration of the plan of care from other disciplines such as physical therapy, occupational therapy, speech therapy, dietetics, or

School of Nursing, Austin Peay State University, 601 College Street, Clarksville, TN 37044, USA
* Corresponding author.
E-mail address: lomaxs@apsu.edu

Nurs Clin N Am 50 (2015) 59–73
http://dx.doi.org/10.1016/j.cnur.2014.10.005
0029-6465/15/$ – see front matter © 2015 Elsevier Inc. All rights reserved.
nursing.theclinics.com

case management. Frontline nurses must transition from working in a silo to working with an interprofessional team.

Learning to function in an interprofessional environment requires an understanding of interprofessional roles and responsibilities and community-oriented/population-oriented care.[2] Frontline nurses are expected to have the required skills for the process of syntheses of evidence in collaboration with other health care members. Nurses are also required to integrate evidence, clinical judgment an interprofessional perspective, and the patient preference in planning, implementing, and evaluating care.[3] Even though theoretic knowledge is important, the participation in collaborative teams provides safe, high-quality, and accountable care.[4] This article overviews the charge for transformation, explains the concept of interprofessional collaborative care, provides examples of interdisciplinary teams in practice for application, and provides resources to improve collaborative care. This article provides a toolkit for frontline nurses to develop interprofessional collaborative care skills.

CHARGE FOR TRANSFORMATION

Patients in the hospital setting are acutely ill and many have complications from chronic illnesses. Their care is complex and reimbursed on a value-based payment system. Quality indicators for reimbursement are evidence-based benchmarks that must be met for full financial reimbursement. High-functioning interprofessional collaborative care is required for patients to have positive outcomes and for achievement of high scores on patient satisfaction surveys. Frontline nurses must respond to the demands for high-quality, safe, and accountable care.

Quality and Safety Education for Nurses

Beginning in 2009 the Quality and Safety Education for Nurses project (QSEN), a part of the American Association of Colleges of Nursing, identified safety competencies for nursing education. One of these competencies was teamwork and collaboration. QSEN asks that nurses function effectively within nursing and interprofessional teams, fostering open communication, mutual respect, and shared decision making to achieve high-quality patient care.[5] The American Nurse Credentialing Center (ANCC), a subsidiary of the American Nurses Association, supports QSEN in their most recent Magnet Application Report and points out that nurses should incorporate interprofessional collaborative practice within their plan of care.[6]

Joint Commission

The US Joint Commission, a nonprofit health care accreditation organization, identified communication errors as the main cause of serious, unexpected patient injuries and improving the effectiveness of communication among health care providers as a 2009 US National Patient Safety Goal. It continues to be a problem in the 2014 US National Patient Safety Goals.[7] Medical errors can be life altering, life threatening, and expensive. Interprofessional communication, teamwork, and collaboration can prevent patient errors but are not being well executed in health care programs throughout the United States.[8] According to Rice and colleagues[9] (2010) interprofessional communication and collaboration are promoted by policy makers as fundamental building blocks for improving patient safety and meeting demands of increasing complex care but are not taught in health care education.

Institute of Medicine

The landmark Institute of Medicine (IOM) 2010 report entitled *Future of Nursing: Leading Change, Advancing Health*, identifies the need for patient-centered care in which the patient and family are integral parts of the team. Evidence shows that patient-centered care leads to greater quality care. In the chapter, "Transforming Leadership," the IOM recommends that nurses be seen as full partners with physicians and other health professional and be involved with redesigning health care.[10] The report requires nurses to take on leadership roles within the health care teams. The IOM report clearly brings to light the critical need for collaboration between health professionals in improving quality and safety in the health care settings. Nurses have a responsibility to gain the skills and abilities to participate as full partners with other health professionals, patients, and their families.[10] Based on the IOM report, nurses must work toward collaboration with multiple health care professionals to provide safe and high-quality care.

UNDERSTANDING INTERPROFESSIONAL COLLABORATIVE CARE

Teamwork, collaboration, and communication are often used synonymously. However, there are subtle differences. Interprofessional teamwork, collaboration, and communication are becoming essential components of patient-centered primary care practice. The term interprofessional is one of the most widely used terms, in conjunction with collaboration, in the health care literature. The term interprofessional is the updated version of older terms such as interdisciplinary, cross-disciplinary, and transdisciplinary.[6]

Teamwork

Effective teams move in a direction, toward goals and objectives.[11] Individuals come together to form teams in an effort to work toward specific outcomes or goals that the teams value. Teams can be interdisciplinary or composed of a single discipline. Taking teamwork to its highest level involves interprofessional teamwork or collaboration. These teamwork behaviors involve collaboration in a patient-centered delivery of care. Collaborative care involves each professional coordinating their care with other health professionals so that deficits, redundancies, and errors are avoided. Nurses should collaborate with others through shared problem solving and shared decision making. This requirement is especially important in circumstances of uncertainty.[12] The Interprofessional Education Collaborative believes that interprofessionals must develop relationship-building values and principles of team dynamics. They also believe that interprofessionals must learn different team roles to deliver patient-centered/population-centered care that is safe, timely, efficient, effective, and equitable.[12] Frontline nurses need to differentiate between teamwork and interprofessional collaboration as follows:

- Teamwork: the combined actions of a group of people, especially when effective and efficient.[13] **Box 1** provides a case report with an example of teamwork in which 3 professionals worked together, communicated with the patient, and answered one of the patients concerns. They were effective and efficient. However, little thought or discussion went into long-term care of this patient.
- Interprofessional collaboration: multidisciplined health care workers partnering with patients, families, caregivers, and communities to deliver safe and high-quality care that empowers and maximizes patient outcomes.[14] **Box 2** provides a case report with an example of differentiation involving interdisciplinary

---

Box 1
Teamwork in collaborative care

Mr Angelo, 89 years old, is a patient on a medical unit. He has a stage 3 ulcer on his leg, is a diabetic, lives alone, and does not like to cook. He is being discharged in a day or two and is concerned that he cannot get around much. The physician arrives to look at the wound and change the dressing. The primary nurse goes to the room to assist and discuss the wound care. The dietitian happens to be on the unit and he comes in to assess the patient's understanding of his diet. The three professionals talk to the patient about his wound and his diet and the patient is given written instructions. The patient asks when he will go home and what help might be available. The physician says he will order home health and the primary nurse says she will get back to the patient with the information.

---

collaboration. The client's care was coordinated with other health professionals so that gaps, redundancies, and errors were avoided. They collaborated with others through shared problem solving and shared decision making, especially in this patient's circumstances of uncertainty and complexity of disease. The thinking, or collaboration, is more planned and long term.

SKILLS FOR THE FORMATION OF INTERPROFESSIONAL COLLABORATION CARE
Teams and Teamwork

Teams are small, complex systems. An important determinant of the team's effectiveness is the interaction among its members. Successful teams typically consist of individuals who respect and value each other contributions and are willing to relinquish some professional autonomy to work effectively with others.[12] Although each individual in the team may be highly skilled, functioning as a team requires more than individual competency. It is difficult to turn a team of experts into an expert team. Four interprofessional collaborative domains or competencies have been established by the Interprofessional Education Collaborative Panel (IPEC) expert panels in 2011. They are Teams and Teamwork, Interprofessional Communication, Values/Ethics for Interprofessional Practice, and Roles/Responsibilities.

If there are the nursing shortages and increasing patient complexity, nursing is called on to develop collaborative solutions. One way to achieve this expectation is through the effective interdisciplinary teams and work groups that can draw on the wide variety of expertise and specialties.[11,15]

Box 2
Interprofessional collaboration

Mr Angelo, 89 years old, is a patient on a medical unit. He has a stage 3 ulcer on his leg, is a diabetic, lives alone, and does not like to cook. He is being discharged in a day or two and is concerned that he cannot get around much. The physician arrives to look at the wound and change the dressing. The primary nurse goes to the room to assist and discuss the wound care. The dietitian happens to be on the unit and he comes in to assess the patient's understanding of his diet. The three professionals talk to the patient about his wound and his diet and the patient is given written instructions. The patient asks when he will go home and what help might be available. The 3 professionals look at each other and the primary nurse says she will get back to the patient.

Once they leave the room the primary nurse asks whether they could all get together the next day for a meeting about the patient's long-term needs. She wants to invite the case manager/social worker, dietician, the wound care nurse, plus the physician. They agree to meet in the morning to plan care for the patient. After an initial discussion with each other the team goes into the patient's room to discuss possibilities with the patient.

Box 3 shows a case report to provide reflection questions to show how frontline nurses can influence patient care as members of interprofessional teams.

The Principle of Synergy in Team Building

The principle of synergy underlies team building. According to Stephen R. Covey[16] in *The 7 Habits of Highly effective People*, synergy is to combine the strengths of people through positive teamwork, thereby achieving goals that no person could have achieved solo. Teamwork requires open-mindedness and a willingness to value differences and interact genuinely. There are 6 basic rules that incorporate several aspects of communication related to synergy and team building:

- Define a clear purpose. Each team member must clearly be knowledgeable about the reason they are together and must be able to articulate the goals, objectives, and purpose of the team.
- Actively listen. Active listening is not judgmental and means being completely focused on what each speaker says. Each team member must be attentive to individual speakers rather than thinking about forming their own responses.
- Maintain honesty. Team members must be objective in their feedback to ideas without belittling the speaker's views.
- Demonstrate compassion. Each team member should listen with a kind heart and an open mind.
- Be flexible. Each team member must be open and flexible to other individuals' perspectives. Everyone works together to accomplish the goal or objective.[15]

Choosing a Team Leader

How do you choose your team leader? Every team needs a leader and, depending on the purpose of the team, it may be the person closest to the situation, the person with the most influence with the institution, or the person who naturally emerges as the leader. Each member of the team has a role and responsibility that coincide with the purpose of the team and should be identified by the team leader or the team. Leading the team is not the easiest thing to do, but neither is being an active, fully participating member of the team. Both require taking risks, including being in a relationship.

Box 3

Case report showing nurse impact on an interprofessional team

Mr Angelo, 89 years old, has been returned to your medical unit. He is a diabetic, lives alone, does not like to cook, and cannot get around much. This admission is his third in 6 months. Since his discharge 3 months ago he has developed some neuropathy and has lost 5.9 kg (13 pounds). His wound is not completely healed. These developments seem to stem from poor nutrition. He is alert and oriented and interested in his care but is depressed about his lack of progress.

1. As you admit this patient, what interdisciplinary team members do you want on the clinical team?

2. What role do you see the physician playing?

3. What team member should hold initial leadership on the team?

4. How will you evaluate the synthesis of the team plan and its impact on the patient's experience?[11]

Phases of Group Formation

There are phases of group formation. Group phases do not necessarily progress in a logical manner. The phases may overlap and/or regress. Group members and the leader should be aware of the phases and their roles in order to move the group forward. The group leader, when forming these groups, should include a variety of people, such as experts, those affected by the issue, people with power to implement the solution, persons with different problem-solving styles, and equal numbers of sensing/thinking and intuitive/feeling individuals. **Table 1** shows an overview of the phases of group formation.

Table 1
Phases of group formation

Name of Phase	Purpose	Possible Actions
Forming or orientation phase	During this phase the group members discover themselves and begin to relate to one another	Group members test each other for appropriate and acceptable behavior; this is the time to exchange information, discover ground rules, size each other up, and determine fit. Implicit norms are avoided because they bring bias to the group process by imposing individual values and beliefs. The leader helps members fit into the group, providing structure, guidelines, and norms, and making members comfortable
Conflict or storming phase	Group members jockey for position, control, and influence	This stage is marked by disputes, confrontations, and disagreements. The leader helps members through this phase, assisting with group roles, rules, assignments, and a common language. The end product is a consolidated identity
Cohesion or norming phase	During this phase the group begins to develop a collective identity	Roles and norms are established with a move toward consensus and objectives. Members reach a common understanding of the nature of the opportunity to reach the group's goals. They diagnose the root cause of the problem, and the deviation from the expected performance. They are open to alternative definitions with multiple views. Morale and trust improve and the negative is suppressed
Working or performing phase	Conflict and dissention are gone and members work with deeper involvement, greater disclosure, and unity	The group is now focused primarily on decision making and productivity
Termination phase	Once goals are fulfilled, the group terminates	The leader guides the members to summarize discussions, express feelings, and make closing statements. The group is reluctant to break up. A celebration helps

Data from Roussel L. Management and leadership for nurse administrators. Burlington (MA): Jones and Bartlett; 2013. p. 213–308; and Huber D. Leadership and nursing care management. 5th edition. St. Louis (MO): Saunders; 2014. p. 128–46.

Group Techniques

Several group techniques have been developed to make groups effective and productive. Among these are the brainstorming, Delphi technique, the nominal group technique, and focus groups.

Brainstorming can be an effective method for generating a large volume of creative ideas. A problem is presented. In brainstorming the goal is to generate as many ideas as possible. One person should record the ideas as presented. Ideas are generated with freedom from critique and judgment. All ideas are welcome, the more the better, and often one idea stimulates another. Members should avoid comments that criticize, such as "That will never work" or "We already tried that." The facilitator keeps the ideas flowing.[17]

The Delphi technique involves systematically collecting and summarizing opinions from expert panels and interested parties through multiple cycles of interviews or questionnaires. The responses are edited, summarized, and refined. A new set of questionnaires is sent to the participants, potentially several times to allow participants to reconsider their responses. The goal is to achieve a consensus. One advantage is that a large number of people may participate without having to meet at the same time, and there are no opportunities for outrageous and unproductive verbal and nonverbal ideas.[18]

The nominal group technique requires team members to provide input into the decision-making process without talking to each other first. Members are divided into small groups. A question or problem is presented as an open-ended question. After a period of silence, team members write down their ideas for the solution to the question or problem. This step can be done before the face-to-face meeting. In a round-robin fashion, members are then asked to share an idea, which is displayed for all to see. Comments and explanations are not welcome at this time. The purpose is to put the ideas in the open for all to see. The next stage allows for questions and explanations of the ideas. The final stage involves ranking options by majority vote. This technique allows equal participation of all team members but is time consuming.

Focus groups are gathered to explore a specific issue. They can be used to evaluate the effects of an intervention, solve a problem, or study new equipment. Under the direction of a moderator the group meets face to face. Members are allowed to validate or disagree with the ideas expressed. Depending on the topic it may be beneficial for the moderator to be a noninvolved person. The moderator must be aware of potential problems inherent in sensitive issues.[19]

Interprofessional Communication

The cornerstone of safe, patient-centered care is successful teamwork, which depends on strong collaborative relationships. Successful collaboration depends on effective communications and is contingent on all parties being available for and receptive toward one another. Effective communication begins with nurses and physicians speaking to one another face to face. In these days of technology, communication is often done via e-mail, texting, computer charting, or phone. Frequent face-to-face interaction of the team members creates ongoing connections and familiarity with one another. Team members who communicate regularly and are in a professional relationship with one another in the good times are more apt to work together smoothly during a crisis. One way to improve communication and collaboration is to provide cross-disciplinary opportunities of shadowing to improve mutual understanding of roles. It is easier to collaborate/communicate with a team member if each clearly understands the colleague's perspective.[20]

In the modern, busy world there are many barriers to clear, focused, effective communication. One such barrier is distractions such as noise, poor lighting, and interruptions by others. Heavy workloads and multitasking can also be distracting. Team members may have highly specialized and technical knowledge bases. The sender and receiver must seek in order for communication to occur. Professional language and jargon may not be similar for all team members. A common language assists in clear understanding of communication. Team members should avoid using jargon. Differences in perception, mental filters, or the way members see the world hinder communication. Messages can be interpreted differently depending on sociocultural, gender, ethnic, and educational differences. In addition, attention should be paid to the emotional status of the person. A person in distress may have difficulty receiving the sender's message. Emotions and problems from home that are brought to the workplace can influence communication and the workplace in a nonproductive way, especially if they go unnoticed. In addition, historical interprofessional and intraprofessional rivalries may keep communication from flowing.[19]

The following communication scripts encourage interprofessional communication or group think:

- To convey interest in what the other person is saying: I see. I get it. I hear what you are saying.
- To encourage individuals to expand further on their thinking: Yes, go on. Tell us more.
- To help individuals clarify the problem in their own thinking: So the problem as you see it is…
- To get individuals to hear what they have said in the way it sounded to others: This is your decision, then, and the reasons are… If I understand you correctly, you are saying that we should…
- To pull out the key ideas from a long statement or discussion: Your major point is… You think that we should…
- To respond to people's feelings more than to their words: You strongly believe that… You do not believe that…
- To summarize specific points of agreement and disagreement as a basis for further discussion: We seem to be agreed on the following points… However, we seem to need further clarification on these points…
- To express a consensus of group feeling: As a result of this discussion, we as a group seem to think that…[19]

Roles and Responsibilities

Roles in any team or group are fluid. Members take on different roles depending on the type of group, group phase, and situation. Group roles may be formal, assigned, or simply assumed by a group member. Formal roles are clearly established by the group leader or the group. Some common fluid roles on a team or group are the so-called devil's advocate, harmonizer, or clarifier. The more formal roles of leader, facilitator, recorder, and timekeeper should be clear to all group members.[21]

Teams are developed to serve differing purposes. Management teams form to manage changes that are complex and demanding. An example of this team is one that considers staffing changes throughout the institution. These teams are led by upper management. Work teams are usually self-managed and have bottom-up communication. These teams have a specific purpose related to the job description and have clearly defined responsibilities. An example of a work team is one that is exploring hourly rounding or fall protocols. Another type of team is a project team that has 1 grand purpose and then is disbanded. An example of this type of team is one that changes the process of electronic charting or initiates interdisciplinary patient rounding.[15]

Value and Ethics Related to Interprofessional Teams

Interprofessional values are an important aspect of any team. Values can be defined as an ongoing belief that a certain mode of conduct or state of existence is personally and socially preferable to the opposite mode of conduct.[22] These values and related ethics are important in creating an interprofessional identity for a team. The values of the leader and the team should be patient centered and grounded in a shared purpose to support the common good in health care. They reflect a shared commitment to creating safe, efficient patient care.

IPEC 2011 has identified a general competency statement on values and ethics related to interprofessional teams. The general competency is to work with individuals of other professions to maintain a climate of mutual respect and shared values. In addition to this shared competency the individual expertise and diversity of each profession must be honored. Traditional ethics and values need to be reimagined into a shared vision for interprofessional collaborative practice. Confidentiality between practitioner and patient is one ethical principle that is already shared among all the professions.[12] The specific competencies related to interprofessional team values are as follows:

- Place the interests of patients and populations at the center of interprofessional health care delivery
- Respect the dignity and privacy of patients and maintain confidentiality in the delivery of team-based care
- Embrace the cultural diversity and individual differences that characterize patients, populations, and health care teams
- Respect the unique cultures, values, roles/responsibilities, and expertise of other health professions
- Work in cooperation with those who receive care, those who provide care, and others who contribute to or support the delivery of prevention and health services
- Develop a trusting relationship with patients, families, and other team members; and high standards of ethical conduct and quality of care in personal contributions to team-based care
- Manage ethical dilemmas specific to interprofessional patient-centered/population-centered care situations
- Act with honesty and integrity in relationships with patients, families, and other team members
- Members to maintain competence in their individual professions appropriate to scope of practice[12]

EXAMPLES OF INTERDISCIPLINARY TEAMS IN PRACTICE
Nursing Care Coordination Teams

Care coordination has been performed by registered nurses and Advanced Registered Nurse Practitioners as a core part of patient-centered care for many years. The American Nurses Association defined care coordination in a White Paper adopting the approaches of the National Quality Foundation and Agency for Healthcare Research and Quality: "Care coordination is (a) a function that helps ensure that the patient's needs and preferences are met over time with respect to health services and information sharing across people, functions, and sites; and (b) the deliberate organization of patient care activities between two or more participants (including the patient) involved in a patient's care to facilitate the appropriate delivery of health care services."[23]

An excellent example of this application and making a difference in patient care is the American Organization of Nurse Executives' Care Innovation and Transformation program. The program started in 2012 had 24 hospital participants involved in a 2-year program to increase patient satisfaction, decrease falls, and reduce nurse turnover and overtime. The Care Innovation and Transformation program showed improvements in patient care through participation of frontline staff on interprofessional teams.[24] The program focuses on health care providers who are closest to patient care. The nurses who are in direct patient care have real-world understanding of what works for patients and what does not improve their care. The interprofessional team listened to the ideas of frontline nurses, bringing confidence and optimism to the team members. Poststudy analysis showed that participating units routinely experienced significant improvements in teamwork and in team cohesion, and decrease in nurse turnover.[24]

The Hospice Team

Hospice care is a family-centered approach that includes, at a minimum, a team of doctors (hospice and personal physician), nurses, home health aides, social workers, chaplains, counselors, and trained volunteers. They work together focusing on the dying person's needs; physical, emotional, or spiritual. The goal is to help keep the person as pain free as possible, with loved ones nearby until death. Team meetings may be held daily or weekly depending on the patient load and client need.

The hospice team develops a care plan that meets each person's individual needs for pain management and symptom control. In many cases, family members or loved ones are the person's primary care givers, and support for the caregivers is discussed in the meetings. Among its major responsibilities, the interdisciplinary hospice team:

- Manages the person's pain and symptoms
- Provides emotional support
- Provides needed medications, medical supplies, and equipment
- Coaches loved ones on how to care for the person
- Delivers special services like speech and physical therapy when needed
- Makes short-term inpatient care available when pain or symptoms become too difficult to manage at home, or the caregiver needs respite time
- Provides grief support to surviving loved ones and friends[25]

Rapid Response Teams

One recommended practice from the Institute for Healthcare Improvement in 2005 was that institutions develop rapid response teams to provide earlier interventions to decompensating patients. Beth Israel Deaconess Medical Center set about identifying and implementing a so-called trigger rapid response team in 2005. A set of triggers was identified so that, when a patient who is not in an intensive care unit (ICU) meets the criteria, there is a standard set of assessments and communication between nurses and physicians. Once a trigger has been identified and communicated, the appropriate team then comes to the bedside for a complete assessment. Teams may consist of ICU nurses, physicians, residents, and/or respiratory therapists. Triggers may include heart rate less than 40 or more than 130 beats per minute, blood pressure decrease less than 90 mm Hg, respiratory rate less than 8 or more than 30 breaths per minute, oxygen saturation less than 90% with oxygen, urinary output less than 50 mL in 4 hours, and any acute change in consciousness or marked nurse concern. After the initiation of the rapid response team the staff at Beth Israel Deaconess Medical Center noticed that the non-ICU unexpected mortality had decreased by more than 50%. The success of this program was credited to a standard set of assessments and a standard language between disciplines. In interdisciplinary rounds it is common to hear, for example, that "Mr S triggered at 1200 for a low blood pressure." For these professionals "trigger" is a new verb that communicates that an action is needed.[26]

TOOLKIT FOR IMPROVING COLLABORATIVE CARE
TeamSTEPPS

Team Strategies and Tools to Enhance Performance and Patient Safety (TeamSTEPPS) is an evidence-based teamwork system designed to optimize patient outcomes by improving communication and teamwork skills among health care professionals. It creates a common language among health care professionals that improves communication. The program includes a comprehensive set of ready-to-use materials and a training curriculum designed to successfully integrate teamwork principles into any health care system. It was developed by the Department of Defense's Patient Safety Program in collaboration with the Agency for Healthcare Research and Quality. Team-STEPPS has 5 key principles based on team structure with 4 teachable-learnable skills: communication, leadership, situation monitoring, and mutual support.[27]

Once the need is assessed the program is tailored to the organization choosing from the multitude of strategies that are available. The several workshops are designed to gain acceptance and support continuance of the skills in the organization.

1. Train-the-Trainer. This 2-day training course is designed to create a cadre of team-work instructors with the skills to train and coach other staff members.
2. TeamSTEPPS Fundamentals. This curriculum includes 4 to 6 hours of interactive workshops for direct patient care providers.
3. TeamSTEPPS Essentials. This curriculum is a 1-hour to 2-hour condensed version of the Fundamentals Course and is specifically designed for nonclinical support staff.[21]

Some of the strategies from the TeamSTEPPS Pocket Guide are listed here:

- Call-Out is used to communicate important or critical information. Call-outs are used during emergent situations in which accuracy is paramount. This process informs all team members of critical assessments simultaneously It helps team members to anticipate the next steps in the situation and directs responsibility to a specific individual who is responsible for carrying out the task.
- Check-Back uses closed-loop communication to ensure that information conveyed by the sender is understood by the receiver as intended. The sender initiates the message, the receiver accepts the message and provides feedback, and then the sender double-checks to ensure that the message was received.
- Handoff: the transfer of information (along with authority and responsibility) during transitions in care across the continuum. It includes an opportunity to ask questions, clarify, and confirm. This process is excellent to use when transferring a patient from one level of care to another to ensure that all areas involving the status and care of the patient are discussed and clear information is exchanged.
- Huddle: a time to gather before or during a crisis to update the health care team on status and reevaluate the plan. Huddle is an ad hoc meeting to reestablish

situation awareness, reinforce plans already in place, and assess the need to adjust the plan.
- Debriefing: a time after an event to review and evaluate actions and results. This informal information is designed to improve the team's performance and effectiveness through lessons learned and reinforcement of positive behaviors.[27]

Situation, Background, Assessment, Recommendation

Miscommunication is the most commonly occurring cause of sentinel events and near misses in patient care. Situation, Background, Assessment, Recommendation (SBAR) is a standard method of communicating between professionals. Patient information can be shared in a concise and structured format. This method of communication was introduced into health care settings in the late 1990s. SBAR can be used for patient hand-off at the end of the shift, communication with physicians, transferring patients from unit to unit, and any time information is to be shared. SBAR again provides a common language for health care providers.

- Situation. What is going on with the patient? "I am calling about Mr Angelo in room 251. Chief complaint is shortness of breath of new onset." In addition, describe the patient situation that has instituted this SBAR communication.
- Background. What is the clinical background or context? "Patient is an 89-year-old diabetic man with stage 3 ulcers and weight loss in the last month. No prior history of cardiac or lung disease. He has been confined to his bed for the last month." This background could include information relevant to the current situation, mental status, current vital signs (all of them), chief complaint, pain level, and physical assessment of the patient.
- Assessment. What do I think the problem is? "Breath sounds are decreased on the right side with acknowledgment of pain. Would like to rule out pneumothorax." This assessment describes the seriousness of the situation and any specific changes in the patient's condition
- Recommendation. What would I do to correct it? Make a suggestion such as a medication, laboratory work, or radiograph. State that "I think that the patient should be assessed now. Are you available to come in?"[6,19,28]

Interprofessional Education Collaborative Panel

The IPEC is composed of the following associations: the American Association of Colleges of Nursing, American Association of Colleges of Osteopathic Medicine, the American Association of Colleges of Pharmacy, the American Dental Education Association, the Association of American Medical Colleges, and the Association of Schools of Public Health. IPEC considers that interprofessional collaborative practice is the key to safe, high-quality, accessible, and patient-centered care.[12] The outcome of this panel was the development of interprofessional collaborative competencies and the encouragement of interprofessional education. These competencies, defined earlier in the article, are Values/Ethics for Interprofessional Practice, Role/Responsibilities, Interprofessional Communication and Teams, and Teamwork.[12] IPEC challenges faculty at various health care schools to plan clinical activities that allow students to engage in interactive learning with each other. Learning together as students facilitates being able to work together in clinical teams in the workforce. To assist in this learning the IPEC panel has identified definitions:

- Interprofessional education: students from 2 or more professions learn collaboratively to improve health outcomes.[14]

> **Box 4**
> **Reflection case report exercise about Mr Angelo (discussed earlier in the article).**
>
> Mr Angelo, 89 years old, has been returned to your medical unit. He is a diabetic, lives alone, does not like to cook, and cannot get around much. This admission is his third in 6 months. Since his discharge 3 months ago he has developed some neuropathy and has lost 6 kg (13 pounds). His wound is not completely healed. These developments seem to stem from poor nutrition. He is alert and oriented and interested in his care but is depressed about his lack of progress.

- Interprofessional collaborative practice: multiple disciplines work together with patients, families, caregivers, and communities to deliver high-quality collaborative care.[14]
- Interprofessional teamwork: the levels of cooperation, coordination, and collaboration characterizing the relationships between professions in delivering patient-centered care.
- Interprofessional team-based care: care delivered by intentionally created, usually small, work groups in health care, that are recognized by other clinicians as well as by themselves as having a collective identity and shared responsibility for a patient or group of patients (eg, rapid response team, palliative care team, primary care team, operating room team).
- Professional competencies in health care: integrated enactment of knowledge, skills, and values/attitudes that define the domains of work of a particular health profession applied in specific care contexts.
- Interprofessional competencies in health care: integrated enactment of knowledge, skills, and values/attitudes that define working together across the professions, with other health care workers, and with patients, along with families and communities, as appropriate to improve health outcomes in specific care contexts.
- Interprofessional competency domain: a generally identified cluster of more specific interprofessional competencies that are conceptually linked and serve as theoretic constructs.[12]

SUMMARY

Several questions were asked about the composition of this interprofessional team (**Box 4**). First, as you admit this patient, what interdisciplinary team members would you want on the clinical team? Mr Angelo has multiple problems that need to be addressed. Outcomes for his plan of care include prevention of readmission to hospital, increase in nutrition for wound healing, increase in his ability to walk, and prevention of further complications of diabetes. From that list the nurse is most likely to want on the team the primary nurse, a social worker or discharge planner, primary physician, dietitian, wound care specialist, physical therapy, a diabetic expert, and the patient and any significant others. What might you add?

The next 2 questions are answered together. They concern the role that you see the physician playing and the team member who should hold initial leadership on the team. The physician is essential on the team to manage the medical care. However, Mr Angelo has many other issues. Because a primary outcome is to prevent readmission to the hospital the social worker or discharge planner should have the overall picture of care and progress and should be in charge. Again, what are your thoughts?

The last question concerns how to evaluate the synthesis of the team plan and its impact on the patient's experience. This is a large team and it may take some time before the members get into the working phase of the relationship. The team must be aware of potential barriers mentioned earlier, especially differing knowledge, use of jargon, and role clashes. To evaluate the impact on the patient experience requires evaluation of the goals and communication with Mr Angelo to see how he views his progress.

A additional word about interprofessional collaboration. When health professionals from differing professions work together to provide patient care, high-quality care is provided and outcomes are achieved. In order for interprofessional collaboration to take place, all health professionals need to make earnest attempts to communicate effectively, value the contributions each member brings to the team, and maintain respect for the roles and individual skill sets each professional brings.

This change will occur over time. Each health care professional has a responsibility and a commitment to interprofessional collaboration. It is hoped that nursing leaders will take a leading role in developing and encouraging such teams.[6]

REFERENCES

1. Edmondson A, Roloff K. Overcoming barrier to collaboration: psychological safety and learning in diverse teams. In: Salas E, Goodwin G, Burke CS, editors. Team effectiveness in complex organizations: cross-disciplinary perspectives and approaches. New York: Psychology Press; 2009. p. 183–208.
2. Suter E, Arndt J, Arthur N, et al. Role understanding and effective communication as core competencies for collaborative practice. J Interprof Care 2009;23:41–51.
3. American Nurses Association. 2008 National Survey of Registered Nurses. US Bureau of Labor Statistic, occupational handbook. Health Aff 2009;28(4):657–68.
4. Gardner D. Ten lessons in collaboration. Online J Issues Nurs 2005;10(1):2.
5. QSEN Institute. Pre licensure competencies. Available at: http://qsen.org/competencies/pre-licensure-ksas/. Accessed June 10, 2014.
6. O'Brien D. Interprofessional collaboration. San Diego (CA): AMN Healthcare, Inc; 2013. Available at: http://www.rn.com/getpdf.php/1892.pdf?Main_Session=0c7d338fb741e35dc663010a8e86bc8b.
7. The Joint Commission Accreditation Program: ambulatory health care national patient safety goals. 2009. Available at: www.jointcommission.org. Accessed June 10, 2014.
8. Institute of Medicine Health professions education. A bridge to quality. Washington, DC: National Academies Press; 2003.
9. Rice K, Zwarenstein M, Conn L, et al. An intervention to improve interprofessional collaboration and communications: a comparative qualitative study. J Interprof Care 2010;24(4):350–61.
10. Institute of Medicine. The future of nursing: leading change, advancing health. Washington, DC: National Academies Press; 2010. p. 221–54.
11. Porter-O'Grady T, Malloch K. Leadership in nursing practice: changing the landscape of healthcare. Sudbury (MA): Jones and Bartlett; 2013. p. 209–74.
12. Interprofessional Education Collaborative Expert Panel. Core competencies for interprofessional collaborative practice: report of an expert panel. Washington, DC: Interprofessional Education Collaborative; 2011.
13. Oxford Dictionaries. 2014. Available at: http://www.oxforddictionaries.com/us/definition/american_english/teamwork. Accessed June 17, 2014.
14. Framework for Action on Interprofessional Education & Collaborative Practice (WHO/HRH/HPN/10.3) This publication is produced by the Health Professions Network Nursing and Midwifery Office within the Department of Human Resources

for Health. Available at: http://www.who.int/hrh/nursing_midwifery/en/ World Health Organization, Department of Human Resources for Health, CH-1211 Geneva 27, Switzerland © World Health Organization 2010, Edited by: Diana Hopkins, Freelance Editor, Geneva Switzerland.

15. Roussel L. Management and leadership for nurse administrators. Burlington (MA): Jones and Bartlett; 2013. p. 213–308.

16. Covey S. The 7 habits of highly effective people. New York: Free Press; 1989.

17. Manktelow J, Carlson J. Brainstorming: generating many radical, creative ideas. Available at: http://www.mindtools.com/. Accessed June 25, 2014.

18. The Delphi Method: achieving well thought-through consensus among experts. Available at: http://www.mindtools.com/pages/article/newTMC_95.htm. Accessed June 25, 2014.

19. Yoder-Wise P. Leading and managing in nursing. 5th edition. St. Louis (MO): Mosby; 2011. p. 345–71.

20. Carbo A, Folcarelli P. Let's talk: building better physician-nurse collaboration forum. In: Lavalley D, editor. Physician-nurse collaboration and patient safety, Vol. 26. 2nd edition. Cambridge (MA): CIRCO; 2008. p. 13.

21. Huber D. Leadership and nursing care management. 5th edition. St. Louis (MO): Saunders; 2014. p. 128–46.

22. Rokeach M. The nature of human values. New York: Free Press; 1973.

23. American Nurses Association. The value of nursing care coordination. (A White Paper of the American Nurses Association). 2012. Available at: http://www.nursingworld.org/carecoordinationwhitepaper. Accessed June 17, 2014.

24. Oberlies A. American Organization of Nurse Executives Care Innovation and Transformation program: improving care and practice environments. J Nurs Adm 2014;44(9):437–40.

25. The National Hospice and Palliative Care Organization. Available at: http://www.nhpco.org/. Accessed June 17, 2014.

26. Folcarelli P, Howell M. Triggers: rapid response at Beth Israel. In: Lavalley D, editor. Physician-nurse collaboration and patient safety, Vol. 26. 2nd edition. Cambridge (MA): CIRCO; Forum 2008. p. 10–2.

27. Pocket Guide: TeamSTEPPS Web site. Available at: http://www.ahrq.gov/professionals/education/curriculum- tools/teamstepps/instructor/essentials/pocketguide.html Publication # 14-0001-2. Accessed September 20, 2014.

28. O'Daniel M, Rosenstein AH. Professional communication and team collaboration. In: Hughes RG, editor. Patient safety and quality: an evidence-based handbook for nurses. Rockville (MD): Agency for Healthcare Research and Quality (US); 2008. Chapter 33. p. 271–84. Available at: http://www.ncbi.nlm.nih.gov/books/NBK2637/http://www.ahrq.gov/professionals/clinicians-providers/resources/nursing/resources/nurseshdbk/index.html.

The Role of Patient-Centered Care in Nursing

Amanda J. Flagg, PhD, MSN, EdM, RN, ACNS-BC, CNE

KEYWORDS

- Patient-/family-centered care • Family at bedside • Bedside report • Holistic nursing
- Patient satisfaction

KEY POINTS

- Patient-/family-centered care is key to patient satisfaction.
- Inclusion of family and friends is needed for increased quality of care.
- Use of a bedside report enhances quality of nursing care delivery.

SCENARIO

Nurse Smith, RN is running behind schedule. This is the third 12-hour shift on a 36-bed medical/surgical unit, and the change-of-shift-report has just been received for 7 patients assigned to her care. The night shift nurse has an appointment and needs to get home immediately. There is little time for questions or verifications of procedures such as early morning blood draws and catheter care necessities. Patient A is scheduled for surgery and is due to be transported at any moment. Problem: the prophylactic antibiotic he was to receive preoperatively has not yet arrived on the unit. Patient B is sleeping, but his glucose reading was 60 at 6:30 AM. Patient C is crying because of poor control of her postsurgical incisional pain, but she is not due for medication for another hour. Nurse Smith's remaining 4 patients will require her already taxed attention to pull her in several other directions within the hour, and there are 2 admissions waiting in the emergency department. Nurse Smith has been assigned to one of them. And the story continues.

INTRODUCTION

This scenario depicts a multitude of challenges and is played out repeatedly in many acute care inpatient facilities across the nation. Nurses like Nurse Smith bear heavy patient loads with limited support systems and ever-increasing responsibilities in the care of patients, particularly those with chronic illness. Health care has become

Disclosure Statement: The author has nothing to disclose.
School of Nursing, Middle Tennessee State University, Box 81, Murfreesboro, TN 37132, USA
E-mail address: Amanda.Flagg@mtsu.edu

progressively more complicated and highly technical and is perceived by many patients to be an impersonal and highly complex system.[1] So where is the patient in all the chaos? How satisfied are patients with nursing care today? What aspects of patient care can be considered in improving the quality of that care that will allow the patient to be seen, heard, and cared for amidst all the noise?

PROBLEM

The effects of changes in the field of health care are reverberating in nursing, which requires the need for increased efficiency in the provision of care. This environment pushes even the most experienced nurse to become more task oriented and less patient focused in a sea of constant admissions and discharges with expectations that patients are to do most of their recovery either in a long-term rehabilitation unit or at home.[2,3] The mantra "doing more with less and less" seems to be the quote of the day, every day.

One form of response to these challenges has echoed in the literature of nursing and other health care professions for several decades; the concept of patient-centered care (PCC). In fact, the Institute of Medicine has placed PCC as 1 of 6 objectives in the improvement of health care quality for the 21st century.[4] So what is PCC and how does it involve nursing care?

Defining Patient-Centered Care

PCC has been depicted as a philosophy, a process, a model, a concept, and a partnership that involves both the patient and health care provider (to include the nurse) arriving at some form of conclusion about the care and treatment of the patient's condition.[5-7] Although there are no definitive definitions of PCC, several attempts have been made to operationalize this concept. A summary of these efforts describing PCC are outlined in **Box 1**.

Kjeldmand and colleagues[12] acknowledged Mead and Bower's[13] early attempts to describe PCC but suggested that the term *patient-centeredness* is central to

---

Box 1
Brief history of patient-centered care

Balint first described PCC in the mid-1950s as a concept of understanding patients as unique beings.[8]

There have been many references to PCC as a philosophy.[9]

a. Mead and Bower (2002) began to form a preliminary framework of patient centeredness as a method of delivering health care to patients by describing 5 distinct dimensions of PCC.[10,11]

   1. Bio psychosocial perspective that takes into account the impact of social and psychological factors of illness

   2. Patient as a unique individual that considers the patient's personal understanding and meaning of illness

   3. Sharing of power and responsibility that considers patients' preferences for information and their participation in decision making

   4. The therapeutic alliance that takes into account the development of common goals and the enhancement of a bond shared between patient and provider

   5. Doctor/nurse as person aspect that addresses the awareness of personal qualities and subjective experiences of the provider within his or her practice setting.

relationship-centered care by acknowledging an ultimate synthesis of both the biomedical and real-world perspectives of both the patient and health care provider. So what is nursing's stand on PCC?

Domains of Patient-Centered Care

Competencies for nursing were analyzed and redefined in 2007 by the Quality and Safety Education for Nurses (QSEN) project that redirected how nurses approach their profession.[1] In this QSEN project, PCC was defined as a competency that recognizes the patient or designee as the source of control and full partner in providing compassionate and coordinated care. This care was based on respect for patients' preferences, values, and needs.[1] **Table 1** outlines additional key dimensions of PCC as it relates to nursing.[1,4,14,15]

Key Factors of a Patient-Centered Care Environment

There are 7 key factors that are imperative to the engagement, support, implementation, and sustainment of PCC.[16,17]

- Leadership involvement, support, and buy-in
- Strategic vision that is clearly defined and operationalized
- Involvement of patients and their families and other support systems
- Involvement of employees to include all health care providers
- Evaluation of and feedback regarding process in place
- Design of the physical environment to be supportive of patients, families, and staff
- Availability of technology that supports communication between patients and health care providers

Barriers to Patient-Centered Care

Although PCC is seen as a positive movement in the future of health care delivery, there are barriers that need to be recognized. Potential barriers include the following.

- No clear definition of PCC
- Lack of educational programs supporting PCC for all health care providers
- Fragmentation of care that focuses on the disease instead of the whole individual
- Staff who are overworked experiencing shortages

Table 1
Sample of dimensions of patient-centered care and nursing

Source	Dimensions
Gerteis et al,[14] 1993	Respect for patients, values, preferences, coordination and integration of care, information, communication, education, comfort, emotional support of family/friends, transition and continuity of care
Institute of Medicine,[4] 2001	Safety, effectiveness, timeliness, equity, and efficiency of care
Watson's ten principles of human science and care[15]	Person-centered nursing conceptual framework: characteristics and attributes of the nurse, context in which care is provided, how care is given, outcomes of care.
QSEN Project, 2007[1]	Patient as source of control, full partner in provision of compassionate care, respect for patient preference, values, and needs.

- Continued dominance of the biomedical mode of practice (doctor and nurse know best)
- Financial costs of educating and recruiting adequate numbers of health care providers in support of PCC

APPLICATION OF PATIENT-CENTERED CARE TO NURSING: HOLISTIC CARE

The philosophy of holistic nursing supports the tenants of PCC that are derived in part from Florence Nightingale who believed in the importance of her patients' conditions through the interaction of their respective environment.[18] Holistic nursing places emphasis on both the environment and treatment of the patient to include patients' uniqueness as human beings along with their cultural views, values, and beliefs.[18,19]

Shared Similarities of Holistic Nursing and Patient-Centered Care

Holistic nursing also encourages nurses to reflect on their own self-care and to engage in PCC that includes the use of such skills as listening and questioning. Takase and Teraoka[20] developed a competency scale to assess and measure Japanese nurses' abilities to cope with ever-increasing complex scenarios similar to the scenario described earlier.[20] The initial testing of this instrument found that 1 of the 5 themes was in full support of adopting ethically oriented practice to include the need for PCC nursing. The 5 themes identified shared similarities between nursing as a philosophy and principles of PCC. These similarities are summarized in **Box 2**.

Holistic nursing values and beliefs are also reflecting of PCC philosophies. They are summarized in **Box 3**.

The combination of PCC and holistic nursing can benefit patients and nurses; however, the inclusion of patients and their families and friends is also considered a positive aspect of these philosophies based on the patients' needs and desires to include them.

PATIENT-CENTERED CARE AND FAMILY-CENTERED CARE

Patient- and family-centered care (PFCC) extends the partnership of patients and health care providers to include families (and friends) at the discretion of the patient involved.[21] The involvement of families encourages the sharing of knowledge and experience in the planning of nursing care for the enhancement and well being of the patient.[22,23] Acute care facilities are engaging in PFCC in several ways to include the provision of the items listed in **Box 4**.

Box 2
Shared nursing interactions using holistic care and PCC

1. Listening to patients' questions, needs, and views

2. Communicating with patients to ensure understanding of their questions, needs, and views

3. Sharing questions, needs, and views with other members of health care teams

4. Establishment of therapeutic relationships with patients and significant others such as families and friends

5. Providing patients and families with needed education regarding their disease processes

6. Evaluating goals of care in accordance with patients' and families' wishes and abilities

7. Providing the best care possible using up-to-date knowledge, competencies, and empathic nursing practice

---

Box 3
Holistic nursing beliefs and PCC philosophies

1. Maintain up-to-date knowledge and competencies
2. Identify gaps in learning and knowledge
3. Reflect on practice
4. Observe objectively, yet compassionately
5. Promote health and well-being of self and others
6. Maintain balance both physically and mentally

PFCC is also mirrored in the practice of decreasing the limitations placed on visiting hours in many facilities. Based on patient and family preference and ability, family members are encouraged to stay with patients overnight and are invited to be involved in some aspects of patient care. Even acutely ill patients are afforded less-restrictive visitation hours in such areas as the emergency department and intensive care units.[24,25] Alternatively, with extended family visiting, consequences that require consideration include the potential of patient exhaustion, unrealistic expectations for perceived needs of patient and family members, and the potential overall effects of such visits on the progress of patient recovery.

FAMILY PRESENCE AT THE BEDSIDE AND BEYOND

Family presence within the PFCC model extends to include not just presence in patient rooms during set visiting hours but during procedures that occur in inpatient and outpatient areas. Depending on the invasiveness of the procedure and patient and family preferences, several research studies have found positive aspects of such practice.[26]

One such procedure is the changing of dressings for severe burn injuries. Because of concerns of increased infection rates and the perception of family members' inability to tolerate observing their loved ones in times of duress, family members are usually not allowed to be present. This often leads to dissatisfaction of care and misperceptions of nursing and medical staff in the eyes of the patient and their loved ones. A study by Bishop and colleagues,[27] found that family presence during a burn wound debridement actually had the opposite effect. In selected cases, patients experienced decreased levels of apprehension and pain.

Conversely, another aspect of including family participation includes pediatric patients. Under the auspices of PFCC, pediatric patients are included in this partnership, particularly in decision-making processes, regardless of their age, based on the extent of their ability and desire to be part of the planning of their care. The same invitation can be extended to the elderly, particularly those patients who have limited cognitive function yet are able to share in basic decision making.

Box 4
Patient- and family-centered care provisions

1. Family information packs concerning location and cafeteria hours
2. Posted photos of all staff members on each inpatient and outpatient unit
3. Resources assisting in the care of the patient at discharge

FAMILY PRESENCE DURING CHANGE-OF-SHIFT REPORT

The presence of family during patient rounds may conjure images of gross violations of Health Insurance Portability and Accountability Act (HIPAA); however, if PFCC is to be respected, the inclusion of patient rounds requires that family presence be not only invited but encouraged. The following tenants are suggestions to consider.[28–36]

- Give patients and families a choice in engaging in rounds.
- Have nurses provide introductions (eg, night shift introduces the day shift nurse and staff).
- Use a circle formation if possible during a report to allow for eye contact to occur.
- Use terminology that all parties can understand.

Benefits of Patient- and Family-Centered Care Rounds

- Increased patient and family satisfaction of care
- Increased communication between patients and nurses
- Decreased confusion regarding discharge planning and teaching
- Opportunities for patient and family education
- Opportunities for discussion and planning of patient care

Barriers to Patient- and Family-Centered Care Rounds

- Limited physical space based on patients' room size and available areas for discreet conversations
- Nursing units' buy-in and use of rounds (eg, are rounds audio-taped? Do nurses round together?)
- Time constraints with change-of-shift report
- Potential for HIPAA violations of patient information

FAMILY PRESENCE DURING CODES

PFCC seems well suited in many health care situations but remains controversial in extreme interactions during lifesaving, resuscitative efforts. Hung and Pang[24] studied family members who were present during successful resuscitative efforts of their loved ones using an interpretive phenomenological approach.[24] **Table 2** summarizes 10 themes that emerged from the data and family member comments reflecting the themes.

Barriers to Family Presence During Codes

Itzhaki and colleagues[37] noted that, in general, lay individuals tended to be more positive toward family presence in a code situation than clinical, staff particularly when the patient survived. Women, both family and clinicians, tended to reflect more negatively in situations in which profuse bleeding was present and resuscitative efforts failed. **Box 5** summarizes barriers that could prevent families from witnessing resuscitation efforts of their family members.

Interventions Used to Embrace and Sustain Patient- and Family-Centered Care

A core competency identified in several studies that supports PFCC is that of communication.[38,39] The following communication strategies are recommended by the Massachusetts Department of Higher Education Nurse of the Future Competency Committee.[40]

- Verbal, written, and electronic versions should be clear and concise.
- Auditory, visual, and tactile forms are important components.

Table 2
Ten themes with examples of participants' responses

Theme	Response
1. Emotional connectedness to the patient	"I was allowed to hold his/her hand"
2. Provision of support to the patient	"I could talk to him/her"
3 Maintaining relationship with patient	"I was allowed to hold his/her hand"
4 Knowing the patient and health conditions	"I could relate aspects of his/her health"
5. Keeping informed of what was going on	"I knew what was being done to save this life"
6. Being engaged in what was going on	"Watching reassured me the right things were being done"
7. Providing information to the resuscitation team	"Could provide the names of medications he/she was taking"
8. Perceived (in)appropriateness	"I was not allowed in the ICU, I felt helpless, alone, discarded"
9. Perceived inconvenience	"I might be in the way of the doctors and nurses—should I be here?"
10. Perceived prohibition	"The door said no entry unless given permission—I just wanted to be there but I don't break rules"

Adapted from Hung M, Pang, MC. Family presence preferences when patients are receiving resuscitation in an accident and emergency department. J Adv Nurs 2010;67(1):56–7.

- Nurses' own communication styles have an impact on the receivers' end of the message.
- Effects of communication can evoke many forms of influence to include spiritual, emotional, and cultural characteristics.
- The right time and setting are imperative considerations.
- The receiver, often the patient or family, should be assessed regarding their ability and readiness to communicate.

Box 5
Barriers to family presence during codes

The patient prefers that family not be present during code situations.

Family members prefer not to or are afraid to observe.

Family members may be concerned or lose control by becoming inconsolable or physically or verbally challenging.

Family members require attention that would detract from patient care.

There is limited physical space in acute care units.

Staff feels family presence is not appropriate.

Staff feels anxious, judged, or concerned with family reactions to their responses under pressure of code situations.

Limited staff is available to allow for adequate support of family witnesses.

Adapted from Itzhaki M, Bar-Tal Y, Barnoy S. Reactions of staff members and lay people to family presence during resuscitation: the effect of visible bleeding, resuscitation outcome and gender. J Adv Nurs 2011;68(9):1967–77.

- Barriers should be observed and considered.
- Rapport should be established between parties.
- Opportunities for questions should be provided.
- Assessment of both verbal and nonverbal behavior should be noted.

Building communication competence leads to PFCC delivery models that increase patient care satisfaction and staff retention and recruitment, decrease length of stay and ED visits, and decrease medication errors.[41] PFCC delivery model components are listed in **Box 6**.

A few facilities are engaging in the concept of PFCC by participating in the Planetree's PCC Hospital Designation Program. Under this model, facilities must adhere to 50 criteria placed under 11 categories to receive such recognition.[42] The 11 categories facilities must meet are as follows.

- Structures and functions needed for development, implementation, and maintenance of PCC
- Human interactions
- Patient education and access to information
- Family involvement
- Nutrition program
- Healing environment
- Arts program to include animal visitation
- Spirituality and diversity
- Integrative therapies to include alternative therapies
- Healthy communities—a plan geared toward the needs of the community at large
- Measurement—use of patient/family satisfaction scores as examples

---

Box 6
Components of Patient- and family-centered care delivery models

1. Coordination of care conference—meeting with all specialties to include patient and family to discuss plan of care initiating discharge planning

2. Hourly rounding (once per hour)—includes pain, elimination, and positioning needs along with other patient/family concerns

3. Bedside report—completed at the bedside with family and friends present at discretion of patient or patient advocate

4. Initializing and use of patient care partner (when available)—a family member, friend, or volunteer in full support of patient's needs and desires

5. Individualized care—Established at admission, to include preferred name, priority of care, learning style, and care partner selection

6. Open medical record policy—allowing patients to document their views at their discretion

7. Opening visiting restrictions—driven by patient or family as applicable in a variety of settings

8. Family presence during resuscitation and other procedures—at discretion of patient as applicable

9. Silence and healing—inviting the patient and family to assess noise level in their environment and to report any discomfort of such to the nurse

Adapted from Hunter R, Carlson E. Finding the fit: patient centered care. Nurs Manage 2014;45:39–43.

Table 3 Sample of studies centered on patient satisfaction	
Article	Findings
Improving patient satisfaction with nursing communication using bedside shift report[33]	Patient satisfaction rate increased from 75% to 87.6%
Patients' perspective on person-centered participation in healthcare: a framework analysis[5]	General attention and interest was felt by patient Patients felt respected Patients felt trust
Efficacy of person-centered care as an intervention in controlled trials—a systematic review[43]	Many studies included the concept of PCC but only a few were actually practicing the model
Effects of patient-centered care on patient outcomes: an evaluation[44]	Patients are demanding more active roles in their care Implementation of PCC increased pt. satisfaction with care
Patient satisfaction as an outcome of individualized nursing care[30]	Positive correlations were found between individualized care and patient satisfaction.

EVALUATION—THE ULTIMATE SCORING CARD

A trend is emerging in the literature associating patient satisfaction of care scores to the delivery of PFCC. Although there are multitudes of variables associated with these forms of measurement, several studies are emerging with such reports, and nursing is helping pave the way for such findings. A small sample of studies is provided in **Table 3**.

Although these articles represent studies exploring concepts of PFCC and patient satisfaction scores in the inpatient setting, outpatient areas are now being included in PFCC models. Most outpatient clinics have associated the reduction of clinic wait times to patient satisfaction scores. Michael and colleagues,[45] also studied the effect of wait times patients experienced in the examination room on satisfaction of overall care.[45] These aspects of care have been identified as key points of interest for patients and clinicians but there are many other variables that require further study within this context of health care delivery.

Wolff and Roter[31] suggested that older patients suffering with chronic illness are more likely to be accompanied to an outpatient visit by either family or friends. They hypothesized that the addition of family members invokes a positive aspect of care by aiding the patient-provider partnership, the exchange of information regarding patient status, and by including family in the decision-making processes. Their study, a meta-analytical review, found that the presence of family should be further studied in hopes of isolating those factors that facilitate decision-making processes. Care of patients with acute and chronic illnesses can be enhanced by understanding the communication processes deemed central to changing health care delivery systems toward a more patient/family focus.

SUMMARY

Now that PCC, holistic nursing, PFCC, bedside rounds, and patient satisfaction scores have been addressed, let's return to the scenario depicting Nurse Smith and her third day of duty to see how these concepts might benefit both the patients placed in Nurse Smith's care and Nurse Smith's practice. Using PFCC:

- Nurse Smith and the night shift nurse would be rounding together, exchanging reports at each patient's bedside.[28–36]
- Any concerns or questions Nurse Smith would have could be efficiently addressed by the night shift nurse, the patient, and a family member if present (based on patient permission).
- Patients' concerns could also be more fully acknowledged, such as patient B's glucose level, and patient C's pain control.
- Nurse Smith's other patients will hear the report on their situations and be given reassurances that Nurse Smith will return after attending to the immediate needs of her first 3 patients. Any requests from these less-critical patients can be answered by appropriately trained delegated personnel.
- A communication board located in each patient room can be updated to include Nurse Smith's name and contact information.[46]
- Hourly rounds will minimally include the checking of patients' pain, elimination, and position changes particularly for those requiring complete, high-level care. Nurse Smith will always ask if there are other concerns or questions.[47]
- Nurse Smith also has the right to ask for additional assistance if the patient load does not allow for all other competencies of nursing care to be carried out according to such examples as QSEN standards, facility policies and procedures, and her Professional Nurse Practice Act.[1]

PFCC does not occur in a vacuum. To function, all health care members from administration to environmental services are part of a team whose central focus is the patient. Nurse Smith is part of a team inclusive of not only health care providers but also the patient, his or her family, and other support systems. Drawing on all parties' experiences to provide care to the patient can only enhance the quality and safety of care that is so critical and so needed yet continues to be so challenging.

REFERENCES

1. Sherwood G, Zomorodi M. A new mindset for quality and safety: the QSEN competencies redefine nurses' roles in practice. Nephrol Nurs J 2014;41(1):15–23.
2. Dabney BW, Tzeng HM. Service quality and patient-centered care. Medsurg Nurs 2013;22(6):359–64.
3. Lusk JM, Fater K. A concept analysis of patient-centered care. Nurs Forum 2013; 48(2):89–98.
4. Institute of Medicine. To err is human: building a safer health system. Washington, DC: National Academies Press; 2000.
5. Thórarinsdóttir K, Kristjánsson K. Patients' perspectives on person-centered participation in healthcare: a framework analysis. Nurs Ethics 2014;21(2):129–47.
6. Burman ME, Robinson B, Hart AM. Linking evidenced-based nursing practice and patient centered care through patient preferences. Nurs Adm Q 2013; 37(3):231–41.
7. Kitson A, Marshall A, Bassett K, et al. What are the core elements of patient-centered care? A narrative review and synthesis of the literature from health policy, medicine, and nursing. J Appl Nutr 2012;69(1):4–15. http://dx.doi.org/10.1111/j1365-2648.2012.06064.x.
8. Balint M. The doctor, his patient, and the illness. London: Pitman Medical; 1964.

9. Lewin SA, Entwistle V, Zwarenstein M, et al. Interventions for providers to promote a patient-centered approach in clinical consultations (Review). Cochrane Database Syst Rev 2005;(4):CD003267.

10. Mead N, Bower P. Patient-centered consultations and outcomes in primary care: a review of the literature. Patient Educ Couns 2002;48:51–61.

11. Slatore CG, Hansen L, Ganzini L, et al. Communication by nurses in the intensive care unit: qualitative analysis of domains of patient-centered care. Am J Crit Care 2012;21:410–8.

12. Kjeldmand D, Holmstrom I, Rosenqvist U. How patient centered am I? A new method to measure patient-centeredness. Patient Educ Couns 2006;62(1):31–7.

13. Mead N, Bower P. Patient-centeredness: a conceptual framework and review of the empirical literature. Soc Sci Med 2000;51:1087–110.

14. Gerteis M, Edgman-Levitan S, Daley J, et al. Through the patient's eyes: understanding and promoting patient-centered care. San Francisco (CA): Jossey-Bass; 1993.

15. Watson J, Lea A. The caring dimensions inventory (CDI): content, validity, reliability and scaling. J Appl Nutr 1997;25(1):87–94.

16. Schaller D. Patient-centered care: what does it take?. Washington, DC: Picker Institute, Oxford and Commonwealth Fund; 2007.

17. Pelzang R. Time to learn: understanding patient-centered care. Br J Nurs 2010; 19(14):912–7.

18. Lange B, Zahourek RP, Mariano C. A legacy building model for holistic nursing. J Holist Nurs 2014;32(2):116–26.

19. Mariano C. An overview of holistic nursing. Imprint 2005;52:48–51.

20. Takase M, Teraoka S. Development of the holistic nursing competence scale. Nurs Health Sci 2011;13:396–403.

21. Duran C, Oman KS, Jordan J, et al. Attitudes toward and beliefs about family presence: a survey of healthcare providers, patients' families, and patients. Am J Crit Care 2007;16(3):270–80.

22. Nykiel L, Denicke R, Schneider R, et al. Evidence-based practice and family presence: paving the path for bedside nurse scientists. J Emerg Nurs 2010; 37(1):9–16.

23. Ciufo D, Hader R, Holly C. A comprehensive systematic review of visitation models in adult critical care units within the context of patient and family centered care. Int J Evid Based Healthc 2011;9:362–87.

24. Hung M, Pang MC. Family presence preference when patients are receiving resuscitation in an accident and emergency department. J Appl Nutr 2010; 67(1):56–67. http://dx.doi.org/10.1111/j1365-2648.2010.05441 x

25. Ewart L, Moore J, Gibbs C, et al. Patient and family centered care on an acute adult cardiac ward. Br J Nurs 2014;23(4):213–8.

26. Bradford KK, Kost S, Selbst SM, et al. Family member presence for procedures: the resident's perspective. Ambul Pediatr 2005;5(5):294–7.

27. Bishop SM, Walker MD, Spivak IM. Family presence in the adult burn intensive care unit during dressing changes. Crit Care Nurse 2013;33(1):14–23.

28. Timonen L, Sihvonen M. Patient participation in bedside reporting on surgical wards. J Clin Nurs 2000;9:542–8.

29. Woodward JL. Effects of rounding on patient satisfaction and patient safety on a medical-surgical unit. Clin Nurse Spec 2009;23(4):200–6.

30. Suhonen R, Papastavrou E, Efstathiou G, et al. Patient satisfaction as an outcome of individualized nursing care. Scand J Caring Sci 2011;26:372–80. http://dx.doi.org/10.1111/j1471-6712.2011.00943.x.

31. Wolff JL, Roter DL. Family presence in routine medical visits: a meta-analytical review. Soc Sci Med 2011;72:823–31.
32. Blakley D, Kroth M, Gregson J. The impact of nurse rounding on patient satisfaction in a medical-surgical hospital unit. Medsurg Nurs 2011;20(6):327–32.
33. Radtke K. Improving patient satisfaction with nursing communication using bedside shift report. Clin Nurse Spec 2013;27(1):19–25.
34. Ferguson LM, Ward H, Card S, et al. Putting the 'patient' back into patient-centered care: an education perspective. Nurse Educ Pract 2013;13:283–7.
35. Santiago C, Lazar L, Jiang D, et al. A survey of the attitudes and perceptions of multidisciplinary team members towards family presence at bedside rounds in the intensive care unit. Intensive Crit Care Nurs 2013;30:13–21.
36. Subramony A, Hametz PA, Balmer D. Family-centered rounds in theory and practice: an ethnographic case study. Acad Pediatr 2014;14:200–6.
37. Itzhaki M, Bar-Tal Y, Barnoy S. Reactions of staff members and lay people to family presence during resuscitation: the effect of visible bleeding, resuscitation outcome and gender. J Appl Nutr 2011;68(9):1967–77.
38. Boykins AD. Core communication competencies in patient centered care. ABNF J 2014;25:40–5.
39. Simmons SA, Sharp B, Fowler J, et al. Implementation of a novel communication tool and its effect on patient comprehension of care and satisfaction. Emerg Med J 2013;30(5):363–70. http://dx.doi.org/10.1136/emermed-2011-200907.
40. Massachusetts Department of Higher Education Nurse of the Future Competency Committee. Nurse of the future nursing core competencies. Boston: Maassachusetts Department of Higher Education; 2010.
41. Hunter R, Carlson E. Finding the fit: patient centered care. Nurs Manage 2014;45:39–43.
42. Frampton SB, Guastello S. Patient-centered care: more than the sum of its parts. Am J Nurs 2010;110(9):49–53.
43. Olsson LE, Jakobsson E, Swedberg K, et al. Efficacy of person-centered care as an intervention in contolled trials – a systematic review. J Clin Nurs 2012;22:456–65. http://dx.doi.org/10.1111/jocn.12039.
44. Sidani A. Effects of patient-centered care on patient outcomes: an evaluation. Res Theory Nurs Pract 2008;22(1):24–37. http://dx.doi.org/10.1891/0889-7182.22.1.24.
45. Michael M, Schaffer SD, Egan PL, et al. Improving wait times and patient satisfaction in primary care. J Healthc Qual 2013;35(2):50–60.
46. Signh S, Fletcher KE, Pandl J, et al. It's the writing on the wall: whiteboards improve inpatient satisfaction with provider communication. Am J Med Qual 2011;26(2):127–31. http://dx.doi.org/10.1177/1062860610276088.
47. Ford BM. Hourly rounding; a strategy to improve patient satisfaction scores. Medsurg Nurs 2010;19(3):188–91.

Transforming Nursing Care Through Health Literacy ACTS

Kempa S. French, RN, MSN, FNP-BC[a,b],*

KEYWORDS

- Health literacy • Patient advocacy • Patient education • Patient-centered care
- Shared decision making • Teach back • Universal health literacy precautions

KEY POINTS

- Limited or low literacy is associated with negative or poor health outcomes.
- All patients, regardless of literacy level, need accessible and actionable health information to make informed decisions about their health.
- Universal Health Literacy Precautions are recommended to meet quality and safety standards for more literate health care systems and providers.
- Front-line nurses can transform their care by using "ACTS" for educational strategies (assess, compare, teach, and survey) and advocacy strategies (assess, collaborate, train, and survey).
- Using ACTS consistently in patient and health system interactions can enhance patient-centered communication and effective care.

INTRODUCTION

After years of trying to conceive, a couple was overjoyed to find out that they were expecting their first child. The diagnosis of an ectopic pregnancy in the young woman's remaining Fallopian tube left the couple devastated by the knowledge that trying for another pregnancy would be futile.

> Craving support and information, (she) waited for the medical professionals that were treating her to offer words of condolences or to give her medical information packets to leaf through. "I left the hospital with 18 staples, empty arms, and a huge hospital bill. Not one person tried to comfort me or say they were sorry for my loss."[1]

Disclosures: K.S. French is the recipient of the 2013 Sigma Theta Tau International/Assessment Technologies Inc. Educational Assessment Grant to support her doctoral research. K.S. French has no proprietary funding to disclose.

a School of Nursing, Austin Peay State University, PO Box 4658, Clarksville, TN 37044, USA; b College of Nursing, Medical University of South Carolina, 99 Jonathan Lucas Street, Charleston, SC 29425, USA

* School of Nursing, Austin Peay State University, PO Box 4658, Clarksville, TN 37044.

E-mail address: frenchk@apsu.edu

http://dx.doi.org/10.1016/j.cnur.2014.10.007
0029-6465/15/$ – see front matter © 2015 Elsevier Inc. All rights reserved.
nursing.theclinics.com

This true-life incident illustrates both opportunities and challenges for front-line nurses when interacting with patients in the current health environment. This young woman received life-saving medical and nursing care, but her educational and emotional needs were not met in her interactions with providers or the health care system. This experience, however, spurred her to seek more information about her diagnosis. She formed an online ectopic pregnancy support group and authored a book sharing information and stories about ectopic pregnancy for other families going through similar situations. The lack of effective health provider communication is not unique to this situation and underscores the urgency for front-line nurses to develop more successful patient-centered communication by incorporating health literacy competencies in all patient interactions.[2]

PROBLEM

Patients with limited or low literacy levels are more likely to report poorer health status levels,[3] use emergency and hospitals more frequently, use preventive health services and self-care management less frequently,[4] and have a 2-fold increased mortality risk for community-dwelling elders[5] compared with those with higher literacy levels.

Limited Literacy Prevalence

The most recent national survey of US literacy levels, the 2003 National Adult Assessment of Literacy, measured the reading proficiencies of a randomized sampling of 16,000 participants and included health-related literacy components.[6] The results suggested that 75 to 80 million (36%) Americans have basic or below basic literacy levels and may have moderate difficulty in correctly following medication instructions or completing consent or insurance forms without assistance. Those groups at greater risk for limited literacy were identified as those older than 65, affected with multiple comorbidities or disabilities, entering school speaking a language other than English, or with lower economic levels. National Adult Assessment of Literacy health literacy assessments were only for written proficiencies and taken out of the context of normal use, which may have limited their generalizability. The health literacy questions did not account for cultural preferences,[7] the effects of provider communication on medication adherence,[8] or comprehension of medical information by the participant.[9,10]

Functional Health Literacy Definition

The 2004 Institute of Medicine consensus report, Health Literacy: A Prescription to End Confusion, defined health literacy as "the degree to which individuals have the capacity to obtain, process, and understand basic health information and services needed to make health decisions.[11(pp34–35)]" This definition reflects past and current health literacy research and practice priorities that emphasize reading skills such as patient reading abilities and the literacy burden of health information.[12,13] These functional literacy-based skills are used by many providers and health systems that seek to "diagnose" patients with limited health literacy through screening and "treat" identified literacy problems by simplifying written and audiovisual health information.

Patient Literacy Screening Tools

Screening for limited literacy may include provider recognition of patient literacy levels through patient behavioral cues or the use of patient screening tools such as the Test of Functional Health Literacy Assessment (TOFHLA), Rapid Estimate of Adult Literacy in Med (REALM), Newest Vital Sign (NVS), or Single Item Literacy Screening (SILS) questions.[14] Patient literacy screening instruments categorize reading abilities to estimate patient literacy levels. Older tools such as TOFHLA or REALM were based on word recognition, numeracy skills, and comprehension formats used in educational settings for student placement purposes. Newer tools attempted to reduce time and administrative burdens in clinical settings by tying literacy levels to common tasks such as reading nutrition labels (NVS) or patient-reported levels of assistance to complete medical forms (SILS).

Limitations of Literacy Screening

Use of screening results involves time and personnel for administration and may not lead to improved patient health outcomes or provider satisfaction with care given even when aware of patient literacy levels. Comparisons of outcomes for 182 diabetic patients with limited literacy seen by 32 physicians with knowledge of their patients' literacy levels versus 31 who did not, noted no significant improvement in patient diabetic control or provider satisfaction with care management.[15] These findings suggest that the time and personnel to administer screenings, document implementation, and follow up with patients may not improve interactions or outcomes for patients or their health care providers.

Health care providers may not always accurately identify low-literacy patients based on their health literacy awareness or literacy-related behavioral cues.[16–18] Dickens and colleagues[19] described these discrepancies when comparing the measured literacy levels of 65 patients hospitalized for congestive heart failure and 30 nurses caring for them on 2 inpatient cardiac units. There was little agreement between the patient's NVS and SILS scores and the nurses' informal literacy assessments ($\kappa = 0.09$). Over- or underestimation of literacy levels may lead nurses to assume that patients fully understand health instructions or that patient knowledge needs are met without additional confirmation. According to these findings, provider knowledge about limited health literacy may not be the most reliable guide for interventions based solely on screening results or behavioral cues indicating limited literacy.

Barriers to Patient Understanding

Americans with lower literacy proficiency may have difficulty navigating the current health care system, but knowledge barriers are not restricted to those at risk for limited literacy or with inadequate access to health care. Functional-based literacy approaches may neglect the health information needs, preferences, and perspectives of the remaining 64% of patients who have adequate or advanced reading levels.[20] Nurses may shortchange patients with adequate or high literacy levels by assuming that those patients can understand and apply complex and potentially unfamiliar medical concepts to their personal health situations.

The functional literacy skills approach has also neglected provider contributions as potential barriers to patient comprehension. Castro and colleagues[9] profiled provider use of medical jargon as observed in 81% of 74 visits between diabetic patients with limited literacy and their providers. Jargon was used an average of 4 times per visit, particularly when making recommendations (37%) or providing patient instructions (29%). The effect of jargon was further evaluated in postvisit telephone calls with a subsample of 19 patients. Respondents had difficulty remembering the meaning of medical terms or jargon used in the initial interaction regardless of whether additional contextual cues were provided by the interviewer (p. S90).[9] Plain language should be the goal for patient-nurse interactions, yet little research exists evaluating nurses' use of medical jargon with patients or the effects of nurses' use of jargon on patient health outcomes.

Additional factors that influence patient comprehension include the underuse of evidence-based health literacy practices reported by providers. Schwartzenberg and colleagues[21] surveyed the health literacy practices of 168 physicians, nurses, and pharmacists attending a health literacy conference. Conference participants reported using provider-centered rather than patient-centered strategies in their patient interactions during the week before the survey. Use of plain language, handing out written materials and speaking slowly more often were mentioned more than health literacy evidence-based practices such as tailoring written materials or instructions to patient-identified preferences or verifying patient comprehension through use of teach-back. Although diabetic control outcomes of those patients were significantly improved when physicians used teach-back techniques to confirm patient comprehension, use of teach-back was only observed for 20% of those interactions.[10] The potential for health improvement was diminished through the inconsistent use of practice standards, such as teach-back, and may be further reduced through lack of provider knowledge about health literacy standards. These barriers to verbal communication may also be worsened if written materials are used as the primary source of health information[12,13]

Interventions such as simplifying written health information may not lead to greater patient comprehension when patients are learning unfamiliar or complex health concepts. Wilson and colleagues[22] piloted an educational intervention to assess maternal comprehension about polio vaccine information with 37 low-income mothers at an urban walk-in immunization clinic. After screening for participant literacy levels, mothers randomly assigned to the control group read standard polio information, whereas the mothers in the experimental group read modified reader-friendly vaccine information. Both groups showed slight improvements in vaccine knowledge, but significant comprehension of key vaccine information was not evident in either group even with the simplified pamphlet.

The limitations of functional literacy-based interventions are seen in the initial patient scenario. The young woman did not have any overt risk factors for limited health literacy, and literacy screening would not have closed her health information gaps. Nurses in this situation missed an opportunity to provide suitable written health information, but written materials alone may not have provided the resources or emotional support to ease her grief and sense of loss. Her reading abilities did not reflect her information-seeking skills, self-motivation, or desire to locate and share health information with others experiencing an ectopic pregnancy. Her needs for accessible and actionable health information were equally as important as for women with low literacy in similar situations. Intervening with simplified materials alone would have provided key information and actions but may not have provided enough information to predict the actions she would have taken without verification or further discussion.

Multidimensional Health Literacy

To address these limitations, health literacy has also been conceptualized as "the wide range of skills and competencies that people develop to seek out, comprehend, evaluate and use health information and concepts to make informed choices, reduce health risks and improve quality of life.[23(pp196–197)]" This more holistic definition builds on a patient's literacy and numeracy skills to include the scientific, civic, and cultural patient influences patients use to translate health information into health-promoting actions. From a multidimensional health literacy perspective, patient health literacy levels are not a single benchmark linked to health risks. Instead, patient and provider health literacies are flexible and dynamic assets characterized by existing experiences and life skills within a range of contexts.[20] When nurses use multidimensional health literacy competencies in practice, they incorporate more patient-centered communication practices with all patients, not just those with limited or low literacy.

Challenges for Front-Line Nurses

Front-line nurses face daily challenges in meeting their professional roles and legal and ethical responsibilities as care providers, educators, and patient advocates. Aging patients with multiple comorbidities, increasing culturally and linguistically diverse populations, technologically complex workloads, and economic pressures may affect the abilities of nurses to communicate safely and effectively with their patients. Although front-line nurses deal with these and other challenges in providing safe and effective care, opportunities also exist for nurses to transform their nursing practice by consistently using health literacy evidence in patient interactions. Nurses can become more effective patient educators by using the ACTS (assess, compare, teach 3, teach-back, and survey) in each patient interaction. Nurses can also use ACTS (assess, collaborate, train, and survey) with patients and peers to advocate for practical improvements in health care systems accessibility. The ACTS acronym can help front-line nurses be effective educators and advocates. The 2 ACTS should take place in all health setting interactions with patients, caregivers, family members, communities, and health systems.

EDUCATION STRATEGIES USING ACTS
Assess Patient Concerns

The first step in assessment is to begin patient interactions by identifying the patient's main concern. By asking the patient to identify their main concern, the focus and priority shifts from being nursing task oriented to a more patient-centered partnership. This patient-directed approach may more effectively target which topics or learning needs are vital to address for the interaction to have the intended outcomes. Asking the patient to voice his or her priority may remove blocks to learning that occur when patients are distracted by anxiety, pain, or issues unrelated to the immediate setting. Querying the patient about their main concern can be done within the context of the nursing task and provides a starting point for additional assessments about available resources or the involvement of significant others in health maintenance activities.

The second assessment step is to discover patients' learning needs and preferences to tailor suitable intervention. Asking patients what their baseline level of knowledge is and how they prefer to learn acknowledges patient or caregiver expertise about their health information and supports their desired level of control in shared decision making.

The third assessment step is to discover core patient values, which will provide cultural, social, and motivational contexts to frame interventions. The nurse should identify potential language, cultural, social, or physical influences, which can be used to work through patient barriers to care or improve patient adherence.

Compare Identified Patient Priorities and Needs with Resources

The comparison of patient-focused assessments with available materials and resources means that nurses use patient-identified learning needs and preferences to match relevant content to patient knowledge gaps. When nurses distill "need-to-know" information from available resources, they target essential concepts to foster greater patient comprehension of health information. The nurse would also account for patient cultural and language variations, sensory alterations, or technological advances to match the diverse range of patient abilities for existing or additional information. This information should be documented in the medical record to ensure that all team members can use this information when providing health services.

Tailoring key information to patient preferences means that nurses can reduce overwhelming and sometimes confusing instructions into easier-to-remember concepts. The emphasis of key information should be on which actions the patient should take and not just on what patients should know. Nurses may also identify unsuitable or poorly matching patient resources, which could be modified or replaced based on patient feedback and nursing appraisal of usefulness over time. The key information would then be available for patients or caregivers to use as augmentation of the originally taught information or for further review in a less distracting environment to enhance adherence to critical health instructions or the follow-up plan of care.

Teach 3, Teach-Back

Teach 3, teach-back means that patients are taught 3 or fewer key actions, health information concepts, or care skills in short segments. Patients then restate the nurse's teaching in their own words or return demonstration of the skill. If patients have difficulty repeating or demonstrating information or skills correctly, then reteaching should be done until all information is repeated correctly. To start the process, nurses should foster a shame-free environment by acknowledging the nurse's responsibility for assuring patient learning in their opening statement. After patients repeat or demonstrate the main concepts or skills, the nurse has immediate feedback about patient misconceptions or difficulties in skill execution. The nurse can then give alternative explanations or modifications quickly to improve comprehension of the desired concepts or skills. This same process should be repeated until the learner has mastered all essential concepts or skills.

One concern that nurses may have about using teach-back is extra time to complete their routine tasks while using this process. These concerns may be allayed by viewing VA Palo Alto Project RED short training videos showing nurses using teach-back when discharging emergency room, mental health, and medical-surgical patients.[24–26] Poor and good examples of nursing communication are presented, but patient comprehension is significantly improved when teach-back strategies are used, although similar nursing time was spent in the demonstrated patient-nurse interactions. Research incorporating teach-back for adults with heart failure[27] and children with complex medication needs[28] supports consistent use of teach-back as leading to better comprehension, higher levels of adherence, and potentially more positive health outcomes.

Survey for Additional Needs

Nurses should survey patients for additional resources or unmet learning needs to close the communication loop. Closed-ended questions such as "Do you have any other questions?" may prematurely end the interaction and increase risks for insufficient information sharing by the nurse and patient frustration with unvoiced or unmet learning needs. The use of open-ended questions keeps the interaction patient focused while allowing for further exploration of patient needs or a natural resolution if concerns have been answered. Although the use of ACTS educational interventions with patients, caregivers, or families can foster health-literate communication, nurses can partner with patients and peers to advocate for a more health-literate organization using ACTS (**Table 1**).[13]

ADVOCACY STRATEGIES USING ACTS
Assess Health Materials and Health Environments

Nurses can advocate for their patients through assessment and selection of suitable health materials for their specific population using identified learning variations and

| Table 1 | | |
| **Education strategies using ACTS** | | |
Intervention	Components	Sample Questions/Nursing Actions
A = Assess	Assess patient main concern	"What is your main concern, as we get ready to talk about your (task, health condition)?"
	Assess patient learning preferences	"What do you know about your health condition?"
		"Everyone has different ways of learning and remembering information. How do you like to learn best?"
	Assess patient values and context	"What do you think is most helpful or most important for you to stay healthy? What keeps you from staying healthy?"
C = Compare	Compare assessment with available resources	Identify and highlight written material, or write down 3 key points to match the patient's concerns and values
		Look for alternative media for patients with sensory alterations, language variations, or technologic proficiencies
T = Teach 3, teach-back	Teach 3 key points using plain language and "chunk and check" Confirm each point for understanding, and reteach if not confirmed	"I want to make sure that I am as clear as possible, so could you share your understanding in your own words" or "Many times, I might go over information really quickly. To make sure I haven't gone too fast, what were 3 important points we talked about?" or "What 3 points will you tell/show your family/significant others about your health condition when you get home?"
S = Survey	Survey for additional questions or concerns	"What other questions or concerns do you have?"

information needs. There may be significant discrepancies, however, between the intents, goals, and perspectives of health information developers, health information providers such as nurses, and the patient population for the desired health information. More than 300 studies have documented significant and ongoing gaps between the reading levels necessary to comprehend most health materials and the reading abilities of the intended audience.[14] Nurses, patients, or other health providers may be minimally involved in the creation or evaluation of health materials, adding to this gap. Developers of health materials may not realize that health information resources are distributed with little additional explanation or confirmation of patient understanding by providers. Most health information available is commercially produced for broad distribution or to meet health system information goals and legal requirements. Nurses may assume that their patients can read and understand complex health information, as seen in discharges focused on getting signatures on the necessary forms and handing out additional reading materials and then stating, "Here, read this information when you get home." Even when simplified or language-specific materials are given, there is no guarantee that someone can read or be able to follow written discharge instructions, despite their verbal fluency or compliant demeanor.

To overcome these assumptions, nurses can use patient education suitability instruments such as the Suitability Assessment of Materials (SAM)[29,30] or Patient

Educational Material Assessment Tool (PEMAT)[30] to gain greater knowledge of material content and context. Assessing the large amount of materials available may appear daunting but is doable if small amounts of materials are evaluated on a regular basis. Nurses may pregroup written materials or online media sites according to very low (2nd grade or less, sensory or language variations), limited (3rd–5th grade), or average (8th grade or higher) suitability levels to more closely match identified patient preferences and abilities. Nurses can then use categorized resources to target patient-identified preferences and values specific to their population. If this process is carried out over time starting with the most frequently used information, benefits may include potential cost savings and reductions of nursing time and effort because of better alignment of patient learning needs with existing resources.

Nurses can also be active participants in assessing their surroundings for user friendliness and accessibility. Most health environments are built with health provider convenience as a priority, and providers may have "expert blind spots" about confusing or difficult-to-understand signs, directions, or physical landmarks.[14] The *Health Literacy Universal Precautions Toolkit* created by Agency for Healthcare Research and Quality [23] contains modules to foster health team member buy-in for the evaluation process and self-assessments to identify strengths and areas for adjustments. Assessment results can then be used as the basis to plan improvements and to invite participation in partnerships to ensure that patient and health care system needs are adequately met.

Collaborate with Patients and Peers

Nurses in collaboration with patients and other peers can work to improve patient education materials. Patients or caregivers who actively participate with nurses in reviewing or modifying patient educational materials may identify information that is more readable, relevant, and actionable.[31] The expertise of language interpreters, medical librarians, social workers, lawyers, or adult educators may also be sought for material analysis or in locating additional resources. Ultimately, these partnerships may also support health system and national goals of having more engaged and health-literate communities or consumers if assessment results are included in health system improvements.[32]

Train with Peers to Implement Health Literacy Competencies

Training all health care team members to use evidence-based health literacy competencies is essential if patient, health system, and national health outcomes are to be achieved. Health provider preprofessional training in plain language, teach-back techniques, tailoring materials, or other health literacy competencies may be minimal or inconsistent across disciplines and insufficient for clinical practice without additional reinforcement.[14,33,34] These deficiencies can be alleviated through regular and standardized training opportunities for all members of health care organizations. Health literacy competencies may require the teaching and reinforcing health provider knowledge, skills and attitudes, and related attributes from health institutions beyond textual modification alone.[11,33] A recent consensus study has proposed health literacy educational competencies and health literacy–related practices for health professionals.[34] When interdisciplinary team members learn and apply health literacy knowledge, skills, and attitudes together, opportunities exist to build stronger team partnerships and gain benefits from sharing information about differing health roles, challenges, and perspectives.

Survey Evidence to Maintain Standards

Routine surveillance of health literacy evidence should be part of health organizational efforts to support patient care safety standards. According to Joint Commission statistics, approximately 60% of all sentinel events can be traced back to communication errors.[35] The Joint Commission added patient- and family-centered communication in 2010 as a National Patient Safety Goal to address these constraints by improving existing communication and cultural competency practices of health facilities. The Commission provided a Roadmap to guide expectations for health system communication competencies when caring for patients with limited English proficiency or with sensory and language variations consistent with the Federal Title VI requirements.[35] Nurses who are involved in health system evaluation and quality improvements may lead organizational changes to meet or exceed Joint Commission accreditation standards and professional benchmarks outlined in the National Action Plan to Improve Health Literacy (**Table 2**).[36]

Table 2
Advocacy strategies using ACTS

Intervention	Components	Nursing Advocacy Actions
A = Assess health materials and environments for user friendliness	Use of readability, suitability instruments with scoring, categorized for future reference Agency for Healthcare Research and Quality Health Literacy Precautions Toolkit	Individual and group evaluation of health material suitability, targeted to population served Health environment assessment using health system evaluation tools
C = Collaborate with patients and peers to advocate for change	Patient and peer input regarding available health materials and health environments	Interviews Focus groups Peer and patient task forces to foster patient-centered environment
T = Teach and practice health literacy competencies	Peer practice to build health literacy competencies and teamwork opportunities	Develop and participate in interdisciplinary continuing education
S = Survey health systems for ongoing integration of evidence	Planned review and analysis of health system environment use of health literacy practices Joint Commission A Roadmap for Hospitals: Advancing Effective Communication, Cultural Competence and Patient- and Family-Centered Care	Participate in review of standards and evidence for accreditation and outcomes

EVALUATION

The National Health Literacy Action Plan details 7 overarching goals to evaluate health literacy clinical practices and guide health literacy research.[36] Support for health information accessibility and usability should occur in all contexts (goal 1), within US health care systems (goal 2) and throughout one's educational path (goal 3). Communities should be empowered to provide health information in nontraditional health settings, such as adult learning programs (goal 4) with the development of broader community-based partnerships (goal 5). Ongoing health literacy research (goal 6) and implementation of evidence-based health literacy practices (goal 7) would continue to refine and improve outcomes for individuals, communities, and health systems to reduce economic, physical, and emotional costs associated with limited health literacy. The assumptions of improvement in the Action Plan or Joint Commission communication standards may not be fully realized without support across the multiple health environments. There are no defined economic, social, or political incentives to implement the Health Literacy Action Plan or Joint Commission patient communication standards, and no timeline or clear benchmarks to evaluate the recommendations or effectiveness if met. Without further research and ongoing health system action, improvements may be minimal or short lived.

SUMMARY

A Universal health literacy precautions approach has been recommended as part of the Health Literacy Action Plan to limit medical errors or harm and enhance communication improvements for a more "health literate society."[2,36] Universal health literacy precautions such as plain language, teach-back, and highlighting or pointing out need-to-know knowledge should be implemented across all health environments by health literacy–proficient providers, actively engaged patients, and involved communities of interest. Nurses are the largest group of health care providers in the United States, and are poised through their daily interactions and relationships with patients, families, and health care systems to push for and integrate universal health literacy precautions.[35,36] Patients of all literacy levels may have difficulty understanding routine health information or instructions because of the innate complexity of medical language, unfamiliar health knowledge concepts, technology barriers, and health care system intricacies.[14,20] Overemphasizing functional literacy skills for assessments or interventions may inadvertently stigmatize those with lower literacy levels[16] or neglect the health information needs of patients with adequate literacy or varying cultural or language backgrounds.[7] Nurses can address these patient barriers to essential health knowledge through support for stronger patient and health system collaborations. When front-line nurses consistently use health literacy ACTS, transformations can occur as the foundation for more effective patient-nurse communication practices.

REFERENCES

1. Sloan R. Life after tragedy. Clarksville (TN): The Leaf Chronicle; 2014. p. A1.
2. Paasche-Orlow MK, Schillinger D, Greene S, et al. How health care systems can begin to address the challenge of limited literacy. J Gen Intern Med 2006;21: 884–7. http://dx.doi.org/10.1111/j.1525-1497.2006.00544.x.
3. Baker DW, Parker RM, Williams MV, et al. The relationship of patient reading ability to self-reported health and use of health services. Am J Public Health 1997;87: 1027–30.
4. Berkman ND, Sheridan SL, Donahue EE, et al. Health literacy interventions and outcomes: an updated systematic review (Evidence Report/Technology Assessment No. 199, Pub No 11–E006). 2011. Available at: http://www.ahrq.gov/downloads/pub/evidence/pdf/literacy/literacyup.pdf. Accessed September 27, 2012 from Agency for Healthcare Research and Quality website.
5. Sudore RL, Yaffe K, Satterfield S, et al. Limited literacy and mortality in the elderly: the Healthy Aging and Body Composition study. J Gen Intern Med 2006;21: 806–12. http://dx.doi.org/10.1111/j.1525-1497.2006.00539.x.

6. Kutner M, Greenberg E, Jin Y, et al. The health literacy of America's adults: results from the 2003 National Assessment of Adult Literacy (NCES 2006 483). Washington, DC: U.S. Department of Education; 2006.

7. Andrulis DP, Brach C. Integrating literacy, culture and language to improve health care quality in diverse populations. Am J Health Behav 2007;31:S122–33.

8. Lemer C, Bates DW, Yoon C, et al. The role of advice in medication errors in the pediatric ambulatory setting. J Patient Saf 2009;5:168–73. http://dx.doi.org/10.1097/PTS.0b013e3181b3a9b0.

9. Castro CM, Wilson C, Wang F, et al. Babel babble: physician's use of unclarified medical jargon. Am J Health Behav 2007;31:S85–95.

10. Schillinger D, Piette J, Grumbach K, et al. Closing the loop: physician communication with diabetic patients who have low health literacy. Arch Intern Med 2003; 163(1):83–90.

11. Nielsen-Bohlman L, Panzer AM, Kindig DA, editors. Health literacy: a prescription to end confusion. Washington, DC: National Academies Press; 2004.

12. Barry M, D'Eath M, Sixsmith J. Interventions for improving population health literacy: insights from a rapid review of the evidence. J Health Commun 2013; 18:1507–22.

13. Brach C, Dreyer B, Schyve P, et al. Attributes of a health literate organization. Discussion paper - working group, institute of medicine. 2012. Available at: http://ww.facesandvoicesofrecovery.org/pdf/eNews/Attributes_of_a_Health_Literate_Organization.pdf. Accessed August 1, 2014.

14. Rudd RE, Keller DB. Health literacy: new directions and research. J Commun Healthc 2009;2:240–8.

15. Seligman HK, Wang FF, Palacio JL, et al. Physician notification of their diabetes patients' limited literacy results: a randomized control trial. J Gen Intern Med 2005;20:1001–7. http://dx.doi.org/10.1111/j.1525-1497.2005.0189.x.

16. Paasche-Orlow MK, Wolf MS. Evidence does not support clinical screening of literacy. J Gen Intern Med 2007;23:100–2. http://dx.doi.org/10.1107/s11606-00700447-2.

17. Bass PJ, Wilson JF, Griffith CH, et al. Resident's ability to identify patients with poor literacy skills. Acad Med 2002;77:1039–41.

18. Turner T, Cull WL, Bayldon B, et al. Pediatricians and health literacy: descriptive results from a national survey. Pediatrics 2009;124:S299–305. http://dx.doi.org/10.1542/peds.2009-1162F.

19. Dickens C, Lambert BL, Cromwell T, et al. Nurse's overestimation of patients' health literacy. J Health Commun 2013;18(Suppl 1):62–9. http://dx.doi.org/10.1080/10810730.2013.825670.

20. Nutbeam D. The evolving concept of health literacy. Soc Sci Med 2008;67: 2072–8.

21. Schwartzenberg JG, Cowett A, VanGeest J, et al. Communication techniques for patients with low health literacy: a survey of physicians, nurses and pharmacists. Am J Health Behav 2007;31:S96–104.

22. Wilson F, Brown DL, Stephens-Ferris M. Can easy-to-read immunization information increase knowledge in urban low-income mothers? J Pediatr Nurs 2006; 21(1):4–12.

23. Zarcadoolas C, Pleasant A, Greer D. Understanding health literacy: an expanded model. Health Promot Int 2005;30(2):195–203. http://dx.doi.org/10.1093/heapro/dah609.

24. Cynosure Health. VA Palo Alto Project RED Mental Health.mp4. 2012. Available at: http://www.youtube.com/watch?v=IWMIFAkBnM8. Accessed August 1, 2014.

25. VAPAHCSvideo. VA Palo Alto Project RED - medical and surgical wards. 2012. Available at: http://www.youtube.com/watch?v=osPwH7gYEU4. Accessed August 1, 2014.

26. VAPAHCSvideo. VA Palo Alto Project RED – Emergency Department. 2012. Available at: http://www.youtube.com/watch?v=GaBxM3BZ3dY. Accessed August 1, 2014.

27. White M, Garbez R, Carroll M, et al. Is "teach-back" associated with knowledge retention and hospital readmission in hospitalized heart failure patients? J Cardiovasc Nurs 2013;28(2):137–46. http://dx.doi.org/10.1097/JCN.0b013e31824987bd.

28. Kornburger C, Gibson C, Sadowski S, et al. Using "teach-back" to promote a safe transition from hospital to home: an evidence-based approach to improving the discharge process. J Pediatr Nurs 2013;28(3):282–91. http://dx.doi.org/10.1016/j.pedn.2012.10.007.

29. Doak CC, Doak LG, Root JH. Teaching patients with low literacy skills. 2nd edition. Philadelphia: J.B. Lippincott; 1996.

30. The patient education materials assessment tool (PEMAT) and user's guide: an instrument to assess the understandability and actionability of print and audiovisual patient education materials. Rockville (MD): Agency for Healthcare Research and Quality; 2013. Available at: http://www.ahrq.gov/professionals/prevention-chronic-care/improve/self-mgmt/pemat/index.html. Accessed August 1, 2014.

31. Nilsen ES, Myrhaug HT, Johansen M, et al. Methods of consumer involvement in developing healthcare policy and research, clinical practice guidelines and patient information material. Cochrane Database Syst Rev 2006;(3):CD004563. http://dx.doi.org/10.1002/14651858.CD004563.pub2.

32. Agency for Healthcare Research and Quality [AHRQ]. Health literacy universal precautions toolkit (AHRQ publications No. 10-0046-EF). Rockville (MD): Department of Health and Human Services (DHHS); 2010.

33. Coleman C. Teaching health care professionals about health literacy: a review of the literature. Nurs Outlook 2011;59:70–8. http://dx.doi.org/10.1016/j.outlook.2010.12.004.

34. Coleman C, Hudson S, Maine LL. Health literacy practices and educational competencies for health professionals: a consensus study. J Health Commun 2013;18(Suppl 1):81–102. http://dx.doi.org/10.1080/10810730.2013.839538.

35. The Joint Commission. Advancing effective communication, cultural competence, and patient- and family-centered care: a roadmap for hospitals. Oakbrook Terrace (IL): The Joint Commission; 2010.

36. U.S. Department of Health and Human Services (DHHS), Office of Disease Prevention and Health Promotion (ODPHP). National action plan to improve health literacy. Washington, DC: Author; 2010.

Cultural Competent Patient-Centered Nursing Care

Linda K. Darnell, MSN, RN,
Shondell V. Hickson, DNP, APN, ACNS-BC, FNP-BC*

KEYWORDS

- Cultural diversity • Cultural competence • Theoretic framework • Ethics
- Cultural tool kits • Cultural assessment • Patient-centered care

KEY POINTS

- Health care has a multicultural environment.
- Behaviors, biases, and attitudes of Health care providers contribute to health care disparities, patient dissatisfaction, and poor patient outcomes.
- Cultural competence is when health care professionals strive to work effectively within the cultural context of an individual, family, and community.
- Cultural diversity is awareness of the presence of differences among patients.
- Patient-centered care is successful when both the nurse and the patient mutually agree to health care needs, knowledge, and experiences.
- The front-line nurse needs to implement cultural awareness, cultural knowledge, cultural skill, and cultural encounter to develop cultural competent care.
- Embracing ethics empowers mutual respect, equality, and trust.
- The National League for Nursing and the Association of Colleges of Nursing provide cultural diversity tool kits for educational resources.
- Becoming a culturally competent front-line nurse meets the challenge to provide patient-centered care for culturally diverse patients, promotes patient satisfaction, and improves health outcomes.

INTRODUCTION

The United States is a melting pot that consists of multiple races, ethnicities, sexual orientations, immigrants, refugees, and patients with disabilities. These changes in the ethnic and cultural composition of the United States population challenges nurses daily to incorporate the diverse needs of their patients into the provision of quality

Disclosure Statement: The authors have nothing to disclose.
School of Nursing, Austin Peay State University, PO Box 4658, McCord 353D, Clarksville, TN 37044, USA
* Corresponding author.
E-mail address: hicksons@apsu.edu

Nurs Clin N Am 50 (2015) 99–108
http://dx.doi.org/10.1016/j.cnur.2014.10.008
0029-6465/15/$ – see front matter © 2015 Elsevier Inc. All rights reserved.

nursing care while facing a shortage of adequate qualified staff to meet these needs.[1] The US Census projects that the minority populations will become the majority by 2042; therefore, professional nurses must demonstrate sensitivity in understanding a variety of cultures to provide optimum and quality care in multiple settings.[2] The composition of the nation's 2.7 million Registered Nurses who provide care in today's health care system consists of 87% Caucasians, 5% African Americans, 4% Asian/Pacific, 2% Hispanics, and 0.5% American.[3] For the current health care staff to meet the demands expected when providing health care services, it is imperative that the nursing staff is culturally competent to meet the needs of a culturally diverse nation while providing culturally appropriate care that will translate into effective outcomes. **Fig. 1** summarizes the United States ethnicities in 2012, demonstrating a need for diverse and culturally competent nurses.

DEFINING CULTURAL COMPETENCE AND CULTURAL DIVERSITY

Cultural competence is when health care professionals strive to work effectively within the cultural context of an individual, family, and community.[4,5] It is the explicit use of culturally based care and health knowledge in a sensitive, creative, and meaningful way to fit the general way of life and needs of individual or groups for their health care needs.[6] Cultural diversity is the awareness of the presence of differences among members of a social group or units.[7] Culture influences patients' perceptions of their health and the methods they pursue to maintain and restore their health.[8] The behaviors, biases, and attitudes of health care providers contribute to health care disparities that are prominent in minority populations and poorer communities. The goal of implementing culturally competent care and recognizing diversity is to reduce health care disparities and remove barriers that may prevent patients from getting well. The

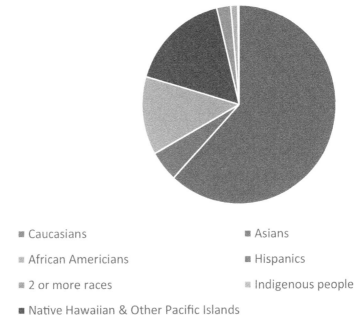

■ Caucasians   ■ Asians

■ African Americans   ■ Hispanics

■ 2 or more races   ■ Indigenous people

■ Native Hawaiian & Other Pacific Islands

Fig. 1. Ethnicities in the United States, 2012. (*Data from* American Association of College of Nurses. Fact sheet: enhancing diversity in the nursing workforce. 2014. Available at: http://www.aacn.nche.edu/media-relations/diversityFS.pdf. Accessed June 10, 2014.)

challenge for the nursing staff is to become knowledgable about diverse cultures and to bring about greater cultural sensitivity and competency while working within the health care system.[9]

THEORETIC FRAMEWORK FOR PRACTICE

The development of the cultural care diversity and universality (CCDU) theory by Madeleine Leininger has gained her the title of the mother of transcultural nursing (TCN). Leininger emphasized that the nurse need not only be a mediator but also knowledgable about clients' culture and diverse factors influencing their needs and ways of life.[10] She depicted the CCDU as a growing body of knowledge for nurses to use and provide proper care for culturally diverse clients. Leininger also implemented the sunrise model, which considers factors such as technological, religious and philosophic, kinship and social, cultural values and ways of life, political and legal, economic, and educational, each forming "sunrays." Each of these dimensions (sunrays) reflects the influences of culturally diverse clients, their families, community, and institutions. Research supports the idea that if attention to diversity is neglected, it can affect the health of patients and the overall quality of health care, which can contribute to an increase in health disparities.[1,11]

MAKING THE CONNECTION WITH THE CULTURALLY DIVERSE PATIENT

The goal of the Transcultural Nursing Society (TNS) is to enhance the quality of culturally congruent, competent, and equitable care that results in improved health and well-being for people worldwide.[10,12] The TNS has promoted the 8 transcultural nursing standards based on Leininger's theory of CCDU. These standards include theoretic foundations of TCN, cultural information gathering, caring and healing systems, cultural health patterns, and caring practices. The Standards for Transcultural Nursing were developed to foster excellence in transcultural nursing practice, provide criteria for the evaluation of transcultural nursing, create a tool for teaching and learning, increase the public's confidence in the nursing profession, and advance transcultural nursing.[13,14] It is important to collaborate with the patient, family members, other health care professionals, healers, and community resources during all phases of this assessment process.[5] The treatment plan is successful when both the nurse and the patient mutually agree to health care needs, knowledge, and experiences. The treatment is unsuccessful if the nurse ignores or contradicts the patient's background, resulting in the patient refusing care or failing to follow prescribed therapy.[15]

Scenario 1: Encountering an Ethnically Diverse Patient

A nurse working at a local hospital on a medical surgical floor was assigned a female patient of Arabic descent. The nurse knocked on the room door and entered the room; she noticed that the patient was alone in the room lying in bed wearing her customary head gear and a hospital gown. The nurse introduced herself and informed the patient that she would perform an assessment and administer scheduled medications. The patient had a language and cultural barrier, and her response was that she was not comfortable taking my medications without her husband being present. The patient further stated, "I'll call you about my medications once my husband gets back." The nurse recognized that the goal in providing culturally competent care is not to change patients or their beliefs but to teach the patients to make educated and safe decisions about their health care. Traditional Arab patients have strict rules regarding the treatment of female patients. Traditional Arab female patients may be accompanied by a male relative, and may not be able or willing to remove certain clothing items when this is necessary for treatment.[16]

DEVELOPING CULTURAL COMPETENCE

Front-line nurses are often challenged to provide physical, holistic, and cost-efficient health care for all cultural populations. The Institute of Health Care Medicine[17] recommends patient-centered care that is respectful of and responsive to individual patient preferences, needs, and values. The need for culturally competent health care providers and organizations is currently well recognized among accrediting and regulatory organizations.[18] Standards of practice for culturally competent nursing care should be refined for all areas of practice, including social justice, critical reflection, TCN knowledge, cross-cultural practice, health care systems and organizations, patient advocacy and empowerment, multicultural workforces, education and training, cross-cultural communication, cross-cultural leadership, policy development, and educational practice and research.[12,14] The front-line nurse needs to implement 4 main components of a person's culture while providing cultural competent care: cultural awareness, cultural knowledge, cultural skill, and cultural encounter.[19] Cultural awareness is a conscious learning of cultural barriers that allows for cultural sensitivity to promote cultural competence and patient-centered care.[20] Cultural knowledge involves understanding major aspects of a culture in relation to aspects of health care practice such as illnesses, health, healing, and nutrition.[19] Cultural skills are the ability to assess and collect cultural information that reduces health care disparities and improves patient satisfaction.[19] Cultural encounter is the direct cross-cultural interaction between people from various diverse backgrounds.[19] **Table 1** summarizes the 4 components needed to provide cultural competent care.

RESPECTING CULTURAL DIVERSITY

As more cultures seek access to health care resources, nurses will be the ones responsible for understanding, facilitating, and integrating traditional culture into modern approaches to health and nursing care.[21] One size does not fit all cultural nursing care for today's front-line nurse. Respecting diversity is essential in health care, and involves the health care provider incorporating the patient's race, ethnicity, culture, life experiences, and religion into the plan of care. Cultural diversity implementations involve the integration of cultural desire, cultural awareness, cultural knowledge, cultural skill, and cultural encounters.[4,13] It is also essential for health care providers to determine whether they comprehend the patient's cultural needs so as to remove any barriers that may affect the patient's outcome. Both the nurse and the client should acknowledge what they find to be different rather than what they find similar in their understanding of the health care needs of the patient, family, and community.

Table 1 Developing cultural competence	
Cultural awareness	Identify one's own cultural background, values, and beliefs, especially in relation to health and health care
Cultural knowledge	Learning the basic general information about predominant culture groups in one's geographic area. Cultural pocket guides can be a good resource
Cultural skill	Be alert for unexpected responses with patients, especially in relation to cultural issues
Cultural encounter	Create opportunities to interact with predominant cultural groups

Data from Lewis SM, Heitkemper M, Dirksen S, et al. Medical-surgical nursing: assessment and management of clinical problems. 7th edition. St Louis (MO): Mosby Elsevier; 2007.

Patients must become involved with their care and work toward following what the nurses recommend for recovery and health maintenance. Finally, the nurse works to negotiate a treatment plan, recognizing that it may be beneficial to incorporate selected aspects of the patient's culture into the patient-centered plan.[5,22]

Scenario 2: Respecting Cultural Diversity

An Advance Practice Nurse (APN) working at a local community clinic often encounters patients who are culturally diverse. This APN, however, has never encountered female patients with genital mutilation. A female Ethiopian patient presented for a well-woman physical that includes a breast examination and a Papanicolaou (Pap) examination. While completing the Pap examination, the APN was astonished to witness genital mutilation. Her first response was to wonder why it is performed and perpetuated, and what values it signifies and sustains. She shared her concerns with the patient who viewed it as a normal aspect of childhood, like a rite of passage. As the APN wrapped up the visit, the patient enquired whether she could bring her daughter to the clinic for the APN to perform the genital circumcision. The APN carefully separated her feelings about the female genital mutilation that may have offended the patient, inhibited further medical care, and impaired the trust and rapport necessary to discuss health issues and the potential harms of continuing the practice. The APN informed the patient that this practice is not done in the United States, and of the complications associated with the practice. The APN also spent time in understanding the patient's culture and the impact genital circumcision may have on the daughter's life. The APN considered that she provided the patient with adequate information and did not offend her.

CODE OF ETHICS AND THE CULTURALLY DIVERSE PATIENT

Morals and ethics are a branch of philosophy. Ethics seeks to provide answers to some of the questions of human conduct that arise in life, and attempts to determine what is right or wrong.[23,24] Application of ethics in the profession of nursing resulted in the development of bioethics. Difficult issues that arise in health care and professional nursing are addressed in ethical values that are based on the nurse's perspective of patient care skills. The principle-based approach to ethics combines elements of both utilitarian and deontology theories, and offers specific guides to action for practice.[15] Four primary principles are identified by Beauchamp and Childress[23] as bioethics approaches: autonomy, nonmaleficence, beneficence, and justice. Many nurses add fidelity, veracity, accountability, privacy, and confidentiality to this list because they play a central role in the tradition of nursing (and medical) ethics and guide the behavior of health care professionals toward patients and their families.[15] The first term, autonomy, depicts a person's right to make an independent decision that affects his or her course of action. Respect for another's autonomy is fundamental to the practice of health care.[24] Through autonomy, patients have a right to make decisions about their health care. The nurse needs to support patients' decisions and choices without overstepping cultural boundaries. The second term, nonmaleficence, refers to doing no harm. The nurse needs to prevent harm or risk to the patient under their care. The ethical mandate is that as nurses we refrain from intentionally inflicting harm.[22] The third term, beneficence, is the obligation to do well, not harm, to other people. In today's health care system we understand that on occasion we unintentionally do harm to patients in the name of care, such as via the side effects of some treatments and medications. Even more problematic is the continued use of medical therapies when they are futile; that is, they do not have the potential for creating a positive outcome but clearly hold potential for adverse outcomes.[22,23] The fourth term, justice, sometimes referred to as fairness, refers to the obligation to treat like cases similarly.[22] Limited resources should be distributed equally relative to demand, meaning that this may involve recognizing subtle instances of bias and discrimination.[15] Finally, fidelity refers to keeping obligations, agreements, commitments, and responsibilities that nurses have made to their selves, the patients, their families, and the communities. Interestingly it is one of the ethical concepts not addressed specifically in some textbooks of nursing ethics.[22] Patients who are entrusted to the nurses' care cannot be abandoned and their needs must always be provided for. Nurses must be faithful to the promise they made to the public to be competent and be willing to use this competence to benefit the patients entrusted to their care.[15]

INTEGRATING CULTURAL DIVERSITY USING THE NATIONAL LEAGUE FOR NURSING AND AMERICAN ASSOCIATION OF COLLEGES OF NURSING TOOL KITS

Current information, easy access, reasoning, and direction for application provide the front-line nurse with methods of nursing care and information for applying skills and techniques in patient-centered care settings. Locating and using these elements in building a set of tools to best provide care at the bedside is the responsibility of today's nursing workforce. Development and utilization of best practices through research and application of the tools learned initially from the kit should be incorporated and evaluated continuously in front-line nursing. In imaging a tool kit, we see a type of box or container in which users store their individual tools or sets of tools they work with on the job. Each tool kit has tools that are new, old, revised, or sharpened constantly, be they individual tools or sets. Just as the National League for Nursing (NLN) and the American Association of Colleges of Nursing (AACN) recognize the need to continue revising and restoring a tool kit, the front-line nurse needs to do the same.

Two prestigious organizations in nursing guidelines and standards, NLN and the AACN, have established tool kits for practice in cultural diversity competencies. The NLN Think Tank on Diversity recommended the development of a tool kit to support administrators and faculty in schools of nursing endeavoring to expand diversity at their institution.[24] The resources in the Diversity Tool Kit come from many disciplines, in addition to higher education nursing education and other groups of health care professionals. The tool kit identifies that quality, safety, and diversity are woven together to provide culturally competent care, and is composed of assumptions, resources, and suggested questions recommended for review. As noted by the American Testing Institute, cultural competence means that nurses understand and address the entire cultural context of each client within the realm of the care they deliver.[25] The AACN provides 6 core graduate cultural competencies for the preparation of the Master's and the doctoral nursing workforce[2]: to prioritize the social and cultural factors that affect health in designing and delivering care across multiple contexts; to construct socially and empirically derived cultural knowledge of people and populations to guide practice and research; to assume leadership in developing, implementing, and evaluating culturally competent nursing and other health care services; to transform systems to address social justice and health disparities; to provide leadership to educators and members of the health care research team in learning, applying, and evaluating continuous cultural competence development; and to conduct culturally competent scholarship that can be used in practice. Nevertheless, competence varies according to standards of practice, different philosophies, and changes over time.[21]

The nursing workforce will need to build on competencies such as the AACN has provided. The AACN has published the Tool Kit of Resources for Cultural Competent

Education for Baccalaureate Nurses, and a cultural diversity tool kit for all levels of nursing. Focusing the tools on the baccalaureate nurse (BSN) is an essential strategy because they will most likely fill most of the front-line nurse positions. Access to the cultural competence education tools is beneficial to both generic graduate and seasoned nurses. Current information, easy access, reasoning, and direction for application will provide the front-line nurse with methods of nursing care and information for application of skills and techniques in patient-centered care settings. Locating and using the tool kit to provide care at the bedside is the responsibility of today's nursing workforce. Development and utilization of best practices through research and application of the tools learned initially from the kit should be incorporated and evaluated continuously on the front line of nursing.

ASSESSMENT OF THE CULTURALLY DIVERSE PATIENT

Berlin and Fowkes[26] designed steps to assess the needs of the culturally diverse patient, recommending that nurses need to listen with regard to whether a patient is from a diverse background or not when providing front-line care. Nurses also should explain what they understand and what they do not with reference to the cultural needs and barriers in health care. Both the nurse and the client must acknowledge what they find to be different, rather than what they find similar, in their understanding of the health care needs of the patient, family, and community. Patients must become involved with their care, and work toward following what the nurse recommends for a patient's recovery and health maintenance.

The mnemonic tool ETHNIC coined by Levine,[27] which means *E*xplanation, *T*reatment, *H*ealers, *N*egotiate, *I*ntervention, and *C*ollaboration, is useful for recollecting the cultural assessment guide. The nurse initiates the assessment by allowing the patient to give an explanation of what they believe is their problem. When the patient is hesitant about explaining problems, the nurse can ask about concerns regarding the problem. Nurses should investigate what has been done by patients to treat their problem before seeking health care. The front-line nurse must determine if the patient has sought other means of a cure or control. Next, the nurse determines whether the patient has sought advice from alternative health practitioners, folk healers, friends, or other individuals who are not health care professionals.[5] The nurse and patient need to negotiate on health care options that can be mutually beneficial to both parties in addition to families and communities. Both nurse and patient need to reach agreement on an intervention that may combine traditional and/or nontraditional health care. It is important to collaborate with the patient, family members, other health care professionals, healers, and community resources during all phases of this assessment process.[5]

To have a successful assessment, both the nurse and the patient should be mutually corresponding and approachable to health care needs, knowledge, and experiences. Successful culturally diverse nursing begins with the awareness of patient's needs and the front-line nurse's obligation to recognize the differences and similarities in health care. Once the diverse needs are noted, an application of current nursing care and skills must be applied by both the care provider and the patient. At this point, knowledge will be incorporated into the plan of care. To achieve a return to patients' health and recovery, the front-line nurse, patient, family, other health care providers, and community will need to reach acceptance of all viewpoints and considerations. Participants must yield to differences in cultural care and find ways to adopt the changes to meet the challenges of patient-centered care. A very important aspect of TCN actions will be the attitude presented by all concerned.[5] No resentment or resistance must be

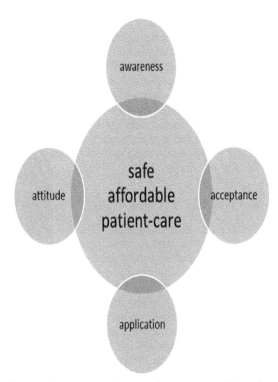

Fig. 2. Quick guide to patient-centered cultural assessment. (*Data from* Cultural competence practice experience of author L.K. Darnell.)

demonstrated or expressed by either participant. **Fig. 2** is a quick guide to patient-
centered cultural assessment for front-line nurses.

Respect for one's differences is reflective of attitude when addressing culturally
diverse health care. Successful cultural nursing care can be rewarding when the 4
A's (awareness, application, acceptance, attitude) are recognized and used in
sequence. Safe, accountable, and quality patient care can be established when recalling the 4 simple needs of the patient and the front-line nurse. According to Taylor and
colleagues,[15] the nurse who recognizes and respects cultural diversity will be better
equipped to exhibit cultural sensitivity and to provide nursing care that accepts the
significance of cultural factors in health and illness.

SUMMARY

Information technologies for today's professional nurses are just a fingertip away. That
being said, the tools needed for culturally diverse patient care should be ones that are
memorable, quickly accessed, and easily recalled. The education department within
the institution needs to develop and integrate cultural diversity awareness programs
so that staff can recognize and demonstrate effective cross-cultural care. It has
been demonstrated that patients feel comfortable and willing to share their cultural
knowledge and values when staff integrate their culture into the plan of care. Providing
culturally competent care does not imply that the nurse should change their beliefs but
rather merge 2 different perspectives for the benefit of optimum patient outcomes. The
nurse must consider both knowledge of self and the patient's culture to fully

comprehend any existing differences. If the nurse is unsure about the patient's background, it is important to inquire rather than stereotype. Although facial expression of shock and anger are difficult to avoid, showing mutual respect for the patient's culture and removing ethnocentrism or imposition will foster a relationship of trust. Patients trust providers who act unselfishly, put patients' interests above their own, and possess the technical competence necessary for proper diagnosis and treatment, at an acceptable cost. Being a culturally diverse health care provider is an excellent asset for any organization, promoting patient satisfaction and improving health outcomes.

REFERENCES

1. Lowe J, Archibald C. Cultural diversity: the intention of nursing. Nurs Forum 2009; 44(1):11–8. http://dx.doi.org/10.1111/j.1744-6198.2009.00122.x.
2. American Association of College of Nurses. Fact sheet: enhancing diversity in the nursing workforce. 2014. Available at: http://www.aacn.nche.edu/media-relations/diversityFS.pdf. Accessed August 2, 2014.
3. U.S Department of Health and Human Services. Implementation guidance on data collection standards for race, ethnicity, sex, primary language, and disability status. 2008. Available at: http://aspe.hhs.gov/datacncl/standards/aca/4302/index.pdf. Accessed August 2, 2014.
4. Campinha-Bacote J. The process of cultural competence in the delivery of healthcare services: a model of care. J Transcult Nurs 2009;13(3):181–4. http://dx.doi.org/10.1177/10459602013003003.
5. Campinha-Bacote J. Delivering patient-centered care in the midst of a cultural conflict: the role of cultural competence. Online J Issues Nurs 2011;16(2). Available at: http://www.nursingworld.org/MainMenuCategories/ANAMarketplace/ANAPeriodicals/OJIN/TableofContents/Vol-16-2011/No2-May-2011/Delivering-Patient-Centered-Care-in-the-Midst-of-a-Cultural-Conflict.html.
6. Leininger MM. Transcultural nursing: concepts, theories, and practices. New York: McGraw-Hill, College Custom Series; 1995.
7. Spencer-Rodgers J, McGovern T. Attitudes toward the culturally different: the role of intercultural communication barriers, affective responses, consensual stereotypes, and perceived threat. International J Intercultural Relations 2002;26(6): 609–31. http://dx.doi.org/10.1016/S0147-1767(02)00038-X.
8. Perez MA, Luquis RR. Cultural competence in health education and health promotion. San Francisco (CA): Jossey-Bass; 2008.
9. Collins SD. Home. 2006. Available at. http://www.nona.org. Accessed August 31, 2014.
10. Sagar PL. Transcultural nursing theory and models: application in nursing education Practice and administration. New York: Springer; 2012.
11. Gilbert MJ, Puebla-Fortier J. The California endowment. 2001. Available at: http://www.calendow.org/. Accessed August 1, 2014.
12. Craven RF, Hirnle CJ. Fundamentals of nursing: human health and function. 7th edition. Philadelphia: Wolters Kluwer Health/Lippincott Williams & Wilkins; 2009.
13. Andrews MM, Boyle JS. Transcultural concepts in nursing care. 6th edition. Philadelphia: Wolters Kluwer Health/Lippincott Williams & Wilkins; 2008.
14. Douglas MK, Rosenkoetter M, Pacquiao DF, et al. Guidelines for implementing culturally competent nursing. J Transcult Nurs 2014;25(2):101–21. Available at: http://www.tcns.org/TCNStandardsofPractice.html.

15. Taylor CR, Lillis C, LeMone P, et al. Fundamentals of nursing: the art and science of nursing care. 7th edition. Philadelphia: Wolters Kluwer Health/Lippincott Williams & Wilkins; 2011.

16. Rabin C. Respecting Muslim patients Needs. New York Times 2010. Available at: http://www.nytimes.com/2010/11/01/health/01patients.html?_r=0.

17. The future of nursing leading change, advancing health advising the nation/ improving health. 2011. Available at: http://www.iom.edu/~/media/Files/ Report%20Files/2010/The-Future-of-Nursing/Future%20of%20Nursing%202010% 20Recommendations.pdf. Accessed August 1, 2014.

18. Dreachslin JL, Gilbert MJ, Malone B. Diversity and cultural competence in health care: a systems approach. San Francisco (CA): JosseyBass; 2012.

19. Lewis SM, Heitkemper M, Dirksen S, et al. Medical-surgical nursing: assessment and management of clinical problems. 7th edition. St Louis (MO): Mosby Elsevier; 2007.

20. O'Donohue WT, Fisher JE. General principles and empirically supported techniques of cognitive behavior therapy. Hoboken (NJ): John Wiley & Sons; 2009.

21. Ray MA. Transcultural caring dynamics in nursing and health care. Philadelphia: F.A. Davis Co; 2010.

22. Ellis JR, Hartley CL. Nursing in today's world: trends, issues, management. Philadelphia: Wolters Kluwer Health/Lippincott Williams & Wilkins; 2008.

23. Beauchamp TL, Childress JF. Principles of biomedical ethics. New York: Oxford University Press; 2001.

24. National League for Nursing. A commitment to diversity in nursing and nursing education. 2010. Available at: http://www.nln.org/facultyprograms/Diversity_ Toolkit/diversity_toolkit.pdf. Accessed August 1, 2014.

25. Wissman J, Knippa A, Assessment Technologies Institute. Fundamentals for nursing. 8th edition. Overland Park (KS): Assessment Technologies Institute; 2008.

26. Berlin E, Fowkes WA. A teaching framework for cross-cultural health care. West J Med 1983;139:934–8. Available at: http://www.pubmedcentral.nih.gov/picrender. fcgi?artid=1011028&blobtype=pdf.

27. Levin S, Like R, Gottlieb J. ETHNIC: A framework for culturally competent clinical practice. New Brunswick (NJ): Department of Family Medicine, UMDNJ-Robert Wood Johnson Medical School; 2000.

Case Management

Judy Woodward, MSN, RN[a],*, Eve Rice, MSN, PNP[b]

KEYWORDS

- Case management ● Disease management ● Health care quality ● Standards of care

KEY POINTS

- The current health care system is fragmented, and case management will be on the front line of necessary change.
- Case management will be an expanded role in the Affordable Care Act initiatives.
- The discipline of case management has standards of practice and credentialing for practice, and is not restricted to one profession.
- Case management has been proved to affect the outcomes of health care.

INTRODUCTION

The future of health care is at a critical point in the United States. The 2001 Institute of Medicine report *Crossing the Quality Chasm* recommended the need for restructuring our current health care system to bring about improvements in safety, effectiveness, patient-centeredness, timeliness, efficiency, and equity.[1] The report further described our care delivery system as fragmented and frustrating for both clients and providers.[1] We have the opportunity to implement change that can bring more quality to patient care, and therefore increase the quality of the lives of our patients.

As we focus more on the specific outcomes and efficiency of health care, one thing becomes very clear: the renewed interest in case management as a strategy to address fragmentation in health care delivery has put it on the front line.[2,3] Case management has been proved to reduce both the length of stay for clients and emergency department (ED) utilization.[3–7] In one study of the use of community-based nurse care-coordination intervention with 57 Medicare clients, monthly Medicare costs were lowered by $686.[5] In another study with the use of community-based nurse case managers, ED encounters were lowered by 29%, inpatient encounters were lowered by 20%, and overnight inpatient days in hospital were lowered by 37%.[4] In the same study, readmission rates were decreased from 70% to 51% over a 3-year period, and 97% of clients had established a relationship with a primary care provider (PCP).[4] In an integrative review of 18 scholarly articles published between 2000 and

[a] Department of Health, Andrew Johnson Tower, 710 James Robertson Parkway, Nashville, TN 37243, USA; [b] School of Nursing, Austin Peay State University, PO Box 4658, Clarksville, TN 37044, USA
* Corresponding author.
E-mail address: Judy.Woodward@tn.gov

Nurs Clin N Am 50 (2015) 109–121
http://dx.doi.org/10.1016/j.cnur.2014.10.009
0029-6465/15/$ – see front matter © 2015 Elsevier Inc. All rights reserved.

nursing.theclinics.com

2013 on nurse-led community-based case management, Joo and Huber[8] concluded that community-based case management is effective in providing quality, patient-centered care, and stated that these benefits should be communicated to health leaders.

Historically our health care system has been reactive instead of proactive in addressing concerns, but all of this is changing today largely because of the Patient Protection and Affordable Care Act, hereafter referred to as the Affordable Care Act (ACA).[9] Case management will become more integral and crucial as structural changes in health care occur.

Case management is not a new idea. In fact case management has been documented in various forms in the United States from the early 1900s, and has strong roots in community and public health.[10,11] In the 1980s the Prospective Payment System was introduced, and case management became widespread and essential to the entire continuum of health care.[11] The Case Management Society of America (CMSA) was founded in 1990, and established the first Standards of Practice for Case Management in 1995.[12]

DEFINITION OF CASE MANAGEMENT

Case management is not a profession, but a fluid and dynamic practice that involves many disciplines and continues to evolve.[13] In fact, the case for moving case management to the advanced practice role is being explored in the nursing profession.[4,13] Although social workers and other health care professionals can become case managers, most case managers are nurses.[11] It is essential that case managers follow their own Practice Act for their state of residence.[11] CMSA supports all of the different disciplines involved in case management, and does not focus on either nursing or social work. Case management translates very easily to nursing for several reasons. A key concept for the practice of case management is the holistic focus on the individual, and this is a fundamental teaching in the nursing discipline.[11] The CMSA defines case management as "a collaborative process of assessment, planning, facilitation and advocacy for options and services to meet an individual's health needs through communication and available resources to promote quality, cost-effective outcomes."[12(p6)] Nurses will quickly recognize the nursing process in this definition of case management. Case management actually parallels the nursing process, and demonstrated later in this article.[14] The American Nurses Credentialing Center expands the CMSA definition: in addition, the case managers "actively participate with their clients to identify and facilitate options and services, providing and coordinating comprehensive care to meet patient/client health needs, with the goal of decreasing fragmentation and duplication of care, and enhancing quality, cost-effective clinical outcomes."[14(p124)] Many organizations have their own definitions of case management, including the National Association of Social Workers, the American Board for Occupational Health Nurses, and the Association of Rehabilitation Nurses.[11]

CURRENT ISSUES RELATED TO CASE MANAGEMENT
The Affordable Care Act and Case Management

Today the current emphasis on both quality outcomes and efficiency in health care is the platform for the ACA, and several parts of the reform legislation affect case management. Case management has always sought to defragment the health care system for clients, and some new provisions of the ACA give care coordination a very prominent role as the central focus of both the medical home model and Accountable Care Organizations (ACOs).[15] The Department of Health and Human Services

(HHS) will be trying some new models of reimbursement and care delivery to determine how providers can improve care while reducing the costs of health care.[2] One major concern is whether the Center for Medicare and Medicaid services (CMS) and the other stakeholders can work cohesively to bring about a change in processes and outcome-measure patient care models.[9] In 2011, HHS proposed some regulations to ACOs, with 65 quality measures that include care coordination.[2] The primary aim for ACOs is the improvement of health in the population by increasing the engagement of clients in making health care decisions and managing their own care, and improving safety and care coordination.[9] Another initiative by the ACA is through the National Academy for State Health Policy (NASHP) for long-term care services. The NASHP is seeking improvement by promoting service coordination and care coordination for this population.[16]

Case management can be a key player in these new measures because they have multiple care-coordination requirements including client preparation for care transition.[2] ACOs will have to meet certain requirements to prove patient-centeredness in care, including a mechanism for the improved coordination of care, which can translate into increased use of case management. For the Medicare community-based care transitions program, facilities that have high readmission rates will be targeted and have financial fines.[2] One hope is that instead of just levying fines to ACOs for 30-day readmissions, strong ACO performance standards can earn financial rewards or incentives.[9] The discharge process will need to be more carefully developed and will need more specific criteria for anticipating and preventing readmission.[9] This approach opens a huge gap in service that can be managed by case managers with extended responsibilities. One tool that is familiar to case managers is predictive modeling (PM), used to help determine which clients are at high risk for hospital admission.[9] PM has long been used by case managers to identify clients who could incur increased medical cost, and therefore need intervention and coordination of care. Now the PM industry is discovering that there are other issues that may be even more significant in predicting readmissions,[9] including clients' own perceptions of their health, functional status, and self-care. Case managers play a unique role in assessing these perceptions because of the relationship they have with clients and their extensive knowledge of the holistic process of client care.[9,14]

The reader should be aware that in the following information on ACA initiatives, case managers are sometimes called by different names, including care coordinators, navigators, discharge planners, and disease managers.[2] Another change proposed by the CMS is to pay physicians for more complex care services starting in 2015.[15] Billable services will include reviewing care plans with the client and arranging community resources. This development will be a growth opportunity for some physicians, who are more used to a plan of care that is medically based instead of the case management "action" plan.[17] The case manager may find himself or herself in the position of educator and coach for the physician who may not be familiar with the essential care-coordination functions.[15] **Table 1** summarizes some of the ACA Care Coordination Initiatives that will affect case management.

Healthy People 2020 and Case Management

One of the overarching goals of Healthy People 2020 is the improvement of "access to comprehensive, quality health care services."[18] This goal seeks to prevent the effects of health care disparities and eliminate barriers to health care. When access to quality health care does not exist, one result is preventable and costly hospital admissions for clients.[18] With this goal, Healthy People 2020 has multiple objectives that translate into

Table 1
Affordable Care Act care coordination initiatives

Initiative	Focus on Case Management
Medicare ACOs	CMS is proposing quality measures that ACOs should meet, and will then be linked to shared savings for the ACOs. Case management will be an essential part of these measures[16]
Patient-centered medical homes	HHS is providing grants for the establishment of patient-centered medical homes that use community-based health teams to provide primary care. Case managers will be required to help coordinate and integrate care
Community-based care transitions	Funding will be available to facilities that have high readmission rates to partner with community-based organizations to provide care transition to target the reduction of admission rates. Case managers will have a central role in this initiative
Independence at home	This initiative will be a team of providers including physicians and nurse practitioners to coordinate care for clients wanting to remain at home. Case management will be part of the team to coordinate services for these clients
Medicare payment bundling	Some eligible providers, which include hospitals, skilled nursing facilities, and home health agencies, can participate in this program. CMS will develop payment methods that will actually pay for care coordination and transitional care services, making case managers essential for this program

Abbreviations: ACOs, accountable care organizations; CMS, Center for Medicare and Medicaid Services; HHS, Department of Health and Human Services.
Data from Franko S, Sminkey P. Center stage in the revolution: a health care reform action guide for the professional case manager. Commission for Case Manager Certification. Issue Brief 2(2):1–8. Available at: http://ccmcertification.org. Accessed August 1, 2014.

opportunity for case management. Healthy People 2020 objectives that relate to case management include:

- Access to Health Services (AHS)-1: Increase the proportion of persons with health insurance
- AHS-5: Increase the proportion of persons who have a specific source of ongoing care
- AHS-6: Reduce the proportion of persons who are unable to obtain or delay in obtaining necessary medical care, dental care, or prescription medicines[18]

Using case management to assist clients in improving access to health care helps to address this goal. Case managers can improve access by these interventions:

- Assisting with access to health insurance coverage, helping a client navigate the current system and make educated choices
- Serve as a liaison to obtain a provider, and assist with improving client-provider communication concerning services. One reference on the Healthy People 2020 site states that a Community Referral Coordinator Program reduced the rate of no-shows at follow-up appointments from 75% to 58%[18]
- Educating clients about services and their disease processes, and helping to increase their ability for self-care and knowledge about when to access their provider or emergency care

CASE MANAGEMENT PRACTICE SETTINGS

Where do case managers practice, and what is their role in patient care? The case manager will serve in any capacity that helps the patient navigate the complex health care system and helps facilitate delivery of care.[11] Although case management can be found in all health care settings, there are differences depending on several factors. The first is the context of the setting. Is this acute or rehabilitation? Wellness or prevention? Mental health or alcohol and drug treatment? The second is the actual health condition and needs of the client and family. Is this a traumatic event or chronic? The third is the type of payment method used. Does the client have Medicaid or Medicare? Is this a workman's compensation case or is the client followed by managed care? The fourth is the actual health care discipline of the case manager. Is the case manager a registered nurse, social worker, or rehabilitation counselor? Using these 4 factors to help stimulate thinking about the care setting, the following sites may use case management, although the list is not inclusive.

- Hospitals to include acute care, transitional care facilities, long-term care facilities, skilled nursing facilities, and rehabilitation facilities
- Ambulatory care or outpatient clinics to include community clinics, such as public health and student health clinics on college campuses
- Public health insurance programs such as Medicare, Medicaid, and the Managed Care Organizations that contract with Medicaid in some states
- Private health insurance programs to include workmen's compensation, occupational health, disability claims, long-term care insurance, and group health insurance
- Private case management companies
- Government-sponsored programs such as correctional facilities, and the Veterans Administration Hospitals and outpatient facilities
- Mental health care facilities to include home health, ambulatory clinics, and day treatment facilities
- Geriatric care facilities to include assisted living and long-term care facilities
- Hospice, palliative care, and respite care facilities and programs
- Physician and medical group practices
- Disease management companies[12]

As health care needs become more complex, the need for case managers will increase and their visibility in all areas will expand.

CASE MANAGEMENT CHARACTERISTICS, KNOWLEDGE, AND SKILL SETS

The case manager is truly a jack-of-all-trades in terms of navigating the complexity of the ever changing health care system for the individual and the family. The new case management roles described earlier will include an even stronger base of clinical skills and liaison skills within our changing health care system.[9] In fact, several articles researched by the authors are calling on the expansion of case management to an advanced practice requirement, owing to the increased complexity of the role.[9] One of the reasons that nurses can transition to the role of case management so effectively is because of the foundational knowledge base of nursing. It is critical for the case manager to understand the disease process, progression of disease, and treatment options.[6,13]

The effective case manager will demonstrate the following skills and qualities: (1) clinical expertise and critical thinking skills, (2) diplomacy, (3) adaptability, (4) excellent organizational skills, (5) knowledge of community resources, (6) the ability to self-direct, (7) assertiveness skills, and (8) attention to detail.[6]

Some of the roles that the case manager will have to assume are as follows.

- *Educator*. One critical component to case management is educating clients and their families about the new disease process, medication, or catastrophic event and rehabilitation. All of the health care information they have been given could be totally unfamiliar to them, and the case manager helps them to understand treatment options to help make informed decisions and locate community resources.
- *Client advocate*. The case manager is continually advocating for clients and their families with the myriad of people and systems clients are thrust into with a new disease process or event. The case manager empowers clients to take charge of their condition, and helps them find ways to manage their disease or event to optimize their quality of life.
- *Facilitator/negotiator*. The case manager must have excellent communication skills to manage all coordination for the client with all health team members. This element is critical in helping avoid fragmentation of services for the client.
- *Planner/coordinator*. The case manager works closely with the client and family to make mutually acceptable goals and the methods used to achieve such goals. This aspect is crucial in helping the client to achieve optimal outcomes and contain costs.[6,9,11]

The case manager has an added difficulty of required communication of sensitive client information. Some communication skill sets that are necessary for the case manager would include conflict management and negotiating skills; motivational interviewing and active listening; and collaboration and team-building communication skills.[11,12] The case manager has to manage all stakeholders in the best interest of the client and family: all of the varied personalities, schedules, and priorities.

CASE MANAGEMENT TOOLS

Case managers rely on many tools to coordinate the care of clients and their families. Because a thorough assessment is critical for the case management process, several types of surveys are used by case managers. Case managers also use systems called clinical pathways and care maps. These tools are sometimes depicted as algorithms, and are useful in helping to proactively identify problems and opportunities for success.[11]

Screening Tools

Case managers use various health-assessment screening tools as information gathering so as to fully understand the client and the best course of planning for education and appropriate resources.[11] A descriptive screening tool will help identify characteristics and preventive health needs that are of greatest need for the client. Predictive tools can show what may happen in a given situation; for example, to show that clients who smoke cigarettes will likely have more upper respiratory infections. Evaluative tools can help the case manager weigh the effectiveness of an intervention; for example, diabetic education and the effect on the hemoglobin A1c.[11] Screening tools used by case managers may include the following.

- The 36-item Short-Form Survey (SF-36) is a multipurpose health survey with 36 questions that has proved to be both reliable and valid. It has functional health and mental health measures, and is generic and not disease specific.

- Patient Activation Measure (PAM) is a 13-item survey that assesses clients' knowledge, skill, and confidence in their ability for self-care. PAM scores can be used to predict health outcomes, including ED usage and medication adherence compliance.
- Health Risk Assessment (HRA) is a lengthy evaluation tool that demonstrates clients' own perception of their health status, and the results are used to predict whether clients have an increased risk of requiring additional care. HRAs are used in several disciplines, and are one of the first assessment tools that a case manager uses in beginning a client's case.[19]
- There are many disease-specific surveys that case managers can use with clients, such as the Beck Anxiety Inventory for anxiety and the Rose Questionnaire Seattle Angina questionnaire.[11]
- PM (see earlier discussion) is also a method used by other disciplines. PM helps to identify clients at high risk for use of medical services. The clients who are identified as high risk by PM are those the case manager will focus on, and may be designated "high touch." High touch has been an effective method for the high-risk client, and includes very frequent contact and, possibly, face-to-face contact. With the industry move to more proactive rather than reactive intervention with clients, PM has become a valuable tool.[19,20] The National Council of Quality Accreditation has added quality initiatives for health plans to participate in to attain a higher accreditation status; health plans are now using PM to help identify those members who are at high risk and are using case management to promote wellness.[19] PM is also being looked at by researchers at the Robert Wood Johnson foundation in hopes that the use of PM can help create virtual clinical trials to help stimulate research and development of new treatments.[19] Historically the industry relied on identification of high-risk clients by providers only, but PM has been shown to be more effective in identifying clients who are at high risk and could benefit by case management.[20]

It must be borne in mind that case management tools alone cannot improve care for the client. Effective change for the client requires the special skill sets, resources, and abilities of the case manager.[19,21]

CASE MANAGEMENT PROCESS

The case management process is carried out within the scope of practice, and includes critical thinking skills and evidence-based practice.[12] One notable facet of the case management process is the fluid and circular nature of the actions. For example, assessment of the client is a continuous process, and if additional needs are recognized they are immediately added to the plan of care; additional goals are then set and monitored, and outcomes evaluated.[12] **Table 2** compares the nursing process with the case management process.

CASE MANAGEMENT STANDARDS OF PRACTICE

The Standards of Practice of the CMSA include the case management process, but also include other facets such as ethics and legal issues.[12] In discussing these standards, the authors also look at some actual cases to see how these standards are translated into practice.

I. *Standard: Client selection for case management.* The case manager has to demonstrate that he or she has used high-risk screening criteria to evaluate the client.[12] One screening tool has already been discussed, the use of PM to

Table 2
Case management in the nursing process

Nursing Process	Case Management Process
Assessment	Client identification: the client can self-refer, or the referral can come from a provider, or they can be identified through methods such as predictive modeling Assessment: case managers complete lengthy intake of identification of needs
Diagnosis	Problem identification/opportunity identification
Planning	Planning: development of case management plan to include mutually agreed-upon goals between the case manager and client/client's family
Implementation	Implementation to include coordination and monitoring client needs/activities: putting the plan into action
Evaluation	Evaluation: have goals been met? Outcomes and possible termination of case if goals are met. An overall goal is to assist the client/client's family to become self-sufficient Note: if client has a chronic disease, disease management will be long term. Disease management is not episodic[6,11,12]

determine risk. These screening criteria will be specific to the area of practice. For example, in one article on trauma case management, the case manager screens not only for the actual critical needs but also for detection of missed injury.[22]

II. *Standard: Client assessment.* Meeting this standard will include demonstration of a thorough physical assessment, medical history, and mental health assessment to include substance abuse and history of abuse or trauma; learning capabilities and literacy level of both client and caregiver; and financial/legal concerns.[12] In one public health study, women receiving Temporary Assistance for Needy Families (TANF) were assessed for depression, substance abuse, and history of trauma and violence.[23] Previously the health behaviors of this population had not been studied effectively.

III. *Standard: Problem/opportunity identification.* The case manager has to document the opportunities for intervention that arise from the barriers identified in the assessment.[12] In a study of women who were victims of domestic violence, the assessment of this population showed that even in crisis, women do demonstrate health-promoting behaviors. The study used motivational interviewing to promote client involvement in the readiness for a behavior change in the plan of care.[24]

IV. *Standard: Planning.* For this standard to be met, the case manager has to demonstrate that the relevant data, including client diagnosis and client preferences, are used and that evidence-based practice is documented.[12] In a community-based case management program in South Korea, the population needs are assessed and the evidence-based practice regarding effectiveness of case management of chronic diseases identified.[25]

V. *Standard: Monitoring.* To meet this standard, the case manager will document ongoing assessment and measure the response of the client to the plan of care. The case manager will continuously assess the client's needs in connection with the plan of care.[12] In one integrative review article of 108 research reports, the investigators stated that the use of case management monitoring of clients with chronic diseases clearly affected the disease progression.[26]

VI. *Standard: Outcomes.* Evaluating whether goals have been met, whether quality of care has been demonstrated, and possibly whether cost-effectiveness has been addressed is required to meet this standard. The case manager uses evidence-based guidelines for the population. The outcomes or evaluation will also assess client satisfaction.[12] In a study of the implementation of a case management process in a rural community setting, case management was found to reduce admissions to the hospital, resulting in enough money saved to hire an advanced practice nurse to run the program.[27] In another study using nurse disease management strategies for hypertensive patients, several risk factors for cardiovascular disease showed significant improvement, and the program was cost-effective.[28,29]

VII. *Standard: Facilitation, coordination, and collaboration.* In meeting the needs of the client, the case manager must demonstrate evidence of collaborative efforts to improve client outcomes, which can include working with several stakeholders at once, from the client's PCP to the local hospital, pharmaceutical companies, and suppliers of durable medical equipment.[12] In the aforementioned rural case management study, the process implementation included working with the hospital, the University of Texas engineering department; and the 3 clinical nurse specialists, who conducted an SWOT (Strengths/Weaknesses/Opportunities/Threats) analysis to facilitate areas for collaboration.[27]

VIII. *Standard: Termination of case.* Not every case is terminated; for example, the ongoing management of a client's chronic disease. For this standard to be met, the case manager has to document the identification of reasons for terminating management of a client, such as reaching mutually agreed-upon goals, client refusal, or client death.[12]

IX. *Standard: Qualifications of case managers.* As in other fields, case managers must be able to demonstrate competence and maintain competence in practice by either: (1) having current, active, and unrestricted licensure or certification in a profession that has case management duties within their scope of practice; or (2) if the state does not require licensure or certification, they must have a baccalaureate or graduate degree in either social work or another health or human services discipline from an institution that is accredited. Case managers must also have completed field experience with supervision as part of their degree.[12]

X. *Standard: Legal.* Case managers must be compliant with any applicable local, state, and federal laws that govern case management practice. The standards also frequently stipulate that case managers are always responsible for working within their scope of practice.[12] This standard lists 2 subcategories under the heading "Legal." (1) Confidentiality and Client Privacy: the case manager must keep up to date with all laws and regulations that affect client privacy and the protection of client information; and (2) Consent for Case Management Services: the case manager has to document evidence that clients and their family/support systems were informed about the services, given the right to refuse services, and given alternatives to case management services.[12]

XI. *Standard: Ethics.* Although this standard could exist under the standard of "Legal," the 5 basic ethical principles are a requirement for case managers to be aware of and to follow in their practice: beneficence, nonmalfeasance, autonomy, justice, and fidelity. This standard also includes an obligation for respectful relationships with coworkers.[12]

XII. *Standard: Advocacy.* This standard is another critical element of the case management process. The case manager should always demonstrate advocacy for the client in all health care services and in promoting self-determination.[12] In one study of a public health nursing case management study, the population consisted of women receiving TANF. Because the welfare reform laws have changed to include lifetime limits for benefit receipt, the health of this population had come to the attention of groups studying health care disparities. The results of this study showed that public health nurse case management intervention was effective in improving health care visit rates for mental health, which resulted in a decrease in depressive symptoms.[23]

XIII. *Standard*: *Cultural competency.* To meet this standard of practice, case managers must be aware of cultural diversity and be able to respond to the needs of these clients. This approach will include an assessment of their specific needs, such as communication resources.[12]

XIV. *Standard*: *Resource management and stewardship.* The case manager will demonstrate adherence to this standard of practice by documenting use of evidence-based guidelines, careful use of resources for the client, and demonstrating the use of the most efficient health care services for the client.[12]

XV. *Standard*: *Research and research utilization.* Case managers will always need to be current with all evidence-based practice and guidelines, including those outside their immediate discipline that can affect the client, and be in compliance with the current standards of practice. When appropriate, case managers will also incorporate meaningful research findings into their practice.[12] In one study published in the *Forum for Health Economics and Policy*, the application of a business model to research financial efficiency from the use of disease management for diabetes demonstrated a saving of approximately $60,000 per patient.[30]

The standards of case management are identified in the following case study of a pediatric client.

CASE STUDY: PEDIATRIC ASTHMA

A pediatric nurse practitioner (PNP) at a local ED identified a client for chronic case management of asthmatic disease. Joe Jones, aged 8 years, has been seen with persistent asthma in the ED as a result of his noncompliance with treatment. He has been seen 10 times in the ED over the winter months in 2013/2014 (*Standard: Client selection process*). The PNP made a referral to Jennifer Patty, a case manager who specializes in pediatric chronic disease management.

The case manager schedules a meeting with Joe and his mother for initial asthma assessment. During this assessment meeting, the case manager obtains a detailed medical history on Joe, and a complete psychosocial history of Joe and his family to include financial history and current insurance coverage. A developmental screening of Joe is also done to include functional and cognitive information. During the assessment, the case manager talks at length with Joe's mother and determines that her health literacy is very low. Joe's mother has very poor understanding of Joe's disease process, medication usage, and compliance (*Standard: Assessment*). The case manager asks about where they live, where Joe goes to school, and the employment status of Joe's mother. The case manager knows the school nurse at Joe's elementary school and makes plans to meet with her.

In reviewing all of the assessment data, the case manager identifies the following problems for Joe (*Standard: Problem identification*):

- Persistent, uncontrolled asthma
- Low socioeconomic status of family
- Low health literacy

- Noncompliance with medication
- Transportation constraints
- Medicaid coverage has not been established for Joe
- No PCP for Joe

Next, the case manager develops an asthma plan for Joe and meets again with Joe and his mother to set mutual goals for the control of Joe's asthma (*Standard: planning*). During this meeting, the case manager completes the Medicaid application for Joe and contacts a PCP who specializes in pediatric asthma (*Standard: Facilitation, coordination, and collaboration; Standard: Advocacy*). The PCP location is on a bus route near Joe's home. The case manager asks Joe's mother about her biggest concerns regarding Joe's health and the family's economic needs. The case manager learns that Joe's mother has inconsistent income from cleaning houses and does not have food stamps, and relies solely on bus transportation. Joe's mother says that every day she is just trying to get through the day and have food on the table. She has not been able to spend time learning about Joe's medication, and states that she knows she needs this information to keep him healthy. She does not verbalize understanding that prevention is a big necessity with asthma management.

The case manager and Joe's mother set the following goals:

- Routine follow-up planning with PCP
- Establish an asthma action plan with school nurse and home
- A reduction of ED visits by 50% over the next 6 months
- Medication regimen will be established and followed

The case manager has frequent contact with Joe's mother over the first 2 months of their case management relationship, providing education about asthma and all medications. The case manager frequently checks with the PCP to ensure that Joe is following his asthma plan and that he is compliant with medications (*Standard: Monitoring*). The case manager contacts the school nurse to discuss Joe's asthma diagnosis and his continuing needs for asthma compliance. The school nurse provides follow-up reports to the PCP about Joe's progress at school. The school nurse monitors his peak flow and administers his daily medication during school hours. The school nurse arranges for Joe to get free breakfast and lunch and to receive the weekend food back-pack from the school each week.

After 6 months, Joe kept all PCP appointments, and demonstrated compliance with all medications with good peak flow readings. He only visited the ED once for an asthma exacerbation during this period. Joe's mother can verbalize understanding of his action plan and disease process (*Standard: Outcomes*). Joe's mother believes he has improved immensely with his asthma, academic status, and behavior. She expresses confidence in being able to identify his asthma triggers before they cause an exacerbation of his asthma. Because Joe has made such good progress, his mother states that her own anxiety has decreased, that she now has a job in the school cafeteria, and has consistent income with health insurance. The case manager is confident with Joe's progress and reduces her communication with Joe's mother to every 6 months, with per diem nurse calls for additional needs.

SUMMARY

This article gives the current definition of case management, includes some current issues that are affecting the practice of case management, and discusses the potential outcomes of these issues. A description of the case management process is detailed in addition to the CMSA Standards of Practice for case managers. A case study in chronic disease management of a pediatric patient with asthma includes a description of the roles, skills, and outcomes of effective case management.

REFERENCES

1. Crossing the quality chasm: a new health system for the 21st century. Institute of Medicine; 2001. Available at: http://www.iom.edu. Accessed August 1, 2014.
2. Franko S, Sminkey P. Center stage in the revolution: a health care reform action guide for the professional case manager. Commission for Case Manager Certification. Issue Brief No date;2(2):1–8. Available at: http://ccmcertification.org. Accessed August 1, 2014.
3. Baguhn B. The case for case management. Healthc Financ Manage 2011;65(12): 40–3 Web.
4. Ulch P, Schmidt M. Clinical nurse specialist as community-based nurse case manager: integral to achieving the triple aim of healthcare. Nurse Leader 2013; 11(3):32–5. Available at: http://www.nurseleader.com.
5. Marek KD, Adams SJ, Stetzer F, et al. The relationship of community-based nurse care coordination to costs in the Medicare and Medicaid programs. Res Nurs Health 2010;33(3):235–42. Available at: http://web.a.ebscohost.com.ezproxy.lib. apsu.edu.
6. Yamamoto L, Lucey C. "Case management "within the walls": a glimpse into the future". Crit Care Nurs Q 2005;28(2):162–78. Available at: http://web.a. ebscohost.com.ezproxy.lib.apsu.edu.
7. Drozda JP Jr, Libby D, Keiserman W, et al. Case management decision support tools: predictive risk report or health risk assessment? Popul Health Manag 2008;11(4):193–6. Available at: http://web.a.ebscohost.com.ezproxy. lib.apsu.edu.
8. Joo JY, Huber DL. An integrative review of nurse-led community-based case management effectiveness. Int Nurs Rev 2014;61(1):14–24. Available at: http:// onlinelibrary.wiley.com.ezproxy.lib.apsu.edu.
9. Meek J. Affordable care act: predictive modeling challenges and opportunities for case management. Prof Case Manag 2012;17(1):15–21. Available at: http:// ovidsp.tx.ovid.com.ezproxy.lib.apsu.edu.
10. Stanhope M, Lancaster J. Foundations of nursing in the community: community-oriented practice. 4th edition. St Louis (MO): Elsevier; 2014.
11. Clinical case management practice. Nursing case management review and resource manual. 4th edition. Nursing Credentialing Center; 2012. Available at: http://www.nursecredentialing.org. Accessed August 1, 2014.
12. Standards of practice for case management. Case Management Society of America; 2010. p. 1–27. Available at: http://www.cmsa.org/portals/0/pdf/ memberonly/standardsofpractice.pdf. Accessed August 1, 2014.
13. Stanton M, Swanson M, Sherrod R, et al. Case management evolution: from basic to advanced practice role. Lippincotts Case Manag 2005;10(6):274–84. Available at: http://ovidsp.tx.ovid.com.ezproxy.lib.apsu.edu.
14. McCullough L. The case manager: an essential link in quality care. Creat Nurs 2009; 15(3):124–6. Available at: http://web.a.ebscohost.com.ezproxy.lib.apsu.edu.
15. Moreo K, Moreo N, Urbano F, et al. Are we prepared for affordable care act provisions of care coordination? Case managers' self-assessments and views on physician roles. Prof Case Manag 2014;19(1):18–26. Available at: http:// ovidsp.tx.ovid.com.ezproxy.lib.apsu.edu.

16. Justice D. States, stakeholders, and climate change: the affordable care act offers a new environment for long-term-care advocacy. Generations 2011;35(1): 32–7. Available at: http://web.a.ebscohost.com.ezproxy.lib.apsu.edu.

17. Birmingham J. Case managers implement "action" plans. Lippincotts Case Manag 2005;10:306–15. Available at: http://ovidsp.tx.ovid.com.ezproxy.lib.apsu.edu.

18. Access to health services. Healthy people 2020. 2014. Available at: www.healthypeople.gov. Accessed August 1, 2014.

19. Hodgman S. Predictive modeling & outcomes. Prof Case Manag 2008;13(1): 19–23. Available at: http://ovidsp.tx.ovid.com.ezproxy.lib.apsu.edu.

20. Freund T, Mahler C, Erler A, et al. Identification of patients likely to benefit from care management programs. Am J Manag Care 2011;17(5):345–52. Available at: http://web.a.ebscohost.com.ezproxy.lib.apsu.edu.

21. Smith A, MacKay S, McCulloch K. Case management: developing practice through action research. Br J Community Nurs 2013;18(9):452–8. Available at: http://web.a.ebscohost.com.ezproxy.lib.apsu.edu.

22. Umbrell CE. Trauma case management: a role for the advanced practice nurse. J Trauma Nurs 2006;13(2):70–3. Available at: http://web.a.ebscohost.com.ezproxy.lib.apsu.edu.

23. Kneipp SM, Kairalla JA, Lutz BJ, et al. Public health nursing case management for women receiving temporary assistance for needy families: a randomized controlled trial using community-based participatory research. Am J Public Health 2011;101(9):1759–68. Available at: http://web.a.ebscohost.com.ezproxy.lib.apsu.edu.

24. D'Amico J, Nelson J. Nursing care management at a shelter-based clinic. Prof Case Manag 2008;13(1):26–36. Available at: http://ovidsp.tx.ovid.com.ezproxy.lib.apsu.edu.

25. Suk G, Ko I, Lee T, et al. Effects of community-based case management by visiting nurses for low-income patients with hypertension in South Korea. Jpn J Nurs Sci 2014;11:35–43. Available at: http://onlinelibrary.wiley.com.ezproxy.lib.apsu.edu.

26. Sutherland D, Hayter M. Structured review: evaluating the effectiveness of nurse case managers in improving health outcomes in three major chronic diseases. J Clin Nurs 2009;18(21):2978–92. Available at: http://web.b.ebscohost.com.ezproxy.lib.apsu.edu.

27. Baldwin K, Black D, Hammond S. Developing a rural transitional care community case management program using clinical nurse specialists. Clin Nurse Spec 2014;28:147–55. Available at: www.cns-journal.com.

28. Cicolini G, Simonetti V, Comparcini D, et al. Efficacy of a nurse-led email reminder program for cardiovascular prevention risk reduction in hypertensive patients: a randomized controlled trial. Int J Nurs Stud 2014;51:833–43. Available at: http://ac.els-cdn.com.ezproxy.lib.apsu.edu.

29. Stafford RS, Berra K. Critical factors in case management: practical lessons from a cardiac case management program. Dis Manag 2007;10(4):197–207. Available at: http://web.b.ebscohost.com.ezproxy.lib.apsu.edu.

30. Beaulieu N, Cutler DM, Ho K, et al. The business case for diabetes disease management for managed care organizations. Forum Health Econ Pol 2006;9(1):37. Available at: http://web.b.ebscohost.com.ezproxy.lib.apsu.edu.

Preventing 30-day Readmissions

Sherri Stevens, PhD, RN*

KEYWORDS

- Readmissions • Discharge teaching • Health literacy • Compliance • Telehealth

KEY POINTS

- Preventing 30-day readmissions is a top priority nationally because of federal guidelines and regulations under the Patient Protection and Affordable Care Act of 2010.
- Improved methods of discharge teaching must be established for patients transitioning out of hospitals and into their homes or the community.
- Reasons for 30-day readmissions include ineffective communication affecting the transition of care, health literacy, and compliance.
- Telehealth and electronic use of health resources enhance new methods of patient treatment and education.

INTRODUCTION

Preventing 30-day readmissions to hospitals is a top priority in the era of health care reform. A national study conducted in 2009 analyzing Medicare data for the year 2003 to 2004 revealed that readmission rates were 19% for Medicare recipients with a cost more than $17 billion annually.[1] Since the Patient Care Affordability Act became law in 2010, requirements for health care facilities to comply with new regulations and guidelines pertaining to readmissions have been established. Recurring readmissions have been problematic through the years, but new regulations will be costly to health care facilities because of payment guidelines. Hospitals are focused on improving the transition of care to avoid 30-day readmissions and provide quality care. Sources have identified patients covered by Medicare and Medicaid as being readmitted at very high rates compared with patients covered by private insurance.[2,3] This article reviews some of the issues concerning discharge planning, compliance, and telemedicine as ways to prevent 30-day readmissions.

Disclosure: None.
Nursing, MTSU, Murfreesboro, TN 37132-0001, USA
* 121 Laural Hill Drive, Smyrna, TN 37167.
E-mail address: sherri.stevens@mtsu.edu

PROBLEM

According to the Affordable Care Act of 2010, Section 3025,[4] criteria for the US Centers for Medicare and Medicaid Services (CMS)[5] define the mandated requirements for decreasing Medicare payments to hospitals with high rates of readmissions. The Hospital Readmissions Reduction Program section of the Affordable Care Act outlines plans for reducing payments to hospitals based on readmissions of acute myocardial infarction (AMI), heart failure (HF) and pneumonia. The financial reductions placed on high rates of readmissions for Medicare recipients began in 2013 with a 1% reduction increasing to 2% in 2014 and 3% by 2015.[6] The Hospital Compare Web site has been developed through efforts from the CMS, the Department of Health and Human Services, and the Hospital Quality Alliance to categorize and publish data regarding 30-day readmissions to hospitals.[7] National data indicate that 1 in 4 patients with HF are readmitted, and that for AMI readmissions are 1 in 5 within 30 days of discharge from a hospital.[1,8] The costs of pneumonia readmissions may exceed $6 billion annually.[9] Readmissions within 30 days can be the result of gaps in the care provided by hospitals as well as the transition process for patients.[1,10,11] There will be new medical conditions added to the 30-day readmission reduction list beginning in 2015, including chronic obstructive pulmonary disease, hip arthroplasty, and knee arthoplasty.[5] Scheduled to be added to the list in 2017 is coronary artery bypass surgery.[5] The readmission penalties to hospitals will affect hospital Medicare reimbursements but will save Medicare millions of dollars.[12] Readmission rates for established criteria have been categorized as quality indicators regarding hospitalizations according to The Hospital Quality Alliance, Institute for Healthcare Improvement, and other organizations.[13] Many health care facilities are scrambling to focus on methods to reduce readmissions but provide quality care in an era of limited financial resources.

From the moment a patient is discharged from a hospital until the patient returns home and begins self-care responsibility is a time of transition. The transition from hospital to home has been classified as a vulnerable time for many patients. During the transition of care, instability and lack of care coordination have contributed to unexpected events affecting the outcome for many patients. On returning home, patients must become responsible for their health and be able to recall all instructions that were given to them while hospitalized. To recall details about care and medications may be difficult for patients after returning to their home environments. It is common for patients to be discharged from health care facilities with intravenous access devices, complex wound care, enteral feeding devices, self-catheterization, surgical drains, and other types of devices that require care management. Patients and family members have the responsibility of learning how to manage the patient as well as the extra equipment, medications, and treatments. During this time of transition patients may fail to fully understand their discharge instructions.

DISCHARGE TEACHING

There are many variables in the concept of discharge teaching. While in hospital, patients are often taught important facts pertaining to disease management, medications, and home care by supporting members of the health care team. Often patients are not in prime learning mode for clearly grasping critical components for maintaining self-care beyond the hospital walls. The acutely ill individual may be recovering from a life-altering event such as an AMI, traumatic injury, or major surgical intervention, and is potentially focused on basic needs such as comfort. It may be difficult for a patient to learn and retain clear details because of physiologic conditions. Although hospital days are limited, discharge teaching must be presented by the health care provider. According to CMS[5] data, average length of hospital short stay decreased from 9.0 days in 1990 to 5.1 days in 2011. A decreased length of stay with an increased acute patient population leaves limited time for educating patients and families.[14]

Family members, significant others, or primary caretakers may be overwhelmed during the hospitalization of a loved one. Comprehension of discharge teaching may be difficult because of extrinsic factors such as stress, jobs, and managing the household responsibilities of a sick patient. It has been noted that patients as well as family members or other caretakers are often not prepared for discharge from the hospital and the transition to home.[15,16] Stressful learning conditions are not beneficial for patients and families.

COMMUNICATION

Communication is necessary in health care at every level and especially in the discharge planning process. Communication has been identified as one of the main reasons for 30-day readmissions. Effective communication can be a determining factor for a successful transition home. Communicating discharge instructions before leaving the hospital may not be perceived or fully understood by the patient and family. Once home, the patient may experience confusion or not be able to recall what was explained before leaving the hospital. The lack of understanding can lead to potential compliance issues because of the uncertainty.[17,18] The lack of communication among health care providers as well as to the patient can contribute to inappropriate care choices that result in readmissions.[19,20]

Communication Barriers Between Health Care Providers and Patients

Communication between health care providers such as primary care physician (PCPs) and other specialists may not be as transparent as it should be regarding patient care. PCPs are often not aware of discharge plans or fail to receive updates and reports pertaining to patient admissions. The lack of communication among health care providers has been identified as contributing to unsuccessful transitions of care.[21,22] A common risk identified in methods to improve discharge coordination and teaching for patients is the lack of communication between the health care providers.[23] It is essential for nurses as well as all members of the health care team to improve communication with patients regarding their transition into the home or community. Although health care providers think that they are teaching effectively, evidence indicates that there is much room for improvement.[1,18] **Table 1** summarizes potential communication barriers that can exist between health care providers and patients.

Poor Communication and Medication Discrepancies

Communication involving medication errors and adverse effects of medications are well documented in the literature.[24–29] **Table 2** summarizes the readmission findings.

Sanderson and colleagues[30] identified a lack of documentation of discharge instructions for a group of patients with coronary heart disease as well as poor patient recall of medications and lifestyle modifications during a telephone survey regarding discharge instructions. Cardiac patients are in 2 of the most readmitted categories, but continue to have inadequate discharge care. Another factor to consider regarding discharge teaching is the elderly population. Elderly individuals may not be able to comprehend discharge instructions or be able to maintain self-care for multiple reasons, such as cognitive limitations, mobility issues, living conditions, and other comorbidities.[31,32] Family and caretakers are often unable to provide constant support

Table 1
Reasons for readmissions: communication

Readmissions Communication	Findings	Investigators
Communication	Poor communication with the patient and among physicians contributes to readmissions	Bell et al,[70] 2009
Ineffective communication Medication instruction	Adverse events such as medication errors involving antibiotics, cardiovascular drugs, and anticoagulants occurred in 1 in 5 patients transitioning to home resulting in readmissions	Forster et al,[19] 2003
Communication among physicians	PCP may not be aware of a patient's admission or receive test results, procedures, discharge summaries in timely manner	Van Walraven et al,[21] 2002
Communication and collaboration between physicians and hospitals	Hospitals and physicians need to communicate and assist with better follow-up care for patients	Jencks et al,[1] 2009
—	Common risks identified for readmissions included poor communication among health care members	Adams et al,[23] 2014

because of work and other responsibilities. Services needed for the elderly may not be available in the community or covered by payment systems. Many elderly patients with chronic health diseases live alone and are not able to resume personal care and activities of daily living after hospitalization.

Table 2
Reasons for readmissions: communication and medication

Communication Readmissions	Findings	Investigators
Medication discrepancies	Medication discrepancies that occur after discharge contribute to readmissions in the elderly population	Lalonde et al,[25] 2008
Medication discrepancies include both system-wide and patient adherence	Medication discrepancies Posthospital medication discrepancies: prevalence and contributing factors	Coleman et al,[24] 2005
Communication and medications	A common system issue involves incomplete discharge instructions, differing information from hospital sources regarding discharge instructions Many medication discrepancies occur after discharge	Broockvar et al,[26] 2006
Medications	Findings indicate a need for better planning and teaching regarding medications	Varkey et al,[27] 2007
Communication Medications Delay to fill prescription	Study identified that patients with AMI filled ordered prescriptions 1 wk after discharge	Jackevicius et al,[28] 2008

Socioeconomic conditions may prevent patients from adhering to discharge instructions, such as not filling prescriptions for medications or failure to attend follow-up visits with physicians. Ho and colleagues[33] reviewed patients after drug-eluting stent placements to determine whether there was a delay in filling prescriptions for clopidogrel once discharged from hospital. Of 7402 patients, 1 in 6 did not fill the prescribed clopidogrel on the day of discharge. The older patients delayed obtaining the prescription, as well as not understanding the importance of the medication. Lack of the prescribed medication can result in poor outcomes, such as occluded stents and eventual hospital readmission. The study clearly indicates a gap in the discharge teaching when the patient does not comprehend the reason and necessity to fill the prescription to preserve the stent. Lack of resources and limited income may also hinder filling new prescriptions ordered at discharge.

HEALTH LITERACY

Health literacy is a major factor that must be considered regarding successful discharge teaching. The Institute of Medicine (2004)[34] defines health literacy as the ability of individuals to process and understand basic health information required for making health decisions. Health literacy can be divided into 4 levels: below basic, basic, intermediate, and proficient. According to the National Assessment of Adult Literacy[35] 59% of adults more than 65 years of age are at below basic or basic levels of health literacy and therefore are only able to understand basic, concrete information. Low health literacy may affect up to 90 million adults in American health care facilities.[36,37] Low health literacy can have a significant impact on knowledge of disease management and understanding of care, which contribute to the frequency of readmissions. A lack of understanding of medication usage, reading labels, proper instructions for taking medications, and filling prescriptions are problems facing many patients with low health literacy. Health literacy can contribute to compliance behaviors because of the lack of understanding of discharge instructions provided in the hospital. Patients with low health literacy may be labeled as noncompliant by hospital staff when in reality they do not understand medical terms and complex explanations of medications.[38] Patients with low health literacy may also show noncompliant behavior because of the inability to understand health-related issues.[39,40]

Patients with low health literacy may not understand printed educational material, because they may think that the message does not apply to them or that the content offered is too vague.[41] **Table 3** summarizes reasons for readmission related to health literacy.

Buckley and colleagues[41] held focus groups with patients for input regarding emergency department printed discharge instructions. The results of the focus groups revealed that words and expressions incorporated into discharge teaching materials written and understood by health care workers were not clear to patients. The participants identified the confusing use of medical terms such as sprain and orthopedist. The participants also thought that using pictures would be beneficial for adhering to instructions. Patient input for writing and designing discharge instructions should be considered more often to gain a better understanding of what patients perceive as important to know. According to the Joint Commission on Accreditation of Healthcare Organizations standards,[42] discharge teaching must be provided and documented in the medical record. Although discharge teaching is provided, health care professionals may not know the literacy level of the patient. Health care providers often present material to patients in medical terms telling them what they need to do without

Table 3		
Reasons for readmission: health literacy		
Health Literacy	Findings	Investigators
Lack of understanding DC instructions	59% of adults more than 65 y old are at below basic or basic levels of health literacy	Kutner et al,[35] 2006
Medication compliance	Patients with low health literacy have a greater rate of not understanding medication	Berkman et al,[36] 2011
Lack of understanding of printed discharge instructions	78% of patients discharged from an ED had difficulty understanding at least 1 area of care pertaining to discharge instructions because of the content	Engel et al,[50] 2009
Poor comprehension of printed ED instructions	Focus groups with patients in EDs reviewed printed discharge instructions. Discharge teaching materials written and understood by health care workers were not clear to patients	Buckley et al,[41] 2012

Abbreviations: DC, discharge instructions; ED, emergency department.

gaining insight into what the patient considers important or understands. In the literature the terms compliant, adherence, and concordance have been used to discuss knowledge comprehension of patients regarding cooperation of health care instructions. Compliance may indicate a choice made by the patient, but it may also be related to low health literacy.[43] Adherence incorporates a patient's agreement to an instruction or recommendation.[44] The concept of concordance allows the health care provider and the patient to share knowledge and work together to establish treatments regarding health care.[45]

In health care facilities there may be discussions regarding who should be responsible for discharge teaching and preparing patients for the transition home. Bedside nurses have long been the primary educators for patients and families. Other health care providers also share the responsibility of participating in the discharge teaching process. Besides nurses, case managers, physicians, hospitalists, and pharmacists may participate in discharge teaching. The interprofessional model is an approach that has been used in some institutions and can be beneficial for patients. The interprofessional model of care consists of multiple health care providers working collaboratively to plan and coordinate care for the patient. Pharmacists are having a greater role in the discharge process by teaching patients and families about medications. Studies indicate that the role of pharmacists in discharge planning can be beneficial for medication counseling.[46]

Nurses spend the most time with patients and families. Hospital staffing and nurse/patient ratios must be considered as variables that affect patient care. Increasing nurse/patient ratios can affect the quality of time nurses are able to spend with patients for education. McHugh and Ma[47] suggest that improving nurses' workloads and work environments can improve patient outcomes and decrease Medicare readmissions. The demanding workload of nurses may interfere with obtaining the discharge needs of patients because of lack of individual time spent per patient.[48,49] Nurses may be rushed through the discharge process and not have adequate time to assess and teach their patients.[49]

Prepackaged discharge instructions have been designed for patients to assist with the transition to home. Preprinted or computerized generic discharge instructions may not be individualized for patients. There is an urgent need to place greater emphasis on individualized teaching when patients receive discharge instructions in the hospital.

The ability to focus on individual patients and their needs for discharge planning may help reduce readmissions.[10]

In a different study reviewing printed discharge instructions, 78% of patients discharged from an emergency department had difficulty understanding at least 1 area of care pertaining to discharge instructions because of the content.[50] Preprinted discharge instructions are often written above the level of understanding of patients.[23] Some research findings confirm that the use of standardized discharge instructions does not decrease hospital readmissions.[51] Generic printed discharge instruction sheets may provide basic information for patients once they return home, but may not include the specific needs of the patient. Comprehensive, patient-specific information, such as health issues, comorbidities, and home medications, may not be included for each patient.[52] Once patients return home they can be overwhelmed and feel uncertain of the discharge instructions pertaining to self-care activities or medications.

Results of a qualitative study with middle-aged women after AMI further show the need for clarity in discharge instructions. After the women in the study were discharged from the hospital they were interviewed regarding their experience of returning home. The women described returning home and feeling uncertain of the meaning of their discharge instructions. There were questions regarding when to resume activities, when to return to work, and how to deal with emotions, and the lack of knowledge created fear and worry about the healing hearts.[53] Most patients receive information in hospital, but have difficulty recalling the information after going home.[54]

Language barriers may also affect the understanding of discharge instructions. Karliner and colleagues,[55] conducted a study to focus on language barriers and understanding of discharge instructions among patients with limited English proficiency from 2 large urban hospitals. Three-hundred and eight Spanish-speaking, Chinese-speaking, and English-speaking patients were recruited from medical surgical floors to participate. Although the patients were provided with interpreters in the appropriate languages, the results of the study revealed low understanding for follow-up appointments (56%) and medication outcomes such as purpose of medication (41%).

With the rate of 30-day readmissions it is evident that health care teams must do better at communicating with patients to facilitate and provide safe transitions home. The elderly population with multiple comorbidities can benefit from better strategic planning for discharge. Successful discharge planning must begin on admission to the facility. New models of care to ensure that earlier collaboration takes place must be driven by evidence.

Postdischarge telephone follow-up may help patients to have the opportunity to review medications or any postdischarge questions. It has been determined that follow-up phone calls to discuss discharge instructions can be an effective method to reduce some readmissions.[17] Follow-up phone calls or nurse visits could enhance learning by reviewing follow-up plans or prescribed home therapies. Patients are often overwhelmed while ill in hospital. In acute settings, patients are in pain, sedated, nauseated, or preparing for daily ordered activities such as ambulation. During the daily hospital routine, multiple health care members may approach the patient with teaching instructions. Patients are discharged quickly, and are often unable to care for themselves fully on returning home, thus relying on family caregivers. Patients may feel inundated with information, and not fully understand or process all of the information. There have been other studies suggesting that follow-up phone calls do not affect readmissions.[14,56,57] Follow-up phone calls combined with other resources may assist patients and families and prevent readmissions.

Some facilities have discharge planning nurses or teams that assist with the discharge process. Other facilities rely on bedside nurses to provide home instructions to patients shortly before they leave the facility. Often patients are instructed to follow up with their primary physicians within a determined time. It has been documented that patients readmitted within 30 days often did not follow up with the PCP.[1] Quality initiatives and new methods of planning patient transitions are needed nationally to prevent an increased rate of readmissions.

COMPLIANCE

Compliance may be defined as the patient not following recommendations of the health care providers. Compliance may include many variables such as age, socio-economic status, available resources, and communication. A lack of understanding of the message is often a contributing factor to unsuccessful compliance with treatment modalities.[58] Reading materials may be written to support generic disease processes and not for each individual, leaving patients confused or unsure of the application. Mixed messages from multiple health care providers may add to the confusion and create compliance issues.

Another important factor in compliance issues is the method or style of teaching. Health care providers must understand the environment and resources of the patient, and how the patient functions in the home and in society. Including the patient in the discharge planning process can create a better understanding of individual needs to avoid potential compliance issues. Culture and diversity must also be considered to improve compliance with treatment modalities once leaving the hospital. According to the literature, many patients do not follow up with appointments per discharge instruction, patients often do not fill prescriptions per discharge instruction, and patients have many issues with medications. Although these topics have been addressed in the context of communication, compliance may be related to health literacy and understanding.[59] Compliance also involves choosing to make lifestyle modifications such as diet and exercise choices for healthy living.

TELEHEALTH

According to the Department of Health and Human Services Medicaid.gov Web site, the definition of Telehealth is "the use of technology to deliver health care, health information or health education at a distance."[60] Telehealth and use of electronic health resources are part of health care reform included in the Affordable Care Act. This form of technology includes e-charts, data systems, digital applications, mobile health apps, and increasing the use of Telehealth to provide health care services to more people.

Telehealth and the ability to use modern technology will be increasingly important in preventing 30-day readmissions and managing chronic health conditions. Some states have enrolled in Telehealth programs and others have not. In order to participate in Telehealth services each state must be comply with CMS guidelines for this service as well as practice within their state practice act.[61] Each state must also provide a plan for how to use the technology among health care workers and patients as well as how to share health information. At present, there are 17 states providing Telehealth services as part of their Medicaid programs. Technology systems and equipment must be established, defined, and available for Telehealth to be successful.

Telehealth services can include using devices such as interactive video conferencing with patients in the home or in rural areas, digital images that can be transmitted from the bedside to other facilities, and online patient engagement.

Technological devices must be able to transmit electronic data via mobile apps, computers, and telephone devices to health care providers. Through a Telehealth program, patient information such as vital signs, glucose monitoring, and medication compliance can be obtained and linked electronically to health care providers.[62] Other countries have been using telemedicine to assist with patient care and help manage costs. Telehealth has been successful in managing patients diagnosed with diabetes and congestive HF, in physical therapy, and in wound care. Advanced practice registered nurses will be needed to implement new technologies for rural health communities in the quest to deliver health care to more people.[63] Telehealth monitoring devices have been used to assist diabetic patients to transmit glycemic data to health care providers and to enhance compliance because of the automated responses and close technical observation of disease management.[62] Rural facilities can transmit data and images to other facilities for treatment options.

In the state of Nebraska, a collaboration of hospitals and health departments formed the Nebraska State Telehealth Network in 2005.[64] This program has been able to provide care for many rural patients, has saved money, and has given health care providers the ability to connect with patients. At present, 80 hospitals are participating in the Nebraska Network and many components of care are being monitored via Telehealth monitoring capabilities, which has resulted in cost savings for the state of Nebraska. The capabilities of Telehealth can enhance the management of chronic diseases and reduce the number of hospital readmissions.[65]

There are barriers to Telehealth, including policy issues concerning patient privacy regarding HIPPA (Health Insurance Portability and Accountability Act) laws and licensing for telemonitoring locations. There are provider and facility regulations that must be established. Reimbursement criteria must meet Medicaid services and federal criteria. Other barriers relevant to Telehealth include the cost. The initial setup and purchasing of equipment can be expensive. Not all states have established Telehealth programs. Health care computer systems and the ability to share and transmit data must be established before initiation of Telehealth programs.

SUMMARY

Reducing readmissions requires introducing new models of discharge planning and transitioning of care from the hospital to the home and community. New models of discharge improvements in the literature include Better Outcomes for Older Adults through Safe Transitions (BOOST)[66] and Re-engineered Discharge (RED).[67] Both programs are evidence-based projects designed to focus on and reduce readmissions.[23] Project RED includes an enhanced discharge assessment with an emphasis on patient and family involvement. BOOST has been designed to identify high-risk elderly patients early in the admission process. Incorporating health coaching into the patient teaching component of hospitalization may allow patients to take an active role in self-care. The health coaching approach allows patients to determine goals and readiness to make lifestyle changes.[68] Health coaching can begin in the hospital and continue in the home for follow-up. Nursing education must also include a greater emphasis on patient teaching, the discharge planning process, and use of community resources to decrease costs.

The economics of readmissions will affect health care facilities greatly in the future. A focus on safety and quality must be emphasized at each facility for improvement. Implementing new programs such as health coaches, and expanding Telehealth and other technological resources can help prevent frequent readmissions to hospital and save money. Community resources and Telehealth may be options to consider for managing at-risk patients who have been discharged. Effective communication and addressing health literacy will improve patient outcomes and decrease readmissions.[69] The future of nursing education must focus on health care reform initiatives and be active in evidence-based solutions to provide quality care.

REFERENCES

1. Jencks SF, Williams MV, Coleman EA. Rehospitalizations among patients in the Medicare Fee-For-Service program. N Engl J Med 2009;360:1418–28. http://dx.doi.org/10.1056/NEJMsa0803563.
2. Podulka J, Barrett M, Jiang J, et al. Readmissions following hospitalization for chronic vs acute conditions 2008. HCUP statistical brief #127. Rockville (MD): Agency for Healthcare Research and Quality; 2012. Available at: http://www.ncbi.nlm.nih.gov/pubmed/?term=Podulka+J%2C+Barrett+M%2C+Jiang+J%2C+Steiner++C.++Readmissions+following+hospitalization+for+chronic+vs+acute+conditions+2008.+HCUP+Statistical+brief+%23127%2C++Rockvale%2C2C+MD%3A+Agency+for+Healthcare+Research+and+Quality%2C+2012. Accessed June 17, 2014.
3. Wier LM, Barrett ML, Steiner C, et al. All cause readmissions by payer and age, 2008. HCUP statistical brief #115. Rockville (MD): Agency for Healthcare Research and Quality; 2011. Available at: http://www.hcup-us.ahrp.gov/reports/statbriefs/sb115.pdf.
4. Healthcare.gov. Patient Protection and Affordability Care Act. Available at: https://www.healthcare.gov/where-can-i-read-the-affordable-care-act/. Accessed July 10, 2014.
5. Centers for Medicare & Medicaid Services, US Department of Health & Human Services. Available at: http://www.cms.gov/Research-Statistics-Data-and-Systems/Statistics-Trends-and-Reports/CMS-Statistics-Reference-Booklet/Downloads/CMS_Stats_2013_final.pdf. Accessed August 4, 2014.
6. Rau J. Medicare revises hospitals' readmissions penalties. Kaiser Health News 2012. Available at: http://www.kaiserhealthnews.org/Stories/2012/October/03/medicare-revises-readmissions+penalties.aspx. Accessed June 30, 2014.
7. Hospital Quality Alliance. Vital new quality data on hospital readmission rates available on hospital compare website. 2009. Available at: http://www.hospitalquality-alliance.org/hospitalqualityalliance/files/090709pressrelease.pdf. Accessed June 20, 2014.
8. Bradley EH, Curry L, Horwitz LI, et al. Contemporary evidence about hospital strategies for reducing 30-day readmissions: a national study. J Am Coll Cardiol 2012;60:607–14. http://dx.doi.org/10.1016/j.jacc.2012.03.067.
9. Mandell LA, Wunderink RG, Anzueto A, et al. Infectious Diseases Society of America/American Thoracic Society consensus guidelines on the management of community-acquired pneumonia in adults. Clin Infect Dis 2007;44:S27–72. http://dx.doi.org/10.1086/511159.
10. Jweinat JJ. Hospital readmissions under the spotlight. J Healthc Manag 2010;55(4): 252–64. Available at: http://www.ncbi.nlm.nih.gov/pubmed/?term=Jweinat+JJ.+Hospital+readmissions+under+the+spotlight.+J+Healthc+Manag.+2010. Accessed July 17, 2014.
11. Shorr AF, Marya D, Zilberberg RR, et al. Remission following hospitalization for pneumonia: the impact of pneumonia type and its implication for hospitals. Clin Infect Dis 2013;1–6. http://dx.doi.org/10.1093/cid/cit254.

12. Fontanarosa PB, McNutt RA. Revisiting hospital readmissions. JAMA 2013; 309(4):398–400. http://dx.doi.org/10.1001/jama.2013.42.
13. Vest JR, Gamm LD, Oxford BA, et al. Determinants of preventable readmissions in the United States: a systemic review. Implement Sci 2010;5:88. http://dx.doi.org/10.1186/1748-5908-5-88.
14. Balaban RB, Weissman JS, Samuel PA, et al. Redefining and redesigning hospital discharge to enhance patient care: a randomized controlled study. J Gen Intern Med 2008;23(8):1228–33. http://dx.doi.org/10.1007/s11606-008-0618-9.
15. Kripalani S, LeFevre F, Phillips CO, et al. Deficits in communication and information transfer between hospital-based and primary care physicians: implications for patient safety and continuity of care. JAMA 2007;297(8):831–41. Available at: http://www.ncbi.nlm.nih.gov/pubmed/?term=Kripalani+S%2C+LeFevre+F%2C+Phillips+CO%2C+Williams+MV%2C+Basaviah+P%2C+Baker+DW.++Deficits+in+communication+and+information+transfer+between+hospital-based+and+primary+care+physicians%3A+implications+for+patient+safety+and+continuity+of+care.+JAMA. Accessed June 17, 2014.
16. Coleman EA, Smith JD, Frank JC, et al. Development and testing of a measure designed to assess the quality of care transitions. Int J Integr Care 2002;2:e02. Available at: http://www.ncbi.nlm.nih.gov/pubmed/?term=Coleman+EA%2C+Smith+JD%2C+Frank+JC%2C+Eilertsen+TB%2C+Thiare+JN%2C+Kramer+AM.++Development+and+testing+of+a+measure+designed+to+assess+the+quality+of+care+transitions.+Int+J+Integr+Care.+2002%3B2%3Ae02. Accessed July 19, 2014.
17. Harrison PL, Hara PA, Pope JE, et al. The impact of postdischarge telephonic follow-up on hospital readmissions. Popul Health Manag 2011;14(1):27–32. http://dx.doi.org/10.1089/pop.2009.0076.
18. Epstein AM. Revisiting readmissions—changing the incentives for shared accountability. N Engl J Med 2009;360(14):1457–9. http://dx.doi.org/10.1056/NEJMe0901006.
19. Forster AJ, Murff HJ, Peterson JF, et al. The incidence and severity of adverse events affecting patients after discharge from the hospital. Ann Intern Med 2003;138:161–7.
20. Moore C, McGinn T, Halm E. Tying up loose ends discharging patients with unresolved medical issues. Arch Intern Med 2007;167:1305–11. Available at: http://www.ncbi.nlm.nih.gov/pubmed/?term=Moore+C%2C+McGinn+T%2C+Halm+E.+(2007)+Tying+up+loose+ends+discharging+patients+with+unresolved+medical+issues.+Arch+Intern+Med.+2007%3B+167%3A+1305-11. Accessed June 14, 2014.
21. Van Walraven C, Seth R, Austin PC, et al. Effect of discharge summary availability during post discharge visits on hospital readmission. J Gen Intern Med 2002; 17(3):186–92. Available at: http://www.ncbi.nlm.nih.gov/pubmed/?term=Van+Walraven+C%2C+Seth+R%2C+Austin+PC%2C+Laupacis+A.+Effect+of+discharge+summary+availability+during+post+discharge+visits+on+hospital+readmission.++J+Gen+Intern+Med.+2002%3B+17(3)%3A+186-92. Accessed June 14, 2014.
22. Roy CL, Poon EG, Karson AS, et al. Patient safety concerns arising from test results that return after hospital discharge. Ann Intern Med 2005;143(2): 121–8.
23. Adams CJ, Stephens K, Whiteman K, et al. Implementation of the re-engineered discharge (RED) Toolkit to decrease all-cause readmission rates at a rural

community hospital. Qual Manag Health Care 2014;23(3):169–77. http://dx.doi.org/10.1097/QMH.0000000000000032.

24. Coleman EA, Smith JD, Raha D, et al. Posthospital medication discrepancies: prevalence and contributing factors. Arch Intern Med 2005;165(16):1842–7. Available at: http://www.ncbi.nlm.nih.gov/pubmed/?term=Coleman+EA%2C+Smith+JD%2C+Raha+D%2C+Min+SJ.+Posthospital+medication+discrepancies%3A+prevalence+and+contributing+factors.++Archives+of++Internal+Medicine.++2005%3B. Accessed August 3, 2014.

25. Lalonde L, Lampron AM, Vanier MC, et al. Effectiveness of a medication discharge plan for transitions of care from hospital to outpatient settings. Am J Health Syst Pharm 2008;65:1451–7. http://dx.doi.org/10.2146/ajhp070565.

26. Broockvar KS, Carlson-LaCorte H, Giambanco V, et al. Medication reconciliation for reducing drug-discrepancy adverse events. Am J Geriatr Pharmacother 2006; 4(3):236–43.

27. Varkey P, Cunningham J, Bispring DS. Improving medication reconciliation in the outpatient setting. Jt Comm J Qual Patient Saf 2007;33(5):286–92. Available at: http://www.ncbi.nlm.nih.gov/pubmed/?term=Varkey+P%2C+Cunningham+J%2C+Bispring+DS.+Improving+medication+reconciliation+in+the+outpatient+setting.+Joint+Commission+Journal+on+Quality+and+Patient+Safety.+2007%3B+33(5)%3A286-92. Accessed July 19, 2014.

28. Jackevicius CA, Tu JV, Demers V, et al. Cardiovascular outcomes after a change in prescription policy for clopidogrel. N Engl J Med 2008;359:1802–10. http://dx.doi.org/10.1056/NEJMsa0803410.

29. Rowe WS, Yaffe MJ, Peoler C, et al. Variables impacting on patients' perceptions of discharge from short stay hospitalization or same day surgery. Health Soc Care Community 2000;8:362–71. Available at: http://www.ncbi.nlm.nih.gov/pubmed/11560706. Accessed July 19, 2014.

30. Sanderson BK, Thompson J, Brown TM, et al. Assessing patient recall of discharge instructions for acute myocardial infarction. J Healthc Qual 2009;6: 25–34.

31. Bobay KL, Jerofke TA, Yakusheva O. Age related differences in perception of quality of discharge teaching and readiness for hospital discharge. Geriatr Nurs 2010;31(3):178–87. http://dx.doi.org/10.1016/j.gerinurse.2010.03.005.

32. Naylor MD, Stephens C, Bowles KH, et al. Cognitively impaired older adults from hospital to home. Am J Nurs 2005;105:52–61. Available at: http://www.ncbi.nlm.nih.gov/pubmed/?term=Naylor+MD%2C+Stephens+C%2C+Bowles+KH+et+al.+Cognitively+impaired+older+adults+from+hospital+to+home.+Am+J+Nurs.+2005%3B+105%3A52-61. Accessed July 19, 2014.

33. Ho MP, Tsai TT, Maddox TM, et al. Delays in filling clopidogrel prescription after hospital discharge and adverse outcomes after drug-eluting stent placement implications for transitions of care. Circ Cardiovasc Qual Outcomes 2010;3: 261–6. http://dx.doi.org/10.1161/CIRCOUTCOMES.109.902031.

34. Institute of Medicine. Health literacy: a prescription to end confusion. Washington, DC: National Academic Press; 2004.

35. Kutner M, Greenberg E, Yin Y, et al. Results from the 2003 National Assessment of Adult Literacy. Washington, DC: National Center for Education Statistics: US Department of Education; 2006.

36. Berkman ND, Sheridan SL, Donahue KE, et al. Low health literacy and health outcomes: an updated systematic review. Ann Intern Med 2011;155:97–107. http://dx.doi.org/10.7326/0003-4819-155-2-201107190-00005.

37. Townsend MS. Patient driven education materials: low literate adults increase understanding of health messages and improve compliance. Nurs Clin North Am 2011;46:367–78. http://dx.doi.org/10.1016/j.cnur.2011.05.011.

38. Coleman EA, Chugh A, Williams MV, et al. Understanding and execution of discharge instructions. Am J Med Qual 2013;28(5):383–91. http://dx.doi.org/10.1177/1062860612472931.

39. Williams MV, Baker DW, Parker RM, et al. Relationship of functional health literacy to patients' knowledge of their chronic disease: a study of patients with hypertension and diabetes. Arch Intern Med 1998;158:166–72. Available at: http://www.ncbi.nlm.nih.gov/pubmed/?term=Williams+MV%2C+Baker+DW%2C+Parker%2C+RM%2C+Nurss+JR.++Relationship+of+functional+health+literacy+to+patients%E2%80%99+knowledge+of+their+chronic+disease%3A+a+study+of+patients+with+hypertension+and+diabetes.+Arch+Intern+Med.+1998%3B+158%3A166-72. Accessed July 18, 2014.

40. Scott T, Gazmararian JA, Williams M, et al. Health literacy and preventive health care use among Medicare enrollees in a managed care organization. Med Care 2002;22(40):395–404.

41. Buckley BA, McCarthy DM, Forth VE, et al. Patient input into the development and enhancement of ED discharge instructions: a focus group study. J Emerg Nurs 2012;1–7. http://dx.doi.org/10.1016/j.jen2011.12.018.

42. The Joint Commission Transitions of Care: The need for a more effective approach to continuing patient care. Available at: http://www.jointcommission.org/assets/1/18/hot_topics_transitions_of_care.pdf. Accessed August 1, 2014.

43. Dracup KA, Meleis AI. Compliance: an interactional approach. Nurs Res 1982;31(1):31–6. Available at: http://www.ncbi.nlm.nih.gov/pubmed/?term=Dracup+KA%2C+Meleis+AI.+Compliance%3A+an+interactional+approach.+Nurs+Res.+1982%3B+31(1)%3A31-6. Accessed July 6, 2014.

44. Bissonnette JM. Adherence: a concept analysis. J Adv Nurs 2008;63(6):634–43. http://dx.doi.org/10.1111/j.1365-2648.2008.04745.x.

45. Flagg AJ. Patient/provider concordance: instrument development [dissertation]. San Antonio (TX): The University of Texas Health Science Center at San Antonio; 2010.

46. Schnipper JL, Kirwin JL, Cotugno MC, et al. Role of pharmacist counseling in preventing adverse drug events after hospitalization. Arch Intern Med 2006;166(5):565–71.

47. McHugh MD, Ma C. Hospital nursing and 30-day readmissions among Medicare patients with heart failure, acute myocardial infarction, and pneumonia. Med Care 2013;51(1):52–9. http://dx.doi.org/10.1097/MLR.0b013e3182763284.

48. Foust JB, Vuckovic N, Henriquez E. Hospital to home health care transition: patient, caregiver, and clinical perspectives. West J Nurs Res 2012;34(2):194–212. http://dx.doi.org/10.1177/0193945911400448.

49. Bowles KH, Foust JB, Naylor MD. Hospital discharge referral decision making: a multidisciplinary perspective. Appl Nurs Res 2003;16(3):134–43. Available at: http://www.ncbi.nlm.nih.gov/pubmed/?term=Bowles+KH%2C+Foust+JB%2C+Naylor+MD.+Hospital+discharge+referral+decision+making%3A+A+multidisiciplinary+perspective.+Applied+Nursing+Research.+2003%3B+16+(3)%2C+134-143. Accessed June 19, 2014.

50. Engel KG, Heisler M, Smith DM, et al. Patient comprehension of emergency department care and instructions: are patients aware of when they do not understand? Ann Emerg Med 2009;53:454–61.e15. http://dx.doi.org/10.1016/j.annemergmed.2008.05.016.

51. Showlater JW, Rafferty C, Swallow N, et al. Effect of standardized electronic discharge instructions on post-discharge hospital utilization. J Gen Intern Med 2011;26(7):718–23. http://dx.doi.org/10.1007/s11606-011-1712-y.

52. Veronovici NR, Lasiuk GC, Rempel GR, et al. Discharge education to promote self-management following cardiovascular surgery: an integrative review. Eur J Cardiovasc Nurs 2014;13(1):22–31. http://dx.doi.org/10.1177/1474515113504863.

53. Stevens S, Thomas SP. Recovery of midlife women from myocardial infarction. Health Care Women Int 2012;33:1096–113. http://dx.doi.org/10.1080/07399332.2012.684815.

54. Gatson M. The psychological care of patients following a myocardial infarction. Prof Nurse 2003;18:625–65. Available at: http://www.ncbi.nlm.nih.gov/pubmed/12861821. Accessed June14, 2014.

55. Karliner LS, Auerbach A, Napoles A, et al. Language barriers and understanding of hospital discharge instructions. Med Care 2012;50(4):283–9. http://dx.doi.org/10.1097/MLR.0b013e318249c949.

56. Walker PC, Bernstein SJ, Jones JN, et al. Impact of a pharmacist-facilitated hospital discharge program: a quasi-experimental study. Arch Intern Med 2009;169(21):2003–10. http://dx.doi.org/10.1001/archinternmed.2009.398.

57. Wong KW, Wong FK, Chan MF. Effects of nurse-initiated telephone follow-up on self-efficacy among patients. J Adv Nurs 2005;49(2):210–22. Available at: http://www.ncbi.nlm.nih.gov/pubmed/?term=Wong+KW%2C+Wong+FKY%2C+Chan+MF.++Effects+of+nurse-initiated+telephone+follow-up+on+self-efficacy+among+patients.+Journal+of+Advanced+Nursing.+2005. Accessed June 14, 2014.

58. Makaryus AN, Friedman EA. Patient's understanding of their treatment plans and diagnosis at discharge. Mayo Clin Proc 2005;80(8):991–4. Available at: http://www.ncbi.nlm.nih.gov/pubmed/?term=Makaryus+AN%2C+Friedman+EA.+Patient%E2%80%99s+understanding+of+their+treatment+plans+and+diagnosis+at+discharge.+Mayo+Clin+Proc%2C+2005%3B+80(8)%3A+991-994. Accessed June 14, 2014.

59. Alikari V, Zyga S. Conceptual analysis of patient compliance in treatment. Health Sci J 2014;8(2):179. Available at: http://connection.ebscohost.com/c/articles/95432725/conceptual-analysis-patient-compliance-treatment. Accessed June 19, 2014.

60. Centers for Medicare & Medicaid Services. 2014. Available at: http://www.cms.gov/Medicare/Medicare-General-Information/Telehealth/index.html. Accessed August 1, 2014.

61. American Telemedicine Association. State Medicaid best practice, remote patient monitoring and home video visits. 2013. p. 1–11. Available at: http://www.americantelemed.org/docs/default-source/policy/state-medicaid-best-practice--remote-patient-monitoring-and-home-video-visits.pdf?sfvrsn=6. Accessed June 18, 2014.

62. Stuckey M, Fulkerson R, Read E, et al. Remote monitoring technologies for the prevention of metabolic syndrome: the Diabetes and Technology for Increased Activity (DaTA) study. J Diabetes Sci Technol 2011;5(4):936–44.

63. Institute of Medicine. The future of nursing: leading change, advancing health. Washington, DC: National Academies Press; 2010.

64. Meyers L, Gibbs D, Thacker M, et al. Building a telehealth network through collaboration: the story of the Nebraska statewide Telehealth Network. Crit Care Nurs Q 2012;35(4):346–52. http://dx.doi.org/10.1097/CNQ.0b013e318266bed1.

65. Bowles KH, Baugh AC. Applying research evidence to optimize telehomecare. J Cardiovasc Nurs 2007;22:5–15.

66. Society of Hospital Medicine. Quality and innovation. 2014. Available at: http://www.hospitalmedicine.org/web/Quality_Innovation/Mentored_Implementatin/Project_BOOST/About_BOOST.aspx. Accessed August 1, 2014.
67. Agency for Healthcare Research and Quality. Advancing excellence in health care. Rockville (MD): National Healthcare Quality & Disparities Reports; 2013. Publication No 12(13)-0084. Available at: http://www.ahrq.gov/professionals/system/hospital/red/toolkit//redtoolkit.pdf. Accessed August 1, 2014.
68. Huffman MH. Health coaching. Home Healthc Nurse 2009;27(8):490–6.
69. Cloonan P, Wood J, Riley JB. Reducing 30-day readmissions health literacy strategies. J Nurs Adm 2013;43:382–7. http://dx.doi.org/10.1097/NNA.0b013e31829d6082.
70. Bell CM, Schnipper JL, Auerbach AD, et al. Association of communication between hospital-based physicians and primary care providers with patient outcomes. J Gen Intern Med 2009;24:381–6.

Culture of Safety

Kristen Hershey, PhD(c), MSN, RN, CNE

KEYWORDS

- Culture of safety • Just culture • Patient safety

KEY POINTS

- A culture of safety is necessary for health care to achieve the success of high-reliability organizations (organizations that have high potential for error, but few adverse outcomes).
- High-reliability organizations have open reporting of error to learn from mistakes, an area that is lacking in health care systems.
- Nurses can take part in transforming the culture at their institution by learning from safety culture principles.

INTRODUCTION

One of the core ethical principles of nursing care is nonmaleficence, or the imperative to do no harm.[1] However, the reality of health care does not always meet this ideal. The problem of health care error was first brought to light by the Institute of Medicine's (IOM) groundbreaking report, *To Err is Human*.[2] In this report,[2] the IOM suggested that health care error was responsible for as many as 98,000 deaths annually in the United States. The IOM recommended that health care change from an individual blame response to error to a system-focused approach. The IOM drew on the history of other high-risk industries to advocate for a culture of safety, in which errors and near misses could be used as opportunities to learn and improve.[2] Many efforts have been initiated since the IOM's 2000 report to decrease the incidence of health care error. However, health care has not yet achieved the success of other industries with high potential for error, such as aviation or the nuclear industry.[3] Chassin and Loeb report that "no hospitals or health care systems have achieved consistent excellence throughout their institutions," and the rate of health care error may be even higher than originally estimated.[3] The Institute for Healthcare Improvement (IHI) estimates that there are 40 to 50 incidents of patient harm per 100 admissions,[4] a frequency that clearly indicates the need for improvement. In this article, the role played by a safe and just culture in promoting safe patient care is described. Information for frontline nurses to enhance the safety culture at their facility and to improve their response to error is also reviewed.

Disclosure: none.
Austin Peay State University, 601 College Street, Clarksville, TN 37044, USA
E-mail address: hersheyk@apsu.edu

Nurs Clin N Am 50 (2015) 139–152
http://dx.doi.org/10.1016/j.cnur.2014.10.011   nursing.theclinics.com

SAFETY CULTURE
High-Reliability Organizations

The Agency for Healthcare Research and Quality (AHRQ) reports that the term culture of safety originated with high-reliability organizations (HROs).[5] An HRO is an organization that operates with a high potential for error but has few adverse outcomes.[6] The nuclear and aviation industries are among the more commonly referenced HROs. The comparison of health care and aviation is useful in showing the disparity between HROs and health care institutions. James[7] estimated that the death rate in the United States caused by hospital-associated preventable harm may be as high as 400,000 people annually. Weick and Sutcliffe[6] pointed out that this number is the equivalent of 2 747 passenger jets full of people crashing every day of the year. A situation like this would be untenable to the aviation industry, yet in health care it is simply business as usual.

According to Weick and Sutcliffe, characteristics of HROs include:

- Preoccupation with failure (being highly aware of all error and potential for error)
- Reluctance to simplify (understanding and appreciating the complexity of the work)
- Sensitivity to operations (awareness of the frontline work being done)
- Commitment to resilience (the capacity to identify, contain, and improve from error)
- Deference to expertise (allowing frontline workers to make decisions and avoiding rigid hierarchies)[6]

These characteristics of HROs are enabled and supported by mutual trust, which Chassin and Loeb[3] identify as a key component of a safety culture.

Characteristics of a Safety Culture

According to the Joint Commission, a safety culture is one that promotes trust and empowers staff to report errors, near misses, and risks. The Joint Commission defines safety culture in health care as "the summary of knowledge, attitudes, behaviors, and beliefs that staff share about the primary importance of the well-being and care of the patients they serve, supported by systems and structures that reinforce the focus on patient safety."[8] It is important to note the emphasis of a safety culture on systems, not only on individual health care workers. However, individual workers affect the safety culture by the contribution of their own attitudes, knowledge, and behaviors.

The system focus in safety culture is key, because problems with safety often originate from the system itself. Reason[9] refers to individual error as active error and systems error as latent error.[9] An active error is one that occurs at the sharp end of health care. This is an error with immediate consequences, committed by a frontline worker. An example is a nurse who failed to check a patient's identification and gave medication to the wrong patient. Latent errors, on the other hand, may be hidden until they combine with other factors.[9] These errors typically involve those removed from direct care, such as managers, administrators, system designers, and maintenance personnel.[9] In the example given earlier, if a faulty or cumbersome barcode scanning process contributed to the nurse not identifying the patient, a system or latent error would be at work. Reason[9] indicates that latent errors are the greatest threat to complex systems and are the root cause of most error. Reason's model for error is often referred to as the Swiss cheese model. Holes represent places where the potential for error exists, but these are often offset by other system and individual defenses. Error reaches the patient only when the holes line up and defenses fail.

Chassin and Loeb[3] identified 3 simple, central attributes of safety culture: trust, report, and improve. In this vision of safety culture, the 3 central attributes are reinforced by one another. As workers trust their peers and management, they feel more comfortable and supported in reporting unsafe conditions. Trust and reporting are strengthened when measures are taken to correct unsafe conditions, and workers are notified of improvements being made.[3] Trust is lacking in many health care systems, which leads to underreporting of error and potential error. The 2013 National Healthcare Quality Report (NHQR) indicates that most health care workers believe that mistakes will be held against them.[10] The report also indicates that more than 50% of health care workers reported no adverse events at their facility in the last 12 months.[10] Given the known rates of health care error, it is highly likely that underreporting accounts for the low number of reported events.

Frankel and colleagues[11] have indicated that accountability is a key factor in safety culture. Accountability occurs when workers are not only able to admit their own concerns but also comfortable monitoring the work of those around them. The simple issue of hand hygiene is 1 example of how accountability can be improved. A recent Centers for Disease Control and Prevention study[12] found that there are more than 200 deaths daily in the United States from hospital-associated infection. This 1 type of adverse event alone accounts for approximately 75,000 preventable deaths per year. Hand hygiene compliance is the most effective way to prevent this type of error, yet compliance rates average only 40%.[3] The Joint Commission Center for Transforming Healthcare lists accountability as a key strategy to help promote hand hygiene compliance.[13] They recommend that every employee, including management, physicians, housekeepers, and chaplains, be held accountable for performing hand hygiene at the appropriate time, as well as helping to monitor the hand hygiene of other employees.[13] Just in time coaching is 1 approach to increasing accountability. For those without access to hospital training on these types of strategies, You Tube videos can help to show this type of coaching in action. The Children's Hospital of Alabama, for example, has a video that models appropriate and inappropriate just in time coaching for health care workers who are not complying with hand hygiene.[14] However, holding others accountable is only 1 facet of accountability. Health care workers must also be willing to accept coaching from others, including patients and families. Both giving and receiving feedback on safety issues is an essential part of safety culture.

Benefits of Creating a Safety Culture

A culture of safety shows a commitment to consistently safe operations, encourages error and near miss reporting, promotes collaboration to find solutions to safety problems, and commits resources to address safety concerns.[5] Instinctively, most health care workers understand that this type of culture improves patient safety and patient outcomes. However, research is still limited as to the effect that culture has on patient safety and outcomes. Part of the problem lies in how progress is measured and tracked. As indicated earlier, the rate of health care error is unknown, and error is probably underreported.[10] Because a safety culture promotes transparency and open reporting, it is likely that reported rates of error and harm will increase initially as safety culture improves. A study by Smits and colleagues[15] confirmed this theory, finding that units that scored higher in certain dimensions of safety culture reported more medication-related events.

Specific and consistent measurement of health care harm is a crucial step in determining the effectiveness of interventions and the impact of a safety culture. The NHQR includes the following measures for the hospital setting:

- Hospital-acquired conditions (includes adverse drug events, falls, pressure ulcers, and other conditions)

- Postoperative sepsis
- Catheter-associated urinary tract infections
- Central line–associated bloodstream infections (CLABSIs)
- Surgical site infection
- Mechanical events associated with central lines
- Obstetric trauma[10]

The Joint Commission[16] concurs that research on the link between culture and patient outcomes is limited and inconclusive; however, they contend that individual case studies of hospitals with improved safety culture indicate that the benefits may be substantial. In 1 instance, they discuss how a hospital system's emphasis on safety culture led to a dramatic decrease in adverse events. An improved focus on safety led to a reduction in 1 type of adverse event, pressure ulcers, to 94% less than the national average.[16]

With Medicare and Medicaid reimbursements being tied to factors such as readmissions and preventable complications, improvements in patient safety are not only good for the patient, they are good for the hospital's bottom line. Improved safety culture has the potential to maximize reimbursement rates, decrease litigation, reduce staff turnover, minimize workman's compensation claims, and improve insurance rates, among other monetary benefits.[16] Frontline nurses can highlight the financial implications of a safety culture when discussing potential safety improvements with management and administration. By appealing to the business case for safety culture, nurses can help to create a safer and more effective health care environment for themselves and their patients.

Measurement of Safety Culture

The Joint Commission[16] requires that hospitals and other organizations they accredit measure their culture of safety regularly. Several tools exist to measure safety culture, but one of the most commonly used measures is the Hospital Survey on Patient Safety Culture (HSOPSC) developed for the AHRQ. The HSOPSC measures safety culture across 12 dimensions:

- Teamwork within units
- Supervisor/manager expectations and actions promoting safety
- Organizational learning and continuous improvement
- Management support for patient safety
- Overall perceptions of patient safety
- Feedback and communication about error
- Communication openness
- Frequency of events reported
- Teamwork across units
- Staffing
- Handoffs and transitions
- Nonpunitive response to errors[17]

The HSOPSC also looks at the overall patient safety grade and number of events reported in the last 12 months.[17]

Composite results for participating hospitals are available at the AHRQ Web site, although few hospitals publish their individual results, and results are often not reported back to hospital staff. Across hospitals, scores are high in areas such as teamwork within units, supervisor expectations, and organizational learning, which range from 81% to 73% positive, respectively.[18] Safety culture dimensions in need of improvement are nonpunitive response to error; handoffs and transitions; and staffing, which range from 44% to 55% positive.[18] These 3 areas in greatest need of improvement are discussed in greater detail in the next section.

ENHANCING SAFETY CULTURE
Nonpunitive Response to Error and a Just Culture

Although a key component of a safety culture is trust, trust cannot be achieved without the assurance that workers will be treated fairly. When the responsibility for latent error falls exclusively on the frontline worker, a safety culture is hindered. The concept of a just culture is used to refer to a fair and reasonable response to error, or what is sometimes referred to as a nonpunitive response to error. The American Nurses Association (ANA) has issued a position statement[19] supporting the concept of just culture in health care and recommending that direct-care nurses advocate for its use in their institutions.

Reason[9] describes a just culture as one in which there is a clear, collective understanding of the line between blameless and blameworthy actions. According to Reason, error occurs when a planned sequence of activities fails to achieve an intended outcome. This situation can occur either because the plan itself was faulty or because there was a problem in the execution of the plan. Failures of execution take the form of slips or lapses; errors in judgment or planning are termed mistakes.[9] Slips, lapses, and mistakes occur every day, and cannot be eliminated completely.[20] An example of a failure of execution is a nurse who intends to remove medication for 1 patient, but types another patient's name into the medication dispensing system. An example of a failure of planning, or a mistake, is not identifying the need to hold a patient's aspirin before surgery. System defenses should be in place to prevent this type of human error from causing harm.[9] Barcode scanners and automatic alerts are examples of defenses to prevent human error.

Marx[20] contended that punishment for slips, lapses, and mistakes has little to no impact on those who did not intend to make an error. In health care, Marx reports, our current system of discipline often places more emphasis on the outcome of the error, rather than the action behind it. An error in which a patient is seriously harmed, even if it was caused by a simple slip or lapse, results in discipline to the health care provider more than reckless conduct that did not result in harm.[20] For example, a nurse who administered a harmful dose of a medication to a patient because of a lapse in attention may be disciplined more harshly than a nurse who administered aspirin instead of acetaminophen and deliberately disregarded safety procedures.

Marx[20] advises a system that bases disciplinary action on the type of behavior rather than the outcome of the error. The 4 types of behavior that Marx identifies are human error, negligence, intentional rule violations, and reckless conduct.[20] As mentioned earlier, human error is not considered an action that can be reduced by punishment. Reporting and tracking incidences of human error may help to create more robust safety systems to prevent such error from causing harm. The second type of behavior, negligence, occurs when an individual should have been aware of the risk but failed to exercise expected care.[20] Marx contends that there are arguments for and against punishing those who have been negligent. However, in HROs, there is extensive research to support a nonpunitive response to this type of error.[20] Intentional rule violations can also provide information to make systems more robust, if there is an open system of reporting. Marx[20] states that in rule-based professions such as medicine and aviation there are many instances in which overlapping rules do not fit the specific circumstances of the job being performed.

Flawed procedures might be overlooked if individuals guilty of work-arounds do not feel comfortable reporting their actions. For example, if nurses are routinely scanning patient barcodes at the nurses' station instead of at the bedside because an insufficient number of mobile computer workstations, the latent issue of inadequate resources should be addressed rather than disciplining the behavior. The final type of behavior, recklessness, is defined as a "conscious disregard of substantial and unjustifiable risk"[20] and must be dealt with by disciplinary action. Even although the term nonpunitive is used frequently in safety culture, experts agree that certain behaviors do require a punitive response. Chassin and Loeb[3] contend that the concept of trust in a safety culture is reinforced when blameworthy acts are dealt with appropriately. Marx also recognizes that even less serious behaviors, such as error, negligence, and rule violations, may require disciplinary measures when they are repetitive. These behaviors also might require remediation, coaching, mentoring, and analyzing the individual's work environment for conditions that promote error.[20]

A just culture is one that promotes trust and enhances reporting. Responding to error by analyzing the behavior, rather than the result, as well as examining system or latent causes for error, gives frontline workers the security to report problems. A safety culture cannot exist without a just culture. A culture that is overly harsh or punitive simply results in errors being hidden and underreported. Safety is 1 area in which the idiom "no news is good news" does not apply.

Handoffs and Transitions

A patient transition occurs when a patient moves from one care setting to another, or from the care of one health care worker to another. Handoffs are the communication between health care workers during these transitions. The period of handoffs and transitions has been documented as an especially dangerous time for patients. It has been estimated that up to 80% of serious medical errors may be related to miscommunication during health care provider handoffs.[21]

The HSOPSC items that measure handoffs and transitions examine health care workers' impression that things fall between the cracks when patients are transferred, that shift changes are problematic for patients, and that important information is lost during shift change or when transferring patients between units.[17] The primary issues affecting handoffs and transitions are communication and teamwork. In reviews of handoff communication, both physicians and nurses are found to omit necessary information 30% or 40% of the time[22,23] and communicate incorrect information approximately 13% of the time.[22] Hilligoss and Cohen[24] indicate that handoffs between units may be even more complex than handoffs within units. Among the reasons for the increase in complexity in between unit handoffs are the lack of established relationships (infrequent communication), power imbalances among units, and the fact that a change in patient status (rather than a preestablished shift change) triggered the transition.

Handoff communication can be improved, but a variety of tools and resources are necessary. Welsh and colleagues[25] point out that there are 21 identified strategies from HROs for reporting processes, but most are not used in health care. Among those most recommended in health care handoffs are face-to-face discussions, opportunities to ask questions, and structured forms. System safeguards can also play a role in handoff communication. Providing staff with shift reports populated with pertinent data from the electronic medical record including up-to-date laboratory results, vital sign trends, intake/output, and other necessary results helps to avoid reliance on memory, which can enhance the accuracy and completeness of a report.[22,25] Structured formats for handoffs include SBAR (situation, background, assessment, and recommendation), PACE (patient/problem, assessment/actions, continuing/ changes, and evaluation), and others.[25] Using a standardized format helps to keep the report on track, providing a report that is both complete and succinct.

Teamwork plays an important role in communication among caregivers. Leape and colleagues[26] indicate that a problem with the current health care culture is that practice occurs in silos, in which nurses, physicians, pharmacists, and others work on their own area, with little communication or teamwork. The Joint Commission warns that poor communication, including intimidating and disruptive behavior, can undermine a culture of safety.[27,28] They state that these behaviors can include refusing to answer questions or impatience with questions, not returning phone calls or pages, and responding condescendingly.[27] Most health care workers have either experienced or witnessed this type of behavior, indicating that it is pervasive in the health care culture.[27] Zero tolerance for disruptive behavior should be in place within institutions. Management and administration should be made aware of all behavior that undermines patient safety. One method that has been recommended to empower staff to speak up is CUS, an acronym for "I am concerned, I am uncomfortable, this is a safety issue."[16] When any staff member speaks up using this type of language, all members of the health care team should listen to their concerns.

Safe Staffing

The HSOPSC items that measure staffing include statements such a: "We have enough staff to handle the workload," "Staff work longer hours than is best for patient care," and "We work in 'crisis' mode." Also included in the HSOPSC is an item related to the use of temporary staff.[17] The Joint Commission recognizes that there is a clear, documented link between insufficient staffing, excessive workloads, worker fatigue, and adverse events. It is reported that nurses who work shifts longer than 12.5 hours are 3 times more likely to make a patient care error.[29] The Joint Commission indicates that staff should be encouraged to report concerns about workplace fatigue and consulted when designing work schedules.[29]

The ANA has introduced the Registered Nurse Safe Staffing Act (H.R. 876/S. 58), which would create legislation requiring hospitals to staff appropriately. Rather than mandated ratios, this act would require individualized unit staffing plans. These plans would be developed by hospital committees made up of more than half direct-care nurses, to ensure that the realities of patient care are taken into account. This legislation would also prohibit nurses from being floated to units in which they are not trained.[30] The ANA indicates that the outcome of this type of legislation would be decreased hospital deaths and adverse events, retaining qualified nurses, and decreasing hospital costs caused by staff turnover and adverse events.[30]

The problems of fatigue and overwork do not only affect patient safety, they create risks for the nurse as well. Fatigue may affect the immune system, metabolism, and the cardiovascular system and impair judgment and performance.[29] Nurses routinely report skipping breaks and meals and working longer hours than scheduled.[29] When nurses do take a break, they often still retain responsibility for their patient, accepting interruptions to answer calls and attend to other patient care obligations.[29] These types of activities put nurses at risk for burnout and occupational injury, as well as health-related problems.[16]

The problem of inadequate staffing can be exacerbated by a culture that does not support patient safety. Leape and colleagues[26] also indicate that there is more to the relationship between safety culture and staffing than simple numbers. They state that "joy and meaning in work" are essential to transforming safety culture. Nurses indicate that the focus on documentation and record keeping, rather than patient care, leads to dissatisfaction and possibly leaving the profession.[26] However, Leape and colleagues also indicate that frontline workers are the best source for ideas on how to improve the work environment.[26] Frontline nurses can advocate for appropriate staffing, both at the unit or hospital level, as well as nationally by supporting their professional organizations and contacting their lawmakers. Nurses should be mindful of their limitations and should decline overtime or additional assignments when fatigued. Frontline nurses should be aware of their own habits and how they affect patient safety. Nurses should take scheduled breaks, practice good sleep hygiene, and encourage other nurses to do the same.[16] To ensure that nurses stay at the bedside, frontline nurses must be willing to voice their ideas about how to improve their individual work setting.

WHEN ERRORS OCCUR

Despite the best efforts and intentions of workers, errors and near misses still occur. When they do occur, it is essential that frontline nurses are aware of best practices in managing error. Two practices are discussed in this section: root-cause analysis (RCA) and supporting the second victim.

Root-Cause Analysis

RCA is a method of analyzing adverse events that originated in HROs but is now used extensively in health care organizations.[31] An RCA looks not only at individual or active errors (asking how an event occurred) but also at system or latent errors (why the event occurred).[16,31] An RCA is a complex process, which involves interviews, record review, and reconstruction of the event by a multidisciplinary team. Factors that should be considered are:

- Institutional/regulatory
- Organizational/management
- Work environment
- Team environment
- Staffing
- Task-related
- Patient characteristics[31]

Nurses involved in RCA should be prepared to look at errors and near misses through the lens of these factors, rather than just identifying the active cause of error.

Promoting open participation in RCA is difficult, because many health care workers have concerns about findings being held against them.[10] Until organizations consistently practice under the principles of just culture, the collection of aggregate data, in which no individual or institution can be identified, is 1 way to mitigate this problem. The AHRQ[10] reports that they have 76 certified Patient Safety Organizations, which collect patient safety reports, which are protected from disclosure but can be used to help learn from adverse events. The Institute for Safe Medication Practices operates a voluntary, national database for reporting medication errors and near misses. Nurses can submit their concerns directly to these types of agencies to help enhance patient safety. Although frontline nurses must be responsible for reporting error and near misses at their own institution as well, anonymous patient safety reports may provide a mechanism for action from error if institutions are focused on blame instead of change.

Everyone involved in adverse events should be involved in RCA, including patients and families. However, Leape and colleagues[26] indicate that patients are typically kept out of analysis of their own adverse events. Historically, hospital systems have discouraged health care workers from discussing mistakes with patients. However, as Leape and colleagues[26] indicate, when open acknowledgment of error is given, along with sincere apologies and a commitment to improve, law suits decrease. Nurses must advocate for patient-centered care to extend to the analysis of adverse events and near misses. Leape and colleagues[26] contend that the patient-centered idea, "nothing about me, without me" should be kept in mind when analyzing safety issues.

Discovering the how and why behind an adverse event is only the first step of an RCA. Corrective action must be implemented and communicated to affect patient safety. An example of this is the Veterans Affairs (VA) medical centers response to rates of suicide in their inpatient facilities.[10] The VA has 3 levels of action from RCAs:

- Stronger actions (simplifying processes, making physical changes)
- Intermediate actions (improving workload, using checklists)
- Weaker actions (policies, training)[10]

By implementing stronger actions, including removing environmental hazards, the risk of having a suicide in a facility decreased by 87% per quarter.[10] Frontline nurses must think about the changes that would result in improvements to safety in their own area. By using the VA example of stronger, intermediate, and weaker actions, interventions with the greatest potential for impact can be given priority.

Chassin and Loeb[3] indicate that a system that conducts analysis of errors and adverse events only is at a beginning stage of safety culture. As an organization becomes more like an HRO, near misses and other potential safety issues are also analyzed for solutions before harm occurs. Leape and colleagues[26] believe that transparency is the single most important attribute of a safety culture. Without this attribute, systems are unable to learn and improve.

The Second Victim

On April 3, 2011, Kimberly Hiatt, a pediatric intensive care nurse with 24 years of experience, took her own life.[32] Hiatt had made a medication error several months before. She administered 10 times the intended dose of calcium chloride to an infant after a misplacing a decimal point during dosage calculation.[33] The patient died 5 days later; however, it is unclear if the overdose was a contributing factor.[33] Although the hospital in which Hiatt worked reported following a just culture model, Hiatt had never had an error in 24 years of employment, and Hiatt reported and took responsibility for her error, she was still immediately escorted from the facility, placed on administrative leave, and later, fired. Further, the state Board of Nursing enacted fines and placed restrictions on her license.[32] Although the outcome of this case is extreme, the response that Kimberly Hiatt encountered after an error is not unusual. Health care workers who are involved in an error often become second victims.

The term second victim was coined by Wu in 2000 and referred to the pain and suffering that physicians face after making a health care error.[34] However, Wu acknowledged that nurses, pharmacists, and other health care workers are also vulnerable to becoming a second victim and may face additional damage because of the hierarchy of the health care system.[24] Seys and colleagues[28] reported that as many as half of all health care workers may experience being a second victim at some point in their career. Wu[34] recommended an open, compassionate response to error to assist second victims and promote patient and worker safety.

Table 1
Online patient safety resources for frontline nurses

Organization	Resources
Agency for Healthcare Research and Quality (http://www.ahrq.gov/)	A federal resource with the mission to make health care safer, higher quality, more accessible, equitable, and affordable. Resources include safety culture assessment tools such as the Hospital Survey on Patient Safety Culture; clinical tools such as the Comprehensive Unit-Based Safety Program, and guidelines for reducing specific instances of patient harm, such as CLABSI. Information is available for patients, health care workers, researchers, and policymakers
Centers for Medicare and Medicaid Services (http://www.cms.gov/)	A federal resource with the aim of better health care at lower cost and improved health. Provides resources to help understand how safety affects cost and quality of care. Links to safety resources are available through the site's *Partnership for Patients*
Institute for Healthcare Improvement (http://www.ihi.org/)	An organization with the mission to improve health and health care worldwide. Resources include white papers to help transmit new information and the IHI Open School. Open School is an outstanding resource to improve safety, understand systems, and enhance leadership. It is free to health care students, and available for a fee to organizations
Institute for Safe Medication Practices (http://www.ismp.org/)	A nonprofit organization devoted to medication error prevention and safe medication use. The Medication Errors Reporting Program (MERP) is a voluntary, confidential reporting system, which allows health care workers to report errors or potentially hazardous conditions. Data are analyzed for system-based problems. Provides medication safety alert newsletters for up-to-date information about potential medication issues
Joint Commission (http://www.jointcommission.org)	An independent, nonprofit organization best known for accrediting hospitals and other health care facilities. The Joint Commission also has a wealth of information related to national patient safety goals, sentinel events, and initiatives such as *Speak Up* to enhance patient involvement in the health care team. Many resources are available for reproduction and use in facilities free of charge
Josie King Foundation (josieking.org)	A nonprofit organization with the mission to prevent individuals from dying or being harmed by medical error. Founded by the mother of a child who died as a result of medical error, it shares this personal story as well as providing resources for families and health care workers to prevent and respond to error
Leapfrog Group (http://www.leapfroggroup.org) (hospitalsafetyscore.org)	A coalition with the goal of improving transparency, quality, and safety in hospitals. Provides a rating system, which is publically available, to give patients information on overall hospital safety grade and other safety information, such as hospital-associated infection, appropriate staffing, and other important safety and quality measures
Medically Induced Trauma Support Services (http://www.mitss.org/)	A nonprofit organization with the mission to "support healing and restore hope" for individuals involved in adverse medical events. Support services are available to health care workers, patients, and families

(continued on next page)

Table 1 (continued)	
Organization	Resources
National Patient Safety Foundation (http://www.npsf.org/)	An organization with the goal of keeping patients and those who care for them free from harm. Provides information for health care workers, including safety blogs and an online learning center (fee). Information for patients includes fact sheets on safety, a universal patient compact, and a postdischarge tool
Robert Wood Johnson Foundation (http://www.rwjf.org/)	A foundation with the goal of improving health and health care for all Americans. Although focused extensively on policy and research, reports such as *Charting Nurses' Future* provide important, pertinent information for frontline nurses

The IHI reported that hospital systems responding to a serious clinical adverse event often have no plan in place for dealing with this type of crisis. Actions are often reactive and not based on a balanced, just culture approach. Excellent tools exist through the IHI and other organizations to help managers and administrators respond to adverse events. However, for the frontline nurse, the best response may be simply providing a compassionate ear.[28,34] Seys and colleagues[28] found that second victims who were able to discuss adverse events with colleagues perceived more support, although discussing clinical error is not a common practice. Recommendations for responding to colleagues who have experienced an error include phrases such as:

- "This must be difficult. Are you okay?"
- "I believe in you"
- "You are a good nurse working in a complex environment"
- "Can we talk about it?"[28]

Overall, avoiding judgment and providing support are key. If crisis plans and support are not available at the health care institution, nurses should also be referred to employee assistance programs or organizations such as the Medically Induced Trauma Support Service or the Institute for Safe Medication Practices (**Table 1**).

Wu[34] has reported that second victims may be defensive or angry, experience stress and burnout, and even resort to alcohol or drug abuse. This situation may put the nurse at even more risk for future error. Creating a defensive environment also does not allow for the nurse at the sharp end of error to contribute to the process of RCA and puts the entire system at risk for error. Responding to second victims with openness and compassion is not only the right thing to do, it is also the safe thing to do.

CULTURE OF SAFETY RESOURCES FOR THE FRONTLINE NURSE
Online Resources

Table 1 provides a list of online culture of safety resources for frontline nurses.

Tips to Empower Safety Culture

Box 1 is a resource for frontline nurses to empower a safety culture.

Box 1
Tips for frontline nurses to improve safety culture

- Practice mindfully
- Report unsafe conditions and errors
- Communicate clearly and respectfully
- Respond to error justly
- Seek and provide feedback
- Recognize limits
- Be part of the solution

SUMMARY

In the 14 years since the publication of the IOM's *To Err is Human*, a great deal of attention has been devoted to developing a culture of safety in health care and creating HROs with consistent records of safety. However, rates of health care error are still unacceptably high and are probably underreported.[3] A top-down approach to creating a culture of safety is often advocated, with leadership and management being key to a successful safety culture. Although a culture of safety does require leadership, and culture is a collective concept, individual behaviors, beliefs, and knowledge contribute to that collective. It is, therefore, the responsibility of the individual nurse to contribute to a culture of safety.

Weick and Sutcliffe[6] delineated the characteristics of HROs that make them so successful. Overarching these characteristics is the idea of practicing mindfully. Although Weick and Sutcliffe discuss this concept primarily in relation to organizations, practicing mindfully can also be considered an overarching principle for individuals to promote safety culture. Practicing mindfully indicates an awareness of potential for error and being alert to one's environment.[6] Relying too heavily on routines, or simply taking a business as usual approach, is the opposite of practicing mindfully.[6] Nurses who practice mindfully can contribute to a culture in which mindful practice is expected and a culture of safety is reinforced.

Safety culture measurements have indicated 3 areas in greatest need of improvement: a nonpunitive response to error; handoffs and transitions; and safe staffing.[18] Frontline nurses can contribute to improvement in these area by reporting errors and near misses, including reporting to national databases that aggregate data. Nurses should be willing not only to give feedback but to receive it as well. All staff have a responsibility for safety, and nurses should be willing to accept coaching when their behaviors are not consistent with safety principles. Communication and teamwork are important aspects of safety culture, and nurses should practice communicating safely and effectively. This communication can include the use of standardized handoff tools and other systems-based approaches to improving handoff communication. Safe staffing should be advocated for at the unit, system, state, and national level. Bedside nurses must be active in their professional organizations and speak out for safe staffing. At an individual level, nurses should be aware of their limits and recognize fatigue and burnout before they cause patient harm. If errors occur, nurses should take part in RCA of the event to enhance future safety.[27] Second victims of health care error must be treated with compassion and given an opportunity to take part in making systems safer.[28,34] Frontline nurses can provide a sympathetic ear to help alleviate the consequences of second victim syndrome.[28] Nurses have an opportunity to be part of transforming culture in every area of the health care system. Those at the sharp end of care have the most to contribute to patient safety solutions and should make their voices heard.

REFERENCES

1. Tong R. New perspectives in healthcare ethics: an interdisciplinary and crosscultural approach. Upper Saddle River (NJ): Pearson; 2007.
2. Institute of Medicine. To err is human: building a safer health system. Washington, DC: National Academies Press; 2000.
3. Chassin MR, Loeb JM. High-reliability health care: getting there from here. Milbank Q 2013;91:459–90.
4. McCannon CJ, Hackbarth AD, Griffin FA. Miles to go: an introduction to the 5 million lives campaign. Jt Comm J Qual Patient Saf 2007;33:477–84.
5. Agency for Healthcare Research and Quality. Patient safety primer: safety culture. Available at: http://psnet.ahrq.gov/primer.aspx?primerID=5. Accessed August 5, 2014.
6. Weick KE, Sutcliffe KM. Managing the unexpected: assuring high performance in an age of complexity. San Francisco (CA): Jossey-Bass; 2001.
7. James J. A new evidence-based estimate of patient harms associated with hospital care. J Patient Saf 2013;9:122–8.
8. The Joint Commission Center for Transforming Healthcare. Facts about the safety culture project. 2014. Available at: http://www.centerfortransforminghealthcare.org/assets/4/6/CTH_SC_Fact_Sheet.pdf. Accessed August 5, 2014.
9. Reason J. Human error. Cambridge (United Kingdom): Cambridge University Press; 1990.
10. Agency for Healthcare Research and Quality. Highlights from the 2013 National Healthcare Quality And Disparities Reports. In: National Healthcare Quality Report. Rockville (MD): US Department of Health and Human Services; 2013. p. 147–72. Available at: http://www.ahrq.gov/research/findings/nhqrdr/nhdr13/2013nhdr.pdf.
11. Frankel AS, Leonard MW, Denham CR. Fair and just culture, team behavior, and leadership engagement: the tools to achieve high reliability. Health Serv Res 2006;41:1690–709.
12. Centers for Disease Control and Prevention. Data and statistics HAI prevalence survey 2014. Available at: http://www.cdc.gov/HAI/surveillance/. Accessed August 5, 2014.
13. The Joint Commission Center for Transforming Healthcare. Hand hygiene storyboard 2014. Available at: http://www.centerfortransforminghealthcare.org/. Accessed August 5, 2014.
14. Children's Hospital of Alabama. Just in time coaching 2012. Available at: https://www.youtube.com/watch?v=NHl3pgCMRmM. Accessed August 5, 2014.
15. Smits M, Wagner C, Spreeuwenberg P, et al. The role of patient safety culture in the causation of unintended events in hospitals. J Clin Nurs 2012;21:3392–401.
16. The Joint Commission. Improving patient and worker safety: opportunities for synergy, collaboration and innovation. Oakbrook Terrace (IL): The Joint Commission; 2012.
17. The Agency for Healthcare Research and Quality. Hospital survey on patient safety culture. Rockville (MD): US Department of Health and Human Services; 2004.

18. The Agency for Healthcare Research and Quality. Hospital survey on patient safety culture 2014 user comparative database report. Available at: http://www.ahrq.org/. Accessed August 5, 2014.

19. American Nurses Association. Position statement: just culture 2010. Available at: http://nursingworld.org/psjustculture. Accessed August 5, 2014.

20. Marx D. Patient safety and the "just culture:" a primer for health care executives. Medical event reporting system–transfusion medicine. New York: Columbia University; 2001.

21. The Joint Commission. Hot topics in healthcare: transitions of care. Available at: http://www.jointcommission.org/assets/1/18/hot_topics_transitions_of_care.pdf. Accessed August 5, 2014.

22. Maughan BC, Lei L, Cydulka RK. ED handoffs: observed practices and communication errors. Am J Emerg Med 2011;29:502–11.

23. Holly C, Poletick EB. A systematic review on the transfer of information during nurse transitions in care. J Clin Nurs 2013;23:2387–96.

24. Hilligoss B, Cohen MD. The unappreciated challenges of between unit handoffs: negotiating and coordinating across boundaries. Ann Emerg Med 2013;61: 155–60.

25. Welsh CA, Flanagan ME, Ebright P. Barriers and facilitators to nursing handoffs: recommendations for redesign. Nurs Outlook 2010;58:148–54.

26. Leape L, Berwick D, Clancy C, et al. Transforming healthcare: a safety imperative. Qual Saf Health Care 2009;18:424–8.

27. The Joint Commission. Sentinel event alert: behaviors that undermine a culture of safety. 2008. Available at: http://www.jointcommission.org/assets/1/18/SEA_40.pdf. Accessed August 5, 2014.

28. Seys D, Scott S, Wu A, et al. Supporting involved health care professionals (second victims) following an adverse health event: a literature review. Int J Nurs Stud 2013;50:678–87.

29. The Joint Commission: Sentinel event alert: health care worker fatigue and patient safety. 2011. Available at: http://www.jointcommission.org/assets/1/18/sea_48.pdf. Accessed August 5, 2014.

30. American Nurses Association. Safe staffing: the registered nurse safe staffing act H.R. 876/S. 58. Available at: http://www.nursingworld.org/SafeStaffingFactsheet.aspx. Accessed August 5, 2014.

31. Agency for Healthcare Research and Quality. Patient safety primer: root cause analysis. Available at: American Nurses Association. Safe staffing: the Registered Nurse Safe Staffing Act H.R. 876/S. 58. Available at: http://psnet.ahrq.gov/primer.aspx?primerID=10#.VASNI1vRZos.email. Accessed August 5, 2014.

32. Aleccia J. Nurse's suicide highlights the twin tragedies of medical errors. NBC; 2011. Available at: http://www.nbcnews.com/id/43529641/ns/health-health_care/t/nurses-suicide-highlights-twin-tragedies-medical-errors/#.VATTzPldUuc.

33. Caldwell SM, Hohenhaus SM. Medication errors and secondary victims. J Emerg Nurs 2011;37:562–3.

34. Wu A. Medical error: the second victim: the doctor who makes the mistake needs help too. BMJ 2000;320:726–7.

Ergonomics

Safe Patient Handling and Mobility

Beth Hallmark, PhD, RN, MSN[a],*, Patricia Mechan, PT, MPH[b], Lynne Shores, PhD, RN[a]

KEYWORDS

- Ergonomics • Safe patient handling and mobility • Nursing care related injury
- High-risk nursing tasks prevention programs
- Safe Patient Handling and Mobility: Interprofessional National Standards
- Bariatric patients • Interprofessional collaborative care

KEY POINTS

- Frontline nurses must ensure that the patient is safe, and follow current evidence-based safety standards and guidelines while protecting themselves from harm.
- The daily work of a frontline nurse requires lifting, pulling, turning, and general moving of patients. These repetitive handling and mobility tasks put them at high risk for a musculoskeletal injury.
- Frontline nurses need ceiling lifts and other state-of-the-art lift equipment for safe handling and mobility of their patients.
- Job-related injuries can be prevented by institutions implementing the 8 Safe Patient Handling and Mobility (SPHM) Interprofessional National Standards, thereby creating a culture of safety.
- Algorithms should be used for assessing patients' needs in the area of SPHM.
- Increased hospitalizations of obese patients put frontline nurses at risk for injury during general care of patients, operating room encounters, and emergency room visits.
- Considering SPHM from an interprofessional perspective, the patient is at the center of the care plan, with essential caregivers all contributing toward reaching the patient's goals. The foundation on which the care plan is built is safety and quality.

INTRODUCTION

Ergonomics intersects several areas of interest to health care providers. Ergonomics involves everything in a nurse's work environment from the design of storage areas, computer work stations, and office seating to caregiving, lifting, and patient handling methods. One very important component in the discussion surrounding ergonomics

Disclosures: None.

[a] Belmont University College of Health Sciences and Nursing, 1900 Belmont Boulevard, Nashville, TN 37212, USA; [b] Consulting, Education, & Clinical Services, Guldmann, 130 Trapelo Road, Second Floor, Belmont, MA 02478, USA

* Corresponding author.

E-mail address: beth.hallmark@belmont.edu

focuses on Safe Patient Handling and Mobility (SPHM). The aim of this review is to investigate current standards of practice in the area of SPHM in addition to outlining evidence-based recommendations for clinical practice.

HISTORY

Creating a culture of safety for patients is a prevalent goal both nationally and internationally; health care providers must ensure that the patient is safe, and follow current evidence-based safety standards and guidelines while also protecting themselves from harm. Both of these goals are a challenge for the health care team. Although the US Bureau of Labor Statistics[1] has reported a downward trend in workplace injury, musculoskeletal injuries remain a great concern for health care systems. In 2012, the US Bureau of Labor Statistics reported that more than 20,000 registered nurses suffered nonfatal work-related injuries involving days away from work while more than 37,000 nursing assistants suffered the same.[1] Approximately 20% of nursing assistants who reported an injury missed more than 31 days of work, and 24% of registered nurses missed the same amount of time.[1] "The most obvious impacts of work injury are those that are quantifiable, such as direct and indirect costs to the hospital, high turnover and staff shortage."[2] The Occupational Safety and Health Administration (OSHA) estimates that $20 billion annually are associated with the direct and indirect costs of back injuries in the health care environment.[3] In the American Nurses Association (ANA) Health and Safety Survey (2011)[4] it is reported that 62% of the 4614 nurses who responded to the survey said that they fear a disabling musculoskeletal injury. **Table 1** summarizes the health and safety concerns of nurses in 2001 and again in 2011. A disabling musculoskeletal injury continues to remain second in rank.

The concern of injury coupled with the statistics surrounding injuries to nurses and nursing assistants make this issue one that cannot be ignored. Educating health care workers and advocating for institutional policies related to SPHM is imperative.

Several organizations have been active in providing advocacy for health care workers at risk for workplace injury: The ANA, the Association of Operating Room Nurses (AORN), Veterans Affairs (VA), the Association of Safe Patient Handling

Table 1 Top 10 health and safety concerns		
Health and Safety Concerns	**2001 (%)**	**2011 (%)**
Acute/chronic effects of stress and overwork	70	74
Disabling musculoskeletal injury	59	62
Contracting an infectious disease	37	43
An on-the-job assault	25	34
Fatigue-related car accident after a shift	19	24
Getting human immunodeficiency virus or hepatitis from a needle stick	45	21
Exposure to hazardous drugs	5	10
Toxic effects from exposure to chemicals	7	9
Developing a latex allergy	21	6
Exposure to smoke from lasers or electrocautery devices	3	5

Data from American Nurses Association. ANA health and safety survey: hazards of the work environment. 2011.

Professionals, and the American Association for Safe Patient Handing and Movement are 5 very active organizations in this push for change. The last 10 to 15 years have seen significant momentum in the area of SPHM. One of the first publications was developed by experts in the Veterans Administration in 2001, a 2-part document entitled *Patient Care Ergonomics Resource Guide: Safe Patient Handling and Movement*.[5] This document was developed to improve the awareness of health care providers regarding methods to help decrease the number of job-related injuries. In 2003, the ANA launched a campaign entitled "Handle with Care," which helped "develop and implement a proactive, multi-faceted plan to promote the issue of safe patient handling and the prevention of musculoskeletal disorders among nurses in the United States."[6] During the same year OSHA published *Guidelines for Nursing Homes, Ergonomics for the Prevention of Musculoskeletal Disorders* specifically for nursing home personnel; in 2009[7] there was an updated version of this document, which is of great value to both nursing homes and inpatient facilities.

More recently in 2011, in collaboration with OSHA, the Association of Occupational Health Professionals published *Beyond Getting Started: A Resource Guide for Implementing a Safe Patient Handling Program in the Acute Care Setting*.[8] This guide focused on equipment selection and evaluation for acute care facilities. A groundbreaking interprofessional document, *Safe Patient Handling and Mobility: Interprofessional National Standards*[9] published by the ANA, but collaboratively authored by multidisciplinary expert groups, was released in 2013, and details 8 program standards related to SPHM. A companion tool, *The Implementation Guide to the SPHM Standards*,[10] considered to be the "how-to" assistance in applying the Standards to one's care setting, was published in 2013. Another important organization in the SPHM movement has been the AORN. Since 2005, when they released their first statement on worker safety, until the present the AORN lobbies for state and federal guidelines for legislation related to SPHM.

Professional organizations and industry have lobbied at both the federal and state levels to advocate for change to protect patients and health care teams. As of mid-2014, 11 states have enacted SPHM laws or resolutions intent on providing recommendations that help guide health care institutions in the development of policies and procedures.[11,12] In addition, there is a federal resolution, House Resolution 2480: Nurse and Health Care Worker Protection Act of 2013, which would amend the Title VXIII of the Social Security Act by requiring standards on SPHM aimed at preventing injury.[13]

The financial and health impact of this topic is vast. Providing an overview of current practices and the evidence to support such practices is imperative in today's ever-changing health care environment. This article provides an overview of these practices and discusses contributing factors to the impact of SPHM.

FACTORS CONTRIBUTING TO NURSING CARE INJURIES AND HIGH-RISK NURSING TASKS

"The Occupational Safety & Health Administration reported that 20% of nurses leave their direct care responsibilities because of work related injuries and risks."[9] The daily work of nurses and nursing assistants requires lifting, pulling, turning, and general moving of patients. Caregiver musculoskeletal injuries are often related to repetitive patient handling and mobility tasks. The National Institute for Occupational Safety and Health (NIOSH) recommends that no caregiver should, in any circumstances, lift more than 35 lb (16 kg).[14–16] Among ergonomics experts, an ideal plan for implementing such a recommendation would be to have ceiling lifts and other state-of-the-art lift equipment available for any patient who needs it according to caregiver assessment. A perceived barrier to obtaining necessary lift equipment for many agencies and organizations is cost; however, the evidence on return on investment (ROI), discussed in depth herein, proves otherwise. Hence, many health care personnel continue to be injured annually while assisting patients. In addition to cost, limited awareness continues to be a factor that prevents progress toward controlling the hazards of unsafe practices.

SAFE PATIENT HANDLING AND MOBILITY RESEARCH AND PROGRAMS

Multiple research studies have documented that implementation of SPHM programs, including lift equipment, are cost-effective for health care agencies. "Organizations estimate that they will save 60% to 80% of worker's compensation costs related to patient mobilization if they have a SPHM program, and will save up to 50% of the cost of replacement staff to fill in for out-of-work or restricted duty staff."[17] A 2013 study by Theis and Finkelstein[18] described the effectiveness of instituting a safe patient handling program, demonstrating that immediately after training there was a significant reduction in the numbers of injuries associated with patient transfers. There was a noted financial impact on the training with a cost/benefit saving for each dollar expended of $3.71.[18] In a recent article published in *Nursing*, Price and colleagues[19] describe the experience of Christiana Care Health System with their Patient Environment, Equipment, Posture, Safety (PEEPS) program. Key elements in the success of this program are adequate equipment in facilities, appropriate training for staff including development of PEEPS team "champions" who serve as program leaders, and clear plans for ongoing education.[19] Wardell[20] reported that the use of safe patient handling equipment for appropriate tasks increased significantly following implementation of the Safe Patient Handling Program (SPHP) at a southern California hospital with approximately 500 beds. "The SPHP included the development of a safe patient handling policy, identification of high risk, high-injury departments to determine their particular lifting and equipment needs, and the purchase of sufficient patient handling equipment and slide sheets."[20]

Using algorithms and the nurses' assessment data for decision making assist the caregivers as they determine the most appropriate equipment needed for the patients.[20] Such algorithms were derived from the Patient Safety Center of Inquiry algorithms that were published in 2001 by Audrey Nelson, an early leader in SPHM. Current algorithms may be found on the Tampa VA VISN 8 (Veterans Integrated Service Networks) safe patient handling Web site (http://www.visn8.va.gov/visn8/patientsafetycenter/safePtHandling/default.asp).[21] Stevens and colleagues[22] demonstrated that use of an SPHP in an acute care hospital setting significantly reduced the number of lost work days, and resulted in a significant reduction in costs related to patient handling injuries.

For more than a decade there have been efforts made toward securing state and federal legislation that would set standards for health care agencies related to provision of SPHM equipment and education for caregivers. There is evidence that implementation of the 2013 ANA Standards will serve to protect both health care workers and patients. There is also some concern that injuries to health care workers that result from patient lifting/transfers/positioning may be lumped with other nonreimbursable events such as health care–acquired infections. The cost of patient handling injuries in terms of dollars, lost work days, and shortened careers has been well documented. In Mayeda-Letourneau's 2014 literature review,[23] findings indicate that: "Reduced work injuries, decreased injury costs, improved patient outcomes validated in research and employees feeling the support of their employer all contribute to a program that moves an organization toward a culture of safety."

It has long been proposed that one method to increase the use of SPHM principles is to teach nursing students about SPHM principles early in their nursing curricula. In 2005, the SPHM Curriculum Module for Nursing Schools was sponsored by the ANA, NIOSH, and the Tampa VA VISN 8. In this research project, 26 schools of nursing participated in a research study that provided instruction in addition to, nursing laboratory experience with, state-of-the-art SPHM equipment and techniques. As part of the instruction, students were advised that after graduation and licensing, they should seek employers who either had SPHM programs in place or plans to institute one in the near future. In 2009, a curriculum was developed by the Centers for Disease Control and Prevention in partnership with the NIOSH, the Veterans Health Administration, and the ANA. The nursing education accrediting bodies have not specifically included SPHM in their accreditation standards but have placed a heavy focus on patient safety and self-care of the nurse. Having accreditation standards for schools of nursing, occupational therapy, and physical therapy that address current information could move schools in the right direction.

One issue that must be taken into consideration is securing the necessary equipment for teaching students. Some universities will have lift equipment in their college of health sciences where nursing students, physical therapy students, and others can learn to use them. For educational institutions that do not have their own equipment, an arrangement with a local hospital for borrowing equipment for a period of instructional time could be considered. Moreover, requests to and collaboration with SPHM technology suppliers and manufacturers can often yield donations or vastly reduced expenses for academic institutions preparing new clinicians.

It is noteworthy that the licensing examination test plan (NCLEX: National Council Licensure Examination) topics for registered nurses historically listed only "body mechanics" when speaking of manual lifting and transfer of clients. Largely as the result of the SPHM trend in recent years, the current NCLEX test plan in the section on Safety and Infection Control lists uses of "safe client handling (body mechanics)" and use of "transfer assistive devices" such as gait/transfer belt, slide board, or mechanical lifts.[24]

Health care institutions of all types can benefit from use of an SPHM program. Examples are hospitals, rehabilitation facilities, ambulatory and same-day care centers, and long-term care facilities. For a facility to be prepared to institute an SPHM program, the 8 SPHM standards outlined in ANA Implementation Manual should be followed.[10] The standards are outlined in the following sections.

SAFE PATIENT HANDLING AND MOBILITY: INTERPROFESSIONAL NATIONAL STANDARDS
Establish a Culture of Safety

The responsibility of the change of any culture begins with the leadership of the organization; establishing a culture of safety in the environment of a health care center is no exception. Experts recommend that efforts center on the establishment of an institutional expectation that the safety of patients and caregivers will consistently be a priority. Organizational leaders should support this culture with the resources needed to firmly establish the culture. For example, staff must be available to teach SPHM principles, and to provide routine, timely follow-up instruction. Within this culture the staff must feel free, without consequence, to report any concerns related to SPHM including the ability to "refuse an assignment due to concern about patients' or their own safety."[25]

Implement and Sustain the Safe Patient Handling and Mobility Program

In preparation for implementing and sustaining an SPHM program, the facility will need to select the SPHM program that best suits the particular care setting. There are numerous health care facilities with fully implemented SPHM programs that could serve as models. For example, the Veterans Administration hospitals in the United States have been some of the early adopters and sustainers of SPHM programs over the last 10 to 15 years. In addition, for-profit and nonprofit hospitals/health care agencies have strong existing SPHM programs. Leaders from well-established programs often have the expertise required by new programs, and can be invited as consultants to assist with initial planning. In addition, there are independent companies whose sole focus is consulting, advising, and developing safety programs in the health care environment, and seeking partnership with such an advisor could be appropriate for some organizations.

As new programs are planned, SPHM standards and NIOSH guidelines should be incorporated. For example, since 2007 NIOSH has advised that no caregiver, regardless of size, gender, or physical condition, should lift more than 35 lb (16 kg). The implications of this one factor alone are tremendous. For example, in the past, when nurses needed to lift a dependent 200-lb (90-kg) patient from a bed to a stretcher, it was acceptable practice to use a turn sheet and enlist the assistance of multiple caregivers on both sides of the bed to perform the lift. That practice is not supported by current evidence. Current best practice would indicate that this patient should be assessed using SPHM algorithms, and consideration given to lifting with a ceiling lift, portable lift, or other appropriate lateral transfer device. Douglas and colleagues[26] describe scenarios whereby algorithms are used for safe patient handling decisions in the home care setting. In a literature review by Lowe and colleagues,[27] the conclusion is made that the home setting requires special consideration when applying safe patient handling principles. However, home health care patients and caregivers could benefit greatly from the use of careful patient assessment and appropriate use of safe patient handling equipment.

Some facilities will want to begin with a pilot unit when implementing an SPHM program. Bariatric units, perioperative areas, and critical care areas are frequently chosen as pilot areas because of the high incidence of caregiver work that involves lifting, positioning, and transferring dependent patients. Safe weight limits for log-rolling is 78 lb (35 kg) by 1 person and 156 lb (70 kg) by 2 persons, and a safe guideline for lifting and holding a leg for less than a few seconds with 2 hands can only be done for patients whose total body weight does not exceed 140 lb (63 kg).[14,28]

An assessment of facility equipment, patient care needs, staff resources, environment of care, and educational needs should be performed. Such an assessment process is often referred to as a risk assessment. Once the organizational risks have been identified, equipment needs are determined, budgetary support is allocated (often over a multiyear plan), and selected leaders along with institutional champions are identified who will have key responsibilities for program success and sustainability. "Champions" are those persons who receive detailed education and hands-on practice that will enable them to instruct other caregivers in all of the facets of the SPHM program. Champions are usually nurses or physical therapists, and ideally have at least part of their ongoing job responsibilities designated to maintenance of the program. Maintenance includes continuing education over time, plans for repair and updating of equipment/supplies, and experts being readily available to assist caregivers with assessing patients' SPHM needs.

Incorporate Ergonomic Design Principles to Provide Safe Environment of Care

Ideally, all care settings would be renovated to incorporate ergonomic design. When this is not possible, it is crucial that ergonomic design be incorporated in all new construction of health care facilities.

Examples include installation of ceiling lifts over inpatient beds and in specialty care areas such as operating rooms, emergency departments, and radiology departments where total patient lifts are frequently performed. It would also include design of patient care areas that allows for the space needed to safely manipulate equipment. In interim circumstances until new construction, several solutions can be implemented that address the ongoing risks for musculoskeletal injury, such as considering proposals to install overhead lifts to determine and compare the real versus perceived expense of integrating in existing facilities; using portable safety technology, and beginning to work on awareness of the safety culture.

Determining the amount and type of equipment is an important early step. Recognizing that a considerable variety of equipment exists, the following could be considered essential categories of equipment.

Total body lift

The preference is a ceiling lift mounted over patient beds (or over operating room tables, x-ray tables, or anywhere caregivers might exceed NIOSH recommended safety limits in the course of patient assistance). Two substantial advantages of the ceiling lift over a floor-based portable lift are that it is always present in the patient's room (the caregiver is not required to retrieve the lift from a storage area), and it is always connected to its power source (it does not need to be charged between uses). Additional important considerations when purchasing lifts are availability and maintenance (cleaning), available storage space, ability of the lift to compatibly interface with existing environment (such as fit under hospital beds), durability, weight capacity, and appropriateness for required care tasks. Marras and colleagues[29] have found that use of ceiling lifts is preferable to floor-based lifts, as they better control the negative biomechanical risks associated with patient lifting and handling, largely because of the need to maneuver the lift with the patient, for example in tight spaces and around corners and doorways. A variety of sizes and styles of slings for use with lifts determines the type of patient care task that can be performed. For example, a seated transfer style sling enables seated transfers, whereas a repositioning sling enables a boost-up in bed or pressure relief turn.

Lateral transfer aids

Two frequently used aids are friction-reducing sheets and air assist devices. In combination with ceiling lifts, lateral transfer devices reduce the workload of transfers from bed to stretcher, stretcher to bed, stretcher to table in the radiology department, and stretcher to table in the operating suite. There are additional lower-tech lateral transfer aids such as improved transfer boards, which have friction-reducing features.

Sit-to-stand lifts (also referred to as standing raising aids)

These lifts are floor-based portable devices used to aid certain patients who have a high risk for falls when moving from the sitting position to the standing position. Sit-to-stand lifts can reduce patient falls and prevent injury to both patients and caregivers when it is necessary to assist an unstable patient to stand from a sitting position and complete stand-pivot transfers required for toileting tasks. Sit-to-stand devices are most often powered, but consideration can be given to nonpowered stand-assist devices, which for patients with appropriate motor ability act as stand-pivot and fall-arrest devices.

Select, Install, and Maintain Safe Patient Handling and Mobility Technology

The achievement of this standard is greatly assisted by writing and defining the scope of work and the minimal standards required for the organization. Organizations should publish requests for proposals criteria, soliciting technology partners. The scope of work will guide the evaluation criteria, and assist in comparing among technology partners and allowing for confident final selection of technology.

Organizations should quantify the costs of ownership (such as maintenance expenses) as part of the ROI calculation. Properly selected well-matched technology will assuredly positively affect the efficacy of an SPHM program, whereas poorly matched technology choices that do not follow a scope-of-work evaluation process could negatively affect an SPHM program.

A technology partner vendor or vendors must be selected through the scope-of-work process. Some institutions have found it helpful to schedule a "vendor fair" at the health care facility, for which several vendors are invited to campus. Caregivers at the facility have an opportunity to experience the equipment as both "patient" and caregiver while hearing the features of the equipment described and demonstrated by product representatives. There are benefits, such as buy-in to the new SPHM program, when the organization seeks input from caregivers regarding the various brands of equipment. Once equipment is installed, maintenance contracts are essential.

Establish a System for Education, Training, and Maintaining Competence

Health care education is recognizing the importance of interprofessional education, and SPHM is no exception. For an institution to effectively implement an SPHM program, all caregivers and team members should be educated using the same nomenclature and standards. One method for incorporating SPHM education is to make it a part of existing annual skills updates for all levels of caregivers. Check-offs on use of SPHM equipment encourages staff to stay current with knowledge and skills. Initial and follow-up instruction should include both didactic and hands-on instruction using the actual equipment that is available in the facility.

Integrate Patient-Centered Safe Patient Handling and Mobility Assessment, Plan of Care, and Use of Technology

The key to this standard is the identification of and concentration on the need of the patient. The establishment of assessment guidelines and identifying a plan of care that is patient specific is essential.[25] Algorithms should be used for assessing clients' needs in the area of SPHM. The changing condition of patients must be a consideration as the assessments are performed, as this may change the needs associated with SPHM. One major advantage of having an SPHM champion in each patient care area of a facility is that this person can become an expert in assessment. The champion can then serve in an advisory or on-call capacity to assist others as they become proficient with assessment, including use of algorithms to determine whether and what type of lift equipment should be used. The system must also include the monitoring of patients' injuries in association with SPHM.[30]

Include Safe Patient Handling and Mobility in Reasonable Accommodation and Postinjury Return to Work

Unfortunately, injuries do occur; an effective SPHM program will include a program to monitor for injury and the ability for staff to return to work once an injury does occur. It is the worker's responsibility to notify the workplace of any injury that happens while "on the job," and the staff member must keep the facility updated on his or her condition and work restrictions. At the same time, the facility must implement a process that provides for a timely return to work while protecting the injured from further harm.

Establish a Comprehensive Evaluation System

This standard addresses the evaluation of the implemented SPHM program at a facility. The evaluation plan should be designed while the SPHM program is being designed. Data should be collected consistently to determine the impact that the SPHM program has on the incidence of caregiver injury, workmen compensation costs, patient injury (such as falls, pressure ulcers, and complications arising from immobility), and the impact on patient and caregiver satisfaction. The use of evidence-based data collection and analysis methods should also be included in the planning.[30] Though essential, the process must not conclude with the data collection; primary to the success of such SPHM programs is the improvements that surround the issues associated with the evaluation data. Once collected, significant changes that are made will benefit the patients, caregivers, and the overall health care system involved.

COMMUNITY CONSIDERATIONS

The Affordable Care Act will affect the care of our patients in many ways, one of which will be that patients will be seen in community settings and more care will be performed in the home or long-term care facilities. The ANA publication *Safe Patient Handling and Mobility: Interprofessional National Standards*[30] addresses the importance of the community setting in the implementation of the SPHM interprofessional standards. The implementation of these standards in the community setting must take into consideration that safety for both the patient and staff is essential. Factors such as constructing new facilities that are prepared to care for patients using SPHM practices, and funding for such programs, must be taken into consideration. Homes may not be adequately designed to care for patients, yet this is where the care must be completed, and the establishment responsible for in-home care must be prepared to provide safe and competent care. Patients and families must be involved in decision making related to SPHM technology. Training for providers of all levels must be implemented, and programs should be evaluated and assessed. The use of SPHM technologies can improve patient outcomes in a variety of settings; however, it is essential to not disregard protocols and standards in all areas of care.

THE BARIATRIC PATIENT AND SAFE PATIENT HANDLING AND MOBILITY

Approximately 78.6 million Americans are obese, accounting for greater than one-third of the population of the United States.[31] Obesity is associated with increased morbidity, increased mortality, and, subsequently, increased admittance to health care facilities.[32] This increase in hospitalization or admittance to facilities in turn puts health care workers at risk of injury during the general care of the patient during operating room encounters and emergency room visits. Obesity is defined by grade according to the patient's body mass index (BMI; calculated as weight in kilograms divided by height in meters squared, ie, kg/m^2). **Table 2** describes typical definitions of obesity.

The issues related to caring for an obese patient are not simply related to ambulation or transfers; simple procedures such as dressing changes may necessitate lifting the limbs of these patients. "One leg of a 350-pound patient can weigh up to 62 pounds."[33] The nationwide epidemic of obesity has placed health care workers at an increased risk for injury associated with the care of these clients. When caring for an obese patient, 3 aspects place the care provider at increased risk: reaching, lifting, and spinal loading all place caregivers at risk of injury.[34] It is difficult to avoid these 3 maneuvers when caring for the obese patient. In addition to the obesity epidemic, the population of nursing staff is aging; the average age of the registered nurse in the United States is 44.6 years. Patient acuity has dramatically increased, and patients are typically dealing with multiple medical issues. All of these factors increase the risk of injury to the patient and caregiver staff.[35] The use of assessment algorithms to determine the needs of patients is essential; included in this assessment should be patients' ability to assist with their mobility, being the true measure for the need to use lift equipment.[36]

Using SPHM equipment provides the caregiver with the means to provide ergonomically safe assistance to these patients. Given that the integration of SPHM technology is required for persons with normal BMI range(s), it is likewise required for persons in high BMI ranges; however, the technology selected for these persons with extended capacity requirements necessitates special consideration. The safe working load (SWL) required for the technology's capacity should be assessed by reviewing the organization's population weight trends. Today's SWL capacities can often exceed 1000 lb (454 kg); however, if such a capacity need is, for example, only 1% of the organization's technology needs while 550 lb (250 kg) or 770 lb (350 kg) fulfilled the remaining 99% of SPHM patient care requirements, then the selection of technology needs should be made accordingly. Such careful selection goes a long way to applying budget resources wisely and not overinvesting in SWL capacity equipment that exceeds the organizational demands.

SPECIALIZED ENVIRONMENTS

Certain specialized units such as the operating room, emergency department, and intensive care unit (ICU) require specialized attention in the discussion surrounding SPHM. As previously mentioned, the AORN has been a leader in advocating for SPHM. The AORN notes 2 specific risks associated with SPHM: (1). repositioning the patient on the operating room table and (2) transferring the patient to the operating

Table 2 Classifications for obesity	
World Health Organization Classifications for Obesity	**Corresponding Body Mass Index (kg/m^2)**
Underweight	<18.50
Normal range	18.50–24.99
Overweight	25.00–29.99
Obesity Class I	30.00–34.99
Obesity Class II	35.00–39.99
Obesity Class III	≥40.00

Data from Institute of NC. WHO classifications for obesity. 2014.

room table. The repositioning of patients on the operating room table and the transfer of the patient to the operating room table both place the staff at risk because of the loads placed on the shoulders and back, and the risk can be decreased by using patient-lifting equipment and friction-reducing devices. Additional risks for injury to the operating room staff include the lifting of patient extremities and the long periods of standing associated with the operating room, causing fatigue which, in turn, also causes the staff an increased risk for patient handling injuries.[37] In addition to the SPHM equipment, the AORN recommends the use of algorithms to determine patients' needs, thus improving patient and staff outcomes. The operating room remains a high-risk area; however, the implementation of recommended standards and protocols can help improve the associated hazards.

The impact of immobilization is not a new discovery; Florence Nightingale discussed the effects long-term immobility in her classic 1898 publication *Notes on Nursing*,[38] and there are countless studies that expand on the important considerations of immobility. The acuity of the patient population and the impact of mechanical ventilation in both the inpatient arena and community setting cannot be ignored. "There appears to be significant potential for harm arising from the current ICU culture of patient immobility and an often excessive or unnecessary use of sedation."[39] In 2011, Morris and colleagues[40] published evidence related to improved outcomes associated with early mobility in the ICU. The effect of mechanical ventilation and sedation, and the evidence to support improved outcomes with increased mobility, support the needs for the establishment of an ICU mobility program. "A 2014 international study of early mobilization practices in 833 IUCs found only 27% had formal early mobility protocols, 21% had adopted mobility practices without a protocol and 52% hadn't incorporated early mobility into routine care practices."[41] The initiation of such programs in the ICU requires buy-in from the administration, demonstration of ROI, and the collaboration of a true interprofessional team. Although there are many considerations specific to the ICU, the use of standards and algorithms to aid in SPHM are essential and should be a part of any early mobility plan without regard to the type of unit. Successful SPHM programs in ICU settings across the United States have seen a cultural change and an improvement in patient outcomes; which is of course the goal.[41] "The greatest impact of early mobilization is through standardized mobility protocols or programs."[42]

Finally, the emergency department has many issues similar to those associated with both the operating room and the ICU. Patients in the emergency department are acutely ill, bariatric patients commonly enter the acute care setting via the emergency department, and the culture of SPHM has not typically been infused throughout the culture of the emergency department. The rapid and emergent pace of the units may be seen as a barrier to the implementation of such programs in the emergency department; the patient's condition may depend on the rapid response of the team. Implementation of the use of algorithms can help determine the appropriate use of SPHM equipment while also considering the greater good of the patient and staff.

INTERPROFESSIONAL CONSIDERATIONS

Considering SPHM from an interprofessional perspective, the patient is at the center of the care plan, with essential caregivers all contributing toward reaching the patient's goals. The foundation on which the care plan is built is safety and quality. All elements of the care plan must be executed according to current evidence-based standards for safety and quality. When considering all levels of patient physical and mobility assistance, the evidence is clear: the historical methods of manual assistance and body mechanics alone no longer constitute what is considered to be safe and/or sufficient quality for the patient and all caregivers.

A key opportunity for interprofessional collaboration at the organizational level is the mutual authorship and definition of mobility assistance parameters and linking of patient mobility needs to the organization's available SPHM technology. Clear understanding and consistent assignment of technology matched to patient needs will assist the entire patient care team as well as the patient. Nurses, therapists, and other team members who assist with various levels of patient mobility can all function under an integrated umbrella of policy, nomenclature, and intradepartmental expectations for patient mobility assistance. One example of such interprofessional success is the Banner Health BMAT (Banner Mobility Assessment Tool for Nurses), which came about as a result of multiyear collaboration between the organization's professionals to achieve a comprehensive and validated mobility assessment system for their patients.[43]

There must be recognition that terminology and different professional perspectives and goals can affect the success of SPHM programs. Interprofessional communication and collaboration in the use of SPHM is a key to the success of the implementation of SPHM policies and protocols. Education together with training will also positively influence the future of such programs.

SUMMARY

The work of many organizations has finally begun to pay off; staff injuries over the last 10 years have steadily declined, staff members are more educated about the use of SPHM technology, structured SPHM programs are more common, and even families and patients are more educated about safe patient care. Nursing must join with the interprofessional team and continue to push for the implementation of standards for SPHM. There is a national push to eliminate manual handling of patients, thus continuing to decrease injury to both patients and staff. The culture of safety must be implemented across the care continuum. It is the "ethical responsibility of every registered nurse to protect the health and safety of patients and self."[30]

REFERENCES

1. Bureau of Labor Statisitcs: Table 18. Number, incidence rate, and median days away from work for nonfatal occupational injuries and illnesses involving days away from work and musculoskeletal disorders by selected worker occupation and ownership, 2012. Available at: http://www.bls.gov/news.release/osh2.t18.htm. Accessed October 22, 2014.
2. Miller K. Risk factors and impacts of occupational injury in healthcare workers: a critical review. Musculoskeletal Medicine 2013;1(1):1–6.
3. Occupational Safety & Health Administration. Safe patient handling. Available at: https://www.osha.gov/SLTC/healthcarefacilities/safepatienthandling.html. Accessed October 22, 2014.
4. American Nurses Association. ANA health and safety survey: hazards of the work environment. 2011. Available at: http://www.nursingworld.org/MainMenu Categories/WorkplaceSafety/Healthy-Work-Environment/SafeNeedles/2011-Health SafetySurvey.html. Accessed October 22, 2014.
5. Department of Veterans Affairs. Patient care ergonomics resource guide: safe patient handling and movement. 2001. Available at: http://www.visn8.va.gov/patientsafetycenter/resguide/ErgoGuidePtOne.pdf. Accessed October 22, 2014.

6. de Castro AB. Handle with care: the American Nurses Association's campaign to address work-related musculoskeletal disorders. Orthop Nurs 2006;25:356–65.

7. Occupational Safety and Health Administration. Guidelines for nursing homes: ergonomics for the prevention of musculoskeletal disorders. 2009. Available at: https://www.osha.gov/ergonomics/guidelines/nursinghome/final_nh_guidelines.html. Accessed October 22, 2014.

8. Occupational Safety and Health Administration. Beyond getting started: a resource guide for implementing a Safe Patient Handling Program in the acute care setting. 2011. Available at: http://www.aohp.org/aohp/Portals/0/Documents/AboutAOHP/BGS_Summer2011.pdf. Accessed October 22, 2014.

9. Oermann M. New standards for safe patient handling and mobility. J Nurs Care Qual 2013;28(4):289–91.

10. Gallagher S. American Nurses Association: implementation guide to the safe patient handling and mobility interprofessional national standards. Silver Spring (MD): Nursing World; 2013.

11. American Nurses Association. Safe patient handling and mobility (SPHM). Silver Spring (MD): Nursing World; 2014.

12. Dawson JM. Embracing safe patient handling. Nurs Manag 2012;43(10):15–7.

13. H.R. 2480. Nurse and Health Care Worker Protection Act of 2013. Available at: Congress.gov. Accessed August 23, 2014.

14. Waters TR, Nelson A, Proctor C. Patient handling tasks with high risk for musculoskeletal disorders in critical care. Crit Care Nurs Clin North Am 2007;19(2):131–43.

15. Beauvais A, Frost L. Saving our backs: safe patient handling and mobility for home care. Home Healthc Nurse 2014;32(7):430–4.

16. Safe Patient Handling Lifting Standards for a Safer American Workforce: Testimony Subcommittee on Employment and Workplace Safety Committee on Health, Education, Labor and Pensions United States Senate. 2010. Available at: http://www.cdc.gov/washington/testimony/2010/t20100511.htm. Accessed October 22, 2014.

17. Celona J. Making the business case for a SPHM program. Am Nurse 2014; 9(Suppl 9):26–9.

18. Theis JL, Finkelstein MJ. Long-term effects of safe patient handing programs on staff injuries. Rehabil Nurs 2013;39:26–35.

19. Price C, Sanderson LV, Talarek DP. Don't pay the price: utilize safe patient handling. Nursing 2013;43(12):13–5.

20. Wardell H. Reduction of injuries associated with patient handling. AAOHN J 2007; 55(10):407–12.

21. Veterans Integrated Service Network. Safe patient handling and movement. 2014. Available at: http://www.visn8.va.gov/visn8/patientsafetycenter/safePtHandling/default.asp. Accessed October 22, 2014.

22. Stevens L, Lamb K, Dasling D. Creating a culture of safety for safe patient handling. Orthop Nurs 2013;32(3):155–66.

23. Mayeda-Letourneau J. Safe patient handling and movement: a literature review. Rehabil Nurs 2014;39:123–9.

24. National Council of State Boards of Nursing. NCLEX test plans. 2014. Available at: https://www.ncsbn.org/nclex.htm. Accessed October 22, 2014.

25. Garcia A. Standards to protect nurses from handling and mobility injuries. Am Nurse Today 2014;9(Suppl 9):11–9.

26. Douglas B, Fitzpatrick D, Golub-Victor A, et al. Should my patient use a mechanical lift? Part 2: algorithm and case application. Home Healthc Nurse 2014;32(3):172–80.

27. Lowe S, Douglas B, Fitzpatrick D, et al. Should my patient use a mechanical lift? A review of the literature. Home Healthc Nurse 2013;31(8):427–32.

28. Waters TR. Recommendations for turning patients with orthopaedic impairments. Orthop Nurs 2009;28(2S):28032.

29. Marras WS, Knapik GG, Ferguson S. Lumbar spine forces during manoeuvring of ceiling-based and floor-based patient transfer devices. Ergonomics 2009;52(3): 384–97.

30. American Nurses Association. Safe patient handling and mobility interprofessional national standards. Silver Spring (MD): Nursing World; 2013.

31. Ogden CL, Carroll MD, Kit BK, et al. Prevalence of childhood and adult obesity in the United States, 2011-2012. JAMA 2014;311(8):806–14.

32. Flegal KM, Kit BK, Orpana H, et al. Association of all-cause mortality with overweight and obesity using standard body mass index categories: a systematic review and meta-analysis. JAMA 2013;309(1):71–82.

33. Gardner LA. Caring for class III obese patients. Am J Nurs 2013;113(11):66–70.

34. Muir M, Archer-Heese G. Essentials of a bariatric patient handling program. Online J Issues Nurs 2009;14(1):1.

35. Fitzpatrick MA. Safe patient handling and mobility: a call to action. Am Nurse 2014;9(Suppl 9):1.

36. Kumpar D. Prepare to care of patients of size. Am Nurse 2014;9(Suppl 9):20–2.

37. AORN. Safe Patient Handling and Movement in the Perioperative Setting Tool Kit 2013. Available at: http://www.aorn.org/Clinical_Practice/ToolKits/Safe_Patient_Handling/Download_the_Safe_Patient_Handling_Tool_Kit.aspx. Accessed August 22, 2014.

38. Nightingale F. Notes on nursing what it is, and what it is not. 1898. Available at: https://archive.org/stream/notesonnursing12439gut/12439.txt. Accessed August 23, 2014.

39. Herridge MS. Mobile, awake and critically ill. CMAJ 2008;178(6):725–6.

40. Morris PE, Griffin L, Berry M, et al. Receiving early mobility during an intensive care unit admission is a predictor of improved outcomes in acute respiratory failure. Am J Med Sci 2011;341(5):373–7.

41. Vollman KM, Bassett R. Transforming the culture: the key to hardwiring early mobility and safe patient handling. Am Nurse 2014;9(Suppl 9):7–10.

42. Pashikanti LV, Von Ah D. Impact of early mobilization protocol on the medical-surgical inpatient population. Clin Nurse Spec 2012;26(2):87–94.

43. Boynton T, Lesly K, Amber P. Implementing a mobility assessment tool for nurses. Am Nurse Today 2014;9(Suppl 9):13–6. Available at: http://www.dli.mn.gov/wsc/PDF/sph_bmat_4_nurses.pdf.

Empowering a Healthy Practice Environment

Jodi Kushner, MSN, RN*, Tasha Ruffin, MSN, RN

KEYWORDS

- Healthy nurse • Healthy work hours • Nurse fatigue • Compassion fatigue
- Shift work sleep disorder • Naps at work • Role conflict • Family and work balance

KEY POINTS

- A healthy nurse balances physical, intellectual, emotional, social, spiritual, personal, and professional well-being to reach self-actualization.
- Lack of self-care can result in obesity and put nurses at risk for medical complications, such as diabetes, hypertension, asthma, musculoskeletal problems, anxiety, and depression.
- A healthy work schedule empowers safety, quality, and patient satisfaction.
- Nurse fatigue puts nurses at risk for an accident, mistake, and error that can have legal ramifications.
- Nurses have an ethical responsibility to consider their fatigue level when accepting overtime hours because their ability to provide safe, quality, and accountable care is compromised.
- Compassion fatigue affects nurses' emotional and physical health and, if not addressed, can result in burnout, job dissatisfaction, decreased productivity, and attrition.
- Shift work sleep disorder occurs when there is a circadian misalignment caused by shift work requiring night shifts, overtime, or extended shifts and puts nurses at risk for extreme fatigue, errors, work-related injury, and certain medical conditions.
- Increased role strain and fatigue can lead to decreased satisfaction in the workforce, which leads to nurses leaving the hospital setting and/or the health care field.
- The personal challenges of a nurse can greatly affect his or her role as a caregiver and are directly related to patient outcomes.
- Using hospital resources can help nurses to overcome some of the challenges of balancing work and home environments.
- Promotion of healthy practices, autonomy, self-worth, and organizational support leads to increased satisfaction, retention, and patient outcomes.

Disclosure: none.
School of Nursing, Austin Peay State University, McCord Room 281, PO Box 4658, Clarksville, TN 37044, USA
* Corresponding author.
E-mail address: politepets@msn.com

Nurs Clin N Am 50 (2015) 167–183
http://dx.doi.org/10.1016/j.cnur.2014.10.013   nursing.theclinics.com

> The key to nursing satisfaction seems to be finding the balance or homeostasis in work and family. Nurses have control over aspects that can affect their level of satisfaction; however, it is also the responsibility of a facility to provide a nurturing, empowering, and supportive environment for their nurses.

INTRODUCTION

As the nursing profession continues to grow and more responsibilities are placed on nurses alone, day-to-day stressors (which may or may not be job related) tend to interfere with nurses' ability to provide for patient safety. Nurses are not only caretakers for patients but also lead lives outside of the work environment. Unfortunately, some of the daily activities and responsibilities of nurses outside of the nursing profession may interfere with patient care outcomes and patient safety. The ability of nurses to balance work and family life is one stressor that leads to sleep deprivation and the lack of caring for one's own well-being, such as unhealthy eating habits and lack of exercise caused by fatigue and exhaustion. It is vital that nurses learn the importance of caring for one's own health first in order to become a more efficient health care professional who cares for others. This healthy lifestyle will help the nurses' ability to make competent decisions, enhance job performance, prevent irreversible mistakes that directly affect patient outcomes, and an overall satisfaction for ones quality of life.

This article provides frontline nurses a tool kit so they can advocate a healthy practice environment. The healthy nurse, healthy work hours, job satisfaction, adequate sleep, power naps at work, and balancing family/work are discussed with recommendations to empower a healthy practice environment. The overweight nurse, nurse fatigue, compassion fatigue, shift work sleep disorder (SWSD), and role strain are discussed as barriers to a healthy practice environment. Case reports with analysis and recommendations are discussed to overcome these barriers. Resources are presented for frontline nurses to develop a tool kit for transforming their environment to a healthy practice environment and to empower them to become healthy nurses.

HEALTHY NURSE

According to the American Nurses Association (ANA), a healthy nurse "focuses on creating and maintaining a balance and synergy of physical, intellectual, emotional, social, spiritual, personal and professional wellbeing."[1(p1)] If balance is achieved and maintained, nurses are empowered to reach self-actualization and function at their maximum potential by

- Providing safe, quality, and accountable patient care
- Establishing a high priority to self-care
- Serving as a role model
- Educating their patients with a patient-centered model
- Advocating for their patients[1]

The Overweight Nurse

Many Americans have stressful jobs that mandate numerous responsibilities. So when speaking about those duties of the nurse, it seems as though the odds are against nurses to live a healthy lifestyle. One of the major problems that nurses face today is practicing what you preach as it pertains to eating healthy and exercising regularly.[2] Unfortunately, with the growing population of overweight nurses, it is rather clear that the demands of work and caring for numerous ill patients have overcome these highly recognized professionals. Many nurses work night shifts in addition to having a strenuous workload. As a result, many depend on the vending machines for various snacks because the cafeteria is closed, which increases the intake of high-fat, sugary items and caffeine.

Not only do some nurses have a poor diet when it comes to working long hours and night shifts but the extra pounds also become a concern when the ability to care for patients is compromised.[3] How can an overweight nurse educate a patient on the importance of a healthy diet and exercising regularly, if she or he is an obese member of society? Some nurses are so large, that it is difficult for them to walk to patients' rooms and back to the nursing station.[4] In addition, overweight nurses risk harming themselves as well as the patients when providing nursing care.[3] Overweight nurses are also at risk for additional health problems that impede their ability to perform specified job requirements.[5] Nurses must learn to remember that they are individuals first and required to take care of themselves before being able to care for patients and their families.[5–8]

Case Report

Nurse Lisa is working full-time and works extra shifts when available. She is also enrolled in an online graduate program full-time. When Lisa comes home from work, she drives through a fast food restaurant for a quick meal and starts her homework when she get home. Her day usually starts at 4:30 AM and ends at 11:00 PM. Over the last few months, Lisa has gained 20 lb and has no energy. She does not have time for herself, hobbies, exercise, or recreation. Lisa is very busy but leads a sedentary lifestyle. At work, Lisa usually eats something from the grill and brings high-calorie snacks back to her unit to eat during the shift. She also drinks high-energy drinks to make it through the shift.

Analysis

Nurse Lisa struggles to balance work and school. She makes poor food choices because of the time constraints from her busy work and school schedule. Nurse Lisa is overwhelmed with her commitments and neglects herself. She thinks she does not have time for healthy lifestyle choices. This imbalance puts nurse Lisa at risk for burnout, errors, obesity, and depression.

Recommendations for Transformation

Nurse Lisa needs to develop a balance between work and school. She also needs to develop an active lifestyle, eat nutritious foods, and exercise. Nurse Lisa can become a healthy nurse by incorporating the following recommendations into her lifestyle:

- Reflect on the complications of obesity, such as diabetes, hypertension, asthma, musculoskeletal problems, anxiety, and depression. Nurse Lisa needs to make a commitment to transform her lifestyle and become a healthy nurse.
- Make a commitment to replace comfort foods of high calories with healthy snacks, such as fruits and raw vegetables at home and work.
- Replace high-energy drinks with water. High-energy drinks can cause unhealthy physiologic changes, such increased heart rate. Blood glucose levels can spike and dip with high amounts of sugar in these energy drinks.

- Replace fast food choices of high calories and high fat with nutritious choices, such as grilled chicken, broiled fish, or salads at work and home. Nurse Lisa needs to analyze food and beverage labels to make healthy choices.
- Develop a self-care program. Nurse Lisa needs to block 2 to 4 hours each week for herself. This time can be spent on a hobby, recreation, or socialization.[9]
- Develop an exercise program. Nurse Lisa can join a wellness center at the hospital or join a gym at a discounted price because of a partnership with the hospital. When nurse Lisa is studying at night, she needs to take a break to walk every 2 hours.
- Commit to a stress management program. Nurse Lisa needs to practice anxiety-reduction measures, such as deep-breathing exercises, taking a relaxing tub bath, and practicing yoga or meditation.
- Develop a time management schedule. Nurse Lisa needs to develop a calendar with commitments for the month and develop a priority of what must be done. If the schedule does not allow for transformation to a healthy lifestyle, nurse Lisa needs to consider not working extra shifts and decreasing her full-time student status to a part-time status.

Resources

The healthy nurse needs to embrace the following motto: take care of you so you can take care of others. This outcome can be met by the nurse modeling healthy behaviors, such as choosing an active lifestyle, exercising, eating nutritious foods, not using tobacco products, and achieving a balance between work and personal life.[1] A valuable resource provided by the ANA, Health Risk Appraisal and Web Wellness Portal, is available to all registered nurses and students to help them become a healthy nurse. The health risk appraisal identifies personal and work environment health, safety, and wellness risks. The nurse can compare their results with ideal standards and national averages.[1] After completion of the survey, a wellness portal is available with tools and resources for the nurse to develop a healthy lifestyle.[1] The Web site can be accessed at www.ahahra.org.

HEALTHY NURSING WORK HOURS

A nurse should have a work schedule that allows adequate rest and empowers the nurse to maintain a healthy nurse lifestyle. Employers not only need to provide nurses with a safe work schedule but also sufficient compensation.[10,11] Healthy nursing work hours empower safety, quality, and patient satisfaction. It also empowers nurse satisfaction. Nurses need to advocate for a healthy work schedule as evidence by the following research findings.

- Safe staffing impacts patient safety and quality of care. Research findings show significant improvements in patient mortality when registered nurse (RN) staffing is increased.[12–16] A review of the literature by Hertel[17] concluded that nurses need to take an active role in safe staffing to promote safe and quality care.
- Safe staffing impacts medical errors. Several research studies concluded that safe staffing and RNs in the nursing staff mix are significantly related to preventing medication errors.[18–21] A research study conducted by the National Institutes of Health concluded that a bachelor's education for nurses reduced hospital deaths.[22]
- Safe staffing impacts nurse retention and satisfaction. Several research studies have found that high patient/nurse ratios are related to burnout and dissatisfaction among RNs.[23–28]

Case Report

Nurse JC works on a busy unit with a high attrition rate. Recently 2 nurses resigned and, because of financial constraints, a decision was made by management not to fill the vacant positions. The nurse manager looked at staffing options and her budget. A decision was made to offer bonus money to existing staff to cover the necessary shifts instead of using an agency nurse or travel nurse. Nurse JC signed up to work 3 extra shifts each week for the next 2 months' schedule, which meant she would be working six 12-hour shifts each week. Nurse JC was appreciative to be given the opportunity to make extra money that was needed in her personal budget, and the nurse manager was grateful she stepped up to the plate and signed up for so many extra shifts. Two weeks into the extra shifts, JC became extremely fatigued and complained her back hurt from transferring patients. JC was transferring a patient from the bed to a chair when she heard a pop in her back resulting in extreme pain. JC was sent to the emergency room and was diagnosed with a lumbar herniated disk that would require surgery. JC would be on workman's compensation and out of work for 4 to 6 weeks. JC was also given an antidepressant for being depressed. The busy unit was now short 3 staffing positions, which meant the remaining nurses had to increase their patient/nurse ratio to care for the patients.

Analysis

Both nurse JC and the nurse manager made staffing decisions that put nurse JC at risk for fatigue, dissatisfaction, burnout, errors, and personal injury. This mutually agreed overtime also put patients at risk for decreased quality of care, safety because of the risk for an error by JC, and dissatisfaction of care received that can impact the patient satisfaction survey scores. Nurse JC continuing to work with extreme fatigue led to a work injury. She will receive a reduced weekly salary while on workman compensation and will lose anticipated income from volunteer overtime. Nurse JC was fortunate that a patient injury or error did not occur. The nurse manager chose a quick fix for the staffing shortage by electing to use existing staff to cover staff needs with bonus incentives. The nurse manager is now faced with an increased staffing shortage and guilt from a staffing decision that resulted in putting nurse JC and her patients at risk.

Recommendations

- The nurse manager needs to provide nurses a safe schedule that might include using agency or travel nurses to meet staffing needs. Staffing decisions need to be evidence based and consider the impact on quality of care and safety.[20]
- Nurse JC needs to accept a work schedule that allows adequate rest between shifts. Nurse JC needs to avoid multiple shifts in a row. She needs to space the shifts to allow for rest.

Resources

Nurses need to advocate for safe staffing by role modeling safe staffing decisions. Nurses should consider joining a committee to develop a safe staffing policy and advocating no mandatory overtime. This policy should incorporate nursing professional organization's position statements, such as the ANA's position on mandatory overtime and nurses' right to refuse an unsafe assignment. Evidence-based staffing grids should also be integrated into the policy. Frontline nurses need to realize this policy formation will impact their practice environment and be active in the policy formation.

NURSE FATIGUE

Nursing is a caring profession that is physically and mentally draining. Most nurses work 12-hour shifts that are challenging and taxing on the body. Overtime demands and the economic need to work a second job add extra stress to the body and mind.[30,31] An imbalance in healthy working hours causes fatigue and even exhaustion. The nurse needs to be aware of the symptoms of fatigue that include slowed reaction time with lapses of attention to detail, compromised problem solving, decreased energy and motivation, and errors of omission.[32] It is important that nurses working with fatigue realize that this puts them at risk for an accident, mistake, and error in which there could be legal ramifications.[33] Nurses have an ethical responsibility to consider their fatigue level when accepting overtime hours because their ability to provide safe, quality, and accountable care is compromised.[34]

In December 2006, the ANA developed position statements in response to nurse fatigue being related to nurse error and compromised patient safety.[35] The ANA urged employers to develop policies and procedures to promote healthy work hours. The position statements include the following:

- Develop a work schedule that allows adequate rest between shifts.
- Provide sufficient compensation in which the nurse does not have to seek supplemental income through overtime or other practices, such as a second job.[35]

Case Report

Nurse Ashley, a new nurse, just came off orientation and was finally allowed to work overtime. She recently bought a new car and moved in an apartment that was causing financial constraints. Ashley was behind in her monthly bills and needed to work extra to get caught up on her bills. She signed up for extra shifts. Nurse Ashley also started working at another hospital in a pro re nata (PRN) position. She was working 5 to 6 shifts a week.

Nurse Ashley went to work and came straight home to go to bed. Within 3 weeks, she was having trouble getting up to work her shifts. She went to work extremely fatigued and irritable, and the quality of her nursing care declined. During one shift, nurse Ashley was experiencing difficulty concentrating and using her clinical reasoning skills. Nurse Ashley made a serious medication error, and her patient ended up in the critical care unit on a mechanical ventilator. An incident report was written, and nurse Ashley was sent home. The family filed a formal complaint and called an attorney with consideration of filing a lawsuit.

Analysis

Nurse Ashley thought she could adapt to working long hours and ignored her extreme fatigue. Nurse Ashley was aware she did not have mental clarity but continued to work even at the risk of an error or personal injury from her extreme fatigue. Nurse Ashley did not report her physical and mental exhaustion to her charge nurse. Her drive for extra money put her patients at risk for compromised quality care and safety. Nurse Ashley's medication error had serious consequences for herself and her patient. She is at risk for a malpractice lawsuit, and her charge nurse along with hospital administration are at risk for being included in the malpractice lawsuit. Nurse Ashley is at risk for legal consequences and will have to live with the guilt that her decision caused serious harm to her patient.

Recommendations

- Administrations and nurses need to develop policies and procedures to promote healthy work hours. The policy needs to limit the number of hours worked per week, and shifts need to be spaced to allow adequate rest.
- Nurses need to have sufficient compensation in which the nurse does not have to seek excessive overtime or work a second job for needed income.
- Nurses need to be aware of the symptoms, consequences, and possible legal ramifications from nurse fatigue.
- Nurses need to follow the ANA's code of ethics, which includes no harm to patients when making overtime decisions and working with extreme fatigue.

COMPASSION FATIGUE

Nursing is a caring profession, and nurses provide patient-centered empathetic care. In the process of caring for patients, nurses can personally experience the pain of their patients and family. This occupational stress is known as compassion fatigue.[36,37] Compassion fatigue affects the nurses' emotional and physical health.[38] Nurses working in specialty areas, such as intensive care, oncology, dialysis, pediatrics, and mental health, are at risk for developing this work-related stress.[39–41] If nurses do not seek help for this continuing stress, burnout, job dissatisfaction, decreased productivity, and attrition can occur.[36,42–44] In discussing compassion fatigue, Lombardo and Eyre[36] point out that compassion fatigue is a form of burnout that affects nurses in caregiving roles.

Burnout results from cumulative stress associated with the demands of daily life. It is a state of physical, emotional, or mental exhaustion related to the inability to cope with one's work environment.[41] Burnout is commonly cited as a reason for leaving the workplace. High patient workloads, multiple deaths, long hours, and shift work can contribute to the development of burnout.[45–47]

Case Report

Nurse Joy is an acute care dialysis nurse at a magnet teaching medical center. It is common for patients to travel from out of town for specialty treatments at this facility. There are also local patients that come to the unit on a regular basis because of specialty treatments not being done in a chronic setting. The nurses in this unit develop supportive and educational relationships with patients and their families. During a treatment of a regular patient, the patient coded and rapid response was called. The patient survived the code but was transferred to the critical care unit with a poor prognosis. The nurses briefly discussed their anxiety and fear of the patient's death after the code. Nurse Joy commented that the patient could not die because she was considered family and she just wanted to go home to cry. The acute care unit was extremely busy, so the nurses had to continue with the next patient needing a treatment. Nurse Joy went home after the shift and had a nightmare about the experience. She not only dreamed about this patient but also other similar experiences she had witnessed over the last 12 months she had worked in the unit. Nurse Joy questioned if she wanted to continue working in this area because of her anxiety and stress she experienced with the types of patients they had in the unit. She also questioned if she wanted to stay in the nursing profession.

Analysis

Nurse Joy works in an acute inpatient dialysis unit where patients are acutely ill and many have poor prognoses. Nurse Joy is repeatedly exposed to end-of-life experiences with decisions made to withdraw care. Return patients frequently ask for nurse Joy to be their dialysis nurse because of her caring and patient-centered empathetic care. The code of a regular patient triggered emotional pain and stress in nurse Joy. Other nurses in the unit also experienced occupational stress but were unable to debrief because of the busy schedule. Nurse Joy is experiencing compassion fatigue. If decompression is not done, nurse Joy is at risk for job dissatisfaction, burnout, and leaving the unit.

Recommendations

It is important that frontline nurses be aware of compassion fatigue and seek resources to help break the continued cycle of occupational stress. The following includes recommendations to prevent burnout and compassion fatigue.

- Promote and participate in opportunities to decompress and share experiences with others, such as debriefing after an end-of-life or stressful experience.
- Schedule monthly Schwartz rounds to combat compassion fatigue. A panel of interdisciplinary caregivers present a patient case followed by a discussion of emotional issues related to the case. Thoughts and feelings are shared in a safe environment with recommendations for decompressing.[45]
- Participate in self-care activities to promote destressing.
- Organizational support can decrease the occurrence of nurse compassion fatigue (appropriate workloads, debriefing, recognition, and emotional support).[48]

ADEQUATE SLEEP

Normally a person requires 7 to 8 hours of sleep, although some people may only require 6 hours and others may require up to 10 hours of sleep. [ac0em][49] The difference in the amount of sleep needed is caused by an individual's intrinsic circadian rhythm being related to the duration and quality of sleep. [acoem][49] Normally the urge to sleep increases late at night, with a peak in the early morning hours. [acoem][49] The National Sleep Foundation recommends that adults get 7 to 8 hours of sleep every night.[49] Unfortunately, with the high demands of balancing family life and working lengthy hours on either day or night shift, nurses fall short of the recommended hours to sleep each night. As a result, many nurses are sleep deprived with impaired functional capabilities and the potential to harm both themselves and patients.[50]

Shift Work Sleep Disorder

Nurses normally work a 12-hour shift; but when you factor in hand-off reports and their commute time to work, this work shift can easily increase to 14 hours. Shift work nurses are vulnerable to significant sleep loss and the inability to have adequate sleep to be refreshed the next day. Nurses that work night shifts and rotating shifts or in emergency departments and critical care are at risk for developing this sleep disorder called SWSD.[51] Nurses with SWSD are at risk for extreme fatigue, errors, work-related injury, and medical conditions, such as diabetes, hypertension, cancer, obesity, and adverse reproductive outcomes caused by sleep deprivation.[52]

SWSD can affect the timing and duration of sleep.[51] In SWSD, there is circadian misalignment caused by shift work requiring night shifts, overtime, or extended shifts that is outside the normal circadian rhythm.[49,52] Circadian signals also control core body temperature and secretion of some hormones, increasing nurses' risk for medical complications.[52] Some nurses are able to adjust to working outside the normal circadian rhythm, whereas others are not with the development of SWSD.[52]

Power Naps

The idea of nurses napping (particularly during a night shift) has been considered by management in many facilities.[53,54] However, with the major impact of health and safety of nursing staff and patients, napping on the job warrants exploration. Two reasons for napping on the clock would include fatigue and shift work (mainly working night shifts).[55,56] Working at night increases the chances of sleep deprivation with a high prevalence of patient errors, near misses, and personal injuries during a specified shift and while driving home.[54] In lieu of this, why would it not be a necessity to have the opportunity for nurses to take a nap on their given break? Nurses have a sworn duty to provide efficient care to those individuals who are in need of medical treatment. For this reason, the responsibility of nurses is to be alert, perform accurate assessments, and remain attentive to make rapid decisions as a result of subtle changes in a patient's condition.[54] Power naps during nurses' breaks and mealtime could refresh nurses and prevent complications from SWSD. Nurses should advocate for a nap policy at their facility.[50,55–57]

Case Report

Nurse AJ is a new nurse that completed her day shift orientation of 6 months and is now being assigned to a night shift schedule. Nurse AJ expressed concern about never working a night shift and the fact that she had always gone to sleep by 8:00 PM. She describes herself as a day person. As nurse AJ transitioned into her night shift schedule, she found herself extremely sleepy at 8:00 PM and had difficulty staying awake until 7:00 AM. Nurse AJ drank several high-energy drinks and ate chocolate candy to help her function during the shift. Nurse AJ had extreme difficulty sleeping during the day and states she only had a few hours of sleep. She came to work with red eyes, extreme fatigue, and low energy. Other nurses told nurse AJ she would get used to it. She also had sleep problems on her days off. Nurse AJ stated she felt like she was in a fog every day. After a month of difficulty sleeping, she went to her doctor for sleep medication. This medication helped some but she felt hungover and had trouble waking up for her night shift. Therefore, she stopped the sleep medication. Nurse AJ became depressed and questioned if she wanted to stay in nursing. She started drinking alcoholic beverages, smoking marijuana, and taking alprazolam (Xanax) for coping and to help her sleep. During a shift, the charge nurse noticed nurse AJ's behavior was strange and her breath smelled of alcohol. Nurse AJ was sent to the emergency department for drug and alcohol screening per hospital policy. She tested positive for cannabis and benzodiazepine, and her blood alcohol content level was 0.7. Nurse AJ was sent home and reported to an impaired nursing program.

Analysis

Nurse AJ had a circadian misalignment from working the night shift and not being able to adjust to the required night shift schedule. Nurse AJ developed SWSD. Nurse AJ did not report this to her nurse manager or charge nurse. Sleep deprivation led her to self-medicate with alcohol, Xanax, and marijuana. Her SWSD put nurse AJ at risk for extreme fatigue, work-place injury, and medication errors. Ineffective coping with sleep deprivation resulted in nurse AJ becoming depressed and turning to drugs that put her and her patients at risk for harm and injury. Nurse AJ made an unethical decision and went to work under the influence of drugs and alcohol. Nurse AJ may be reported to her board of nursing with the impaired nurse referral. She may also be required to attend a hearing about her unprofessional behavior and risk of harm to her patients. An impaired nursing program can rehabilitate her and empower her to return to the workforce.

Recommendations

- Because of the risk of extreme fatigue, work-place injury, errors, and certain medical conditions, it is important for frontline nurses to be knowledgeable about SWSD.
- If a nurse exhibits symptoms of SWSD, the nurse should report this problem to the unit manager or charge nurse. The administration should respond to the risks associated with SWSD by arranging a change to the nurse's shift to accommodate his or her normal circadian sleep cycle. This shift change could involve transferring the nurse to another unit or putting him or her on a list for the next opening for the shift needed.
- Advocate for the development of a nap policy. Instead of negative consequences from a nurse napping while at work, develop a policy that allows power napping during meal times and breaks. Propose a business plan for a quiet room in the facility to accommodate napping.[54,57,58]

Resource

A grant to the American Nurses Foundation allowed funding to develop an on-demand webinar on SWSD for nurses that also provides continuing nurse education (CNE) credit. This tool-kit resource educates nurses about the sleep disorder, provides assessment tools, and discusses nonpharmacologic and pharmacologic management.[51] This webinar is valuable for all frontline nurses to evaluate themselves for SWSD.

BALANCED WORK AND FAMILY LIFESTYLE

With the growing demands on nurse professionals, chances are their daily activities and household responsibilities are hectic before clocking in to work long hours for their employer.[59,60] Often times, work is more likely to affect ones family life than vice versa.[59] Nurses are often faced with a work-family conflict that causes them to leave the work force and focus primarily on their households.[61] A work-family conflict describes the struggle to balance work and family; undertaking one role produces a challenge to perform the responsibilities of the other.[61] One of these conflicts is the struggle to balance work and child care. A conflict between personal households and an employer makes it difficult for nurses to perform their job responsibilities while focusing on the patients and providing quality nursing care in a safe environment.[60]

Role Strain

Role strain and fatigue are directly linked to satisfaction. Nurses who are experiencing role strain and/or fatigue report higher levels of dissatisfaction in their jobs. Role strain is often associated increased workloads, decreased autonomy, and a perception of inadequate support from supervisors. According to Lambert and Lambert[62] (2001), role strain "has been conceptualized as the consequence of disparity between an individual's perception of the characteristics of a specific role and what is actually being achieved by the individual currently carrying out the specific role."[62(p161)] Nurses who experience role strain report feelings of decreased levels of confidence, self-esteem, sense of control, and self-worth. Role strain is exacerbated with conflicts between work and home responsibilities. Nurses can feel guilt when neglecting home responsibilities to meet work responsibilities. The following factors are triggers for role strain[62]:

- Work environmental factors[62]
  - Low job control, high work demands, providing poor quality care
  - Dealing with death and dying on a frequent basis (ie, hospice, oncology, emergency department, or intensive-care-unit nursing)
  - Poor working relationships with coworkers, supervisors, and physicians, difficult family members, and clients/patients
  - Low organizational commitment and support
- Influencing and predicting factors[62]
  - Ability to manage job-induced tension
  - Autonomy
  - Physiologic hardiness, self-esteem, and social intimacy
  - Caring for chronically ill and terminal patients
  - Disengagement, distrust, reevaluating one's career
  - Imbalance in work and home
  - Lack of empathy and poor communication
- Physiologic factors[62]
  - Blood pressure, heart rate, epinephrine levels
  - Perceived control at work

Job Satisfaction

Job satisfaction in nursing seems to be directly linked to the intent to leave or stay in a job. Facilities with nurses that report higher levels of job satisfaction seem to have higher retention rates.[44,63] Nurse satisfaction has been defined by the presence of fulfillment. Fulfillment is attained through autonomy, meaning, and a positive and supportive work environment. Facilities that either have magnet status or embody the principles of a magnet hospital have demonstrated higher nurse satisfaction and retention rates.[64] The principles required by the American Nurse Credentialing Center for magnet status involve quality leadership, organizational structure, management style, policies, models of care, quality of care, quality improvement, consultation and resources, autonomy, community, nursing image, nurses as teachers, interdisciplinary relationships, and professional development.[64] The areas of criteria are often referred to as the *forces of magnetism*. Nurses find meaning and satisfaction in environments that provide opportunities for autonomy, involvement, group cohesion, and organizational support.[43]

Job dissatisfaction can occur when nurses are unable to find meaning or satisfaction in their workplace. Job dissatisfaction is as follows:

- Decreased satisfaction can lead to a nurse leaving his or her job and possibly the nursing profession.
- It is affected by workloads, organizational support, and peer support.
- Decreased satisfaction is often accompanied by role strain, nurse fatigue, and/or burnout.

Nurse satisfaction can be empowered when nurses

- Participate in activities that promote autonomy, involvement, and leadership, such as facility nursing councils or committees.[65,66]
- Work in magnet hospitals report higher levels of satisfaction.
- Meaningfulness and satisfaction occur in environments that are learning focused and possess cohesive management and teamwork with sufficient patient-contact time.[67]

Work and family balance can occur when

- Nurses are unable to self-schedule.
  - Nurses' inability to request specific shifts interferes with the balance of work and family.
  - Nurses required to work requested hours can cause dislike in the job and reflect on job performance and satisfaction.
- Nurses are unable to find adequate child care for the hours worked.
  - Often times nurses must leave the profession because of the inability of finding child care for the shifts worked (weekends and night shifts).
  - Nurses must work undesired shifts because of child care availability.
- Nurses are unable to spend time with family.
  - Nurses miss valuable time with spouses and/or children because of the long hours and various shifts.

Work and family balance can occur when

- Facilities can provide support systems/programs for nurses balancing work and family.
- Facilities can allow nurses to self-schedule in order to meet the needs of their family.
- Facilities can provide child care at work.

Case Scenario and Implementation of Strategies

Sue is a 32 year old who has been an RN for 3 years. She works on the medical-surgical floor, which has been receiving oncology/hospice overflow for the past 3 months. Sue is married and has 2 grade-school children. When Sue was hired, she requested to work primarily weekends. Her average patient load is 6 to 7 patients.

Problem

Sue has begun to dread the weekends and working. She finds herself irritable with her children and husband during the week. Sue has also gained 15 pounds over the past 3 months. During the week, Sue does not feel like cooking as much as she used to and is picking up fast food more frequently. On days that Sue works, she will pick up something to eat on her way home and goes to bed shortly after arriving home.

At work, Sue is feeling like she is overwhelmed and cannot manage her patient load. She is finding herself short with patients, family members, and her coworkers. Sue feels emotionally exhausted and frustrated. She is unhappy about her weight gain and feels that, by working almost every weekend, she is missing out on valuable family time. Sue is seriously considering leaving her job and beginning to wonder if nursing is really for her. Sue's nurse manager notices the change in her and decides to talk to her about it.

Sue and her nurse manager meet. Sue voices her concerns about working every weekend. She tells her nurse manager that she is missing all of her children's extracurricular activities. Sue's nurse manager agrees to look at the schedule to see what changes she can make for the next schedule. She tells Sue that she is a good nurse and she would like to keep her around. The nurse manager also asks if there are any other issues Sue would like to talk about. Sue decides to share her feelings of being overwhelmed and feeling like she is not providing good care.

Recommended Lifestyle Changes

Sue's nurse manager suggests that Sue take time for herself and her family. She also suggests that Sue become involved in some of the nursing committees in the hospital.

This involvement may help Sue feel an increased sense of control, autonomy, and self-esteem. Sue thanks the nurse manager and considers the suggestions.

Implementation of Lifestyle Changes

Sue decides that she needs to make herself and her family a priority again. She decides to start exercising and eating better. Sue begins cooking more and bringing leftovers to work with her. Sue begins to lose the weight and has been able to attend some of her children's activities. She also decides to join the policy review committee at the hospital. Sue is beginning to feel less anxious about working and feeling an increased sense of control and self-worth. Sue no longer feels like she selected the wrong career.

Evaluation of the Scenario

Sue experienced many of the stressors that are common to many bedside nurses. She works 12-hour shifts on a busy floor with a patient population that can require high emotional demands. Sue felt overwhelmed, stressed out, and dissatisfied with her job. The demands of her job placed a strain on her family life, which made her feel inadequate in her job and at home. Sue attempted to compensate for her feelings of inadequacy by eating more, which led to her weight gain. Sue realized that she needed to make some changes in order to make her situation better. She had to use the resources around her to empower herself.

Sue had to make the choice to gain back the control over her workplace and home environment. The positive choices she made allowed her to find meaning and satisfaction in her job again. Taking control of her ability to cope with her work environment and home life provided Sue with what she needed, a healthier prospective and approach. Many times options are available; however, one may not realize what those options are until they ask. Sue's ability to communicate with her nurse manager about her family needs not only addressed her concerns but also improved her satisfaction and willingness to remain in her current position. Sue's choice to eat healthier improved her overall health, which improved her abilities at work and also the quality of time she spends with her family. Sue is no longer too tired to interact with her family. Achieving her family and work balance provides Sue with the ability to manage her work stressors more effectively.

SUMMARY

Many nurses face multiple challenges outside the work environment. Not only do nurses juggle the demands of caring for many patients but they also must maintain their households and care for their families. However, several nurses forget about one of the most important aspects of their job requirements: caring for themselves first. It is essential for nurses to understand that in order to provide the best possible care for their patients, they must first care for themselves. This care involves healthy food choices, an adequate amount of sleep, and finding an effective way of managing the stressors of daily life. The ability to balance work and family is an important goal to achieve. Nurses who have achieved balance are able to provide their patients with quality care. They are able to focus their attention and energy on caring for their patients and their needs. There are certain factors or stressors that cannot be changed. The only way to change the number of assigned patients or the patient population is to physically change the work environment by changing floors or facilities. Role strain and nurse fatigue are factors that are linked to decreased satisfaction. Finding methods to address role strain and nurse fatigue is important for both nurses and facilities to consider.

Facilities should provide support for nurses and staff, whereas nurses must also identify ways of coping on their own. It is important for nurses and hospital administrators to be aware of the factors that promote retention and satisfaction in nursing. Knowing the environmental factors that promote satisfaction allows nurses to look for those qualities in their future employer. It also provides a guideline for administrators on practices that will retain nurses. The key to nursing satisfaction seems to be finding the balance or homeostasis in work and family. Nurses have control over aspects that can affect their level of satisfaction; however, it is also the responsibility of a facility to provide a nurturing, empowering, and supportive environment for their nurses.

REFERENCES

1. American Nurses Association. Healthy nurse. Available at: http://www.nursing world.org/MainMenuCategories/WorkplaceSafety/Healthy-Nurse. Accessed August 15, 2014.
2. Blake H, Malik S, Mo P, et al. 'Do as i say, but not as i do': are next generation nurses role models for health? Perspect Pubic Health 2011;131(5):231–9.
3. Durning M. Can fat nurses be good nurses? Scrubs: a nurse's guide to good living 2012.
4. Patterson C. Nurses must be fit to fight: big bodies may hold big hearts, but obese health workers are in no shape to tackle NHS problems [comment]. The Guardian; 2014. Available at: http://www.theguardian.com/commentisfree/2014/aug/01/nurses-obesity-fitter-nhs. Accessed August 15, 2014.
5. Katrandjian O. Study finds 55 percent of nurses are overweight or obese. World News 2012.
6. Naish J. Tackling a weighty issue. Nurs Stand 2012;26(23):20–2.
7. The Press Association. Overweight nursing and medical staff should slim, says NHF chief. Nurs Times 2014. Available at: www.nursingtimes.net30. Accessed August 15, 2014.
8. Trossman S. An issue of weight. The American nurse. 2013. Available at: http://www.theamericannurse.org/index.php/2013/03/01/an-issue-of-weight/. Accessed August 25, 2014.
9. Grindel C, Hagerstrom G. Nurses nurturing nurses: outcomes and lessons learned. Medsurg Nurs 2009;18(3):183–94.
10. Bae SH. Presence of nurse mandatory overtime regulations and nurse and patient outcomes. Nurs Econ 2013;31(2):59–68.
11. Maben J, Latter S, Clark J. The sustainability of ideals, values and the nursing mandate: evidence from a longitudinal qualitative study. Nurs Inq 2007;14(2):99–113.
12. Nicely K, Sloane D, Aiden L. Lower mortality for abdominal aortic aneurysm repair in high-volume hospitals is contingent upon nursing staffing. Health Serv Res 2012;48(3):972–91. http://dx.doi.org/10.1111/1475-6773.12004.
13. Rogowski J, Staiger D, Patrick T, et al. Nurse staffing and NICU infection rates. JAMA Pediatr 2013;167:445–50.
14. Shekelle P. Nurse patient ratios as a patient safety strategy. Ann Intern Med 2013; 158(5):404–10.
15. Spetz J, Harless D, Herrera C, et al. Using minimum nurse staffing regulations to measure the relationship between nursing and hospital quality of care. Med Care Res Rev 2013;70(4):380–99.
16. West E, Barron D, Harrison D, et al. Nursing staffing, medical staffing, and mortality in intensive care: an observational study. Int J Nurs Stud 2014;51(5): 781–94.

17. Hertel R. Healthcare Reform and Issues in Nursing Regulating patient staffing: a complex issue. Med-Surg Matters 2012;21(1):3–7.
18. Duffin C. Increase in nurse numbers linked to better patient survival rates in ICU. Nurs Stand 2014;28(33):10.
19. Frith K, Anderson E, Tseng F, et al. Nursing staffing is an important strategy to prevent medication errors in community hospitals. Nurs Econ 2012;30(5): 288–94.
20. International Council of Nurses. ICN forum: nurse staffing cuts pose risk to patients, society. 2013. Available at: http://www.ich.ch/images/stories/documents/pillars/sew/Communique_WFF_2013.pdf. Accessed August 15, 2014.
21. Nurse staffing ratios. AORN J 2013;97(5):604, 538.
22. National Institutes of Health. Nurse staffing and education linked to reduced mortality. 2014. Available at: http://www.nih.gov/news/health/feb2014/ninr-26.htm. Accessed August 15, 2014.
23. Aiken LH, Clark SP, Sloan DM, et al. Hospital nurse staffing and patient mortality, nurse burnout, and job dissatisfaction. JAMA 2002;288(16):1987–93.
24. Arling G, Muellar C. Nurse staffing and quality: the unanswered question. J Am Med Dir Assoc 2014;15(6):376–8.
25. Mark B, Spetz J, Reiter K, et al. California's minimum nurse staffing legislation: Results from a natural experiment. Health Serv Res 2013;28(2):435–54.
26. McKenna E, Clement K, Thompson E, et al. Using a nursing productivity committee to achieve cost savings and improve staffing levels and staff satisfaction. Crit Care Nurse 2011;31(6):55–65.
27. Ramson K, Dudjak L, August-Brady M, et al. Implementing an acuity-adaptable care model in a rural hospital setting. J Nurs Adm 2013;43(9):455–60.
28. Tellez M. Work satisfaction among California registered nurses: a longitudinal comparative analysis. Nurs Econ 2012;30(2):73–81.
29. Berger A, Hobbs B. Impact of shift work on the health and safety of nurses and patients. Clin J Oncol Nurs 2005;10(4):465–71.
30. Duddle M, Boughton M. Intraprofessional relations in nursing. J Adv Nurs 2007; 59(1):29–37.
31. Bae SH. Nurse overtime, working conditions, and the presence of mandatory nurse overtime regulations. Workplace Health Saf 2012;60(5):205–14.
32. Barker L, Nussbaum M. Fatigue, performance and the work environment: a survey of registered nurses. J Adv Nurs 2011;67(6):1370–82.
33. American Nurses Association. Nursing fatigue. Available at: http://www.nursingworld.org/MainMenuCategories/WorkplaceSafety/Healthy-Nurse-Environment. Accessed August 15, 2014.
34. American Nurses Association. Work environment. Available at: http://www.nursingworld.org/MainMenuCategories/WorkplaceSafety/Healthy-Nurse-Environment. Accessed August 15, 2014.
35. American Nurses Association. Position statement: assuring patient safety: the employers' role in promoting healthy nursing working hours for registered nurses in all roles and settings. 2006. Available at: http://www.nursingworld.org/MainMenuCategories/Policy-Advocacy/Positions-and-Resolutions/ANAPositionStatements/Position-Statements-Alphabetically/AssuringPatientSafety.pdf. Accessed August 15, 2014.
36. Lambardo B, Eyre C. Compassion fatigue: a nurse's primer. Online J Issues Nurs 2011;16(1). http://dx.doi.org/10.3912/OJIN.Vol16No01Man03.
37. Sado B. Reflecting on the concept of compassion fatigue. Online J Issues Nurs 2011;16(1). http://dx.doi.org/10.3912/OJIN.Vol16No02Man01.

38. Harr C. Promoting workplace health by diminishing the negative impact of compassion fatigue and increasing compassion satisfaction. Social Work & Christianity 2013;40(1):71–88.

39. Abendroth M, Flannery J. Predicting the risk of compassion fatigue a study of hospice nurses. J Hosp Palliat Nurs 2006;8(6):346–56. Available at: http://journals.lww.com/jhpn/Abstract/2006/11000/Predicting_the_Risk_of_Compassion_Fatigue__A_Study.7.aspx.

40. Aytekin A, Kuguoglu S, Yllmaz F. Burnout levels in neonatal intensive care nurses and its effects on their quality of life. Aust J Adv Nurs 2013;31(2):39–47.

41. Potter P, Deshields T, Divanbeigi J, et al. Compassion fatigue and burnout prevalence among oncology nurses. Clin J Oncol Nurs 2010;14(5):56–62. Available at: http://ons.metapress.com/content/r744058h42804261/.

42. Lavoie-Tremblay M, Wright D, Desforges N, et al. Creating a healthy workplace for new-generation nurses. J Nurs Scholarsh 2008;40(3):290–7.

43. Lavoie-Tremblay M, Paquet M, Duchesne MA, et al. Retaining nurses and other hospital workers: an intergenerational perspective of the work climate. J Nurs Scholarsh 2010;42(4):414–22.

44. MacKusick C, Minick P. Why are nurses leaving? Findings from an initial qualitative study on nursing attrition. Medsurg Nurs 2010;19(6):335–40. Available at: https://test.amsn.org/sites/default/files/documents/practice-resources/healthy-workenvironment/resources/MSNJ_MacKusick_19_06.pdf.

45. Thompson A. How Schwartz rounds can be used to combat compassion fatigue. Nurs Manag (Harrow) 2013;20(4):16–20.

46. Hairr D, Salisbury H, Johannsson M, et al. Nurse staffing and the relationship to job satisfaction and retention. Nurs Econ 2014;32(3):142–7.

47. Bogaert P, Kowalski C, Weeks SM, et al. The relationship between nurse practice environment, nurse work characteristics, burnout and job outcome and quality of nursing care: a cross-sectional survey. Int J Nurs Stud 2013;50(12):1667–77.

48. Mitka M. Nursing overtime. JAMA 2007;297(22):2465.

49. National Sleep Foundation. How much sleep do we really need? Available at: http://sleepfoundation.org/how-sleep-works/how-much-sleep-do-we-really-need. Accessed August 15, 2014.

50. Alsppach G. Napping on the night shift. Crit Care Nurse 2008;28(6):12–9. Available at: http://ccn.aacnjournals.org/content/28/6/12.short.

51. American Nurses Association. Shiftwork sleep disorder. Available at: http://nursingworld.org/HomepageCategory/NursingInsider/Archive-1/2013-NI/Feb-2013-NI/Free-SWSD-CE.html. Accessed August 15, 2014.

52. Lerman SE, Eskin E, Flower DJ, et al. Fatigue risk management in the workplace. J Occup Environ Med 2012;54(2):231–58.

53. Edwards MP, McMillan DE, Fallis WM. Napping during breaks on night shift: critical care nurse manager's perceptions. Dynamics 2013;24(4):30–5.

54. Fallis W, McMillan D, Edwards M. Napping during night shift: practices, preferences, and perceptions of critical care and emergency department nurses. Crit Care Nurse 2011;31(2):e1–11. Available at: http://ccn.aacnjournals.org/content/31/2/e1.short.

55. McMillan D, Fallis W. Benefits of napping on night shifts. Nurs Times 2011;107(44):12–3.

56. Silva-Costa A, Rotenberg L, Griep R, et al. Relationship between sleeping on the night shift and recovery from work among nursing workers – the influence of domestic work. J Adv Nurs 2010;67(5):972–81.

57. Farmilo K. Power napping for nurses: an underutilized strategy for staying sharp and engaged in the course of a shift. Am J Nurs 2014;114(5):11.

58. Geiger-Brown J, Rogers VE, Trinkoff AM, et al. Sleep, sleepiness, fatigue and performance of 12-hour-shift nurses. Chronobiol Int 2012;29(2):211–9.

59. Grzywacz JG, Frone MR, Brewer CS, et al. RNs struggle to balance work and home life. Quantifying work- family conflict among registered nurses. Res Nurs Health 2006;36(12):33.

60. Marks L. Balancing work and caregiving. Career Plann Adult Dev J 2008;23(4): 52–9. Available at: http://www.questia.com/library/journal/1P3-1497416101/balancing-work-and-caregiving#/.

61. Fujimoto T, Kotani S, Suzuki R. Work-family conflict of nurses in Japan. J Clin Nurs 2008;17:3286–95. Available at: http://onlinelibrary.wiley.com/doi/10.1111/j.1365-2702.2008.02643.x/abstract;jsessionid=CF9662103827BAA45D1839307416A23C.f01t01?deniedAccessCustomisedMessage=&userIsAuthenticated=false.

62. Lambert V, Lambert C. Literature review of role stress/strain on nurses: an international perspective. Nurs Health Sci 2001;3:161–72. Available at: http://onlinelibrary.wiley.com/doi/10.1046/j.1442-2018.2001.00086.x/abstract?deniedAccessCustomisedMessage=&userIsAuthenticated=false.

63. Ferlise P, Baggot D. Improving staff nurse satisfaction and nurse turnover use of a closed-unit staffing model. J Nurs Adm 2009;39(7–8):318–20.

64. ANA Healthy Nurse ANCC. ANCC magnet recognition program. 2014. Available at: http://nursecredentialing.org/magnet.

65. DiMeglio K, Padula C, Piatek C, et al. Group cohesion and nurse satisfaction examination of a team-building approach. J Nurs Adm 2005;35(3):110–20. Available at: http://journals.lww.com/jonajournal/Abstract/2005/03000/Group_Cohesion_and_Nurse_Satisfaction__Examination.3.aspx.

66. Roulin N, Mayor E, Bangerter A. How to satisfy and retain personnel despite job-market shortage multilevel predictors of nurses' job satisfaction and intent to leave. Swiss J Psychol 2014;73(1):13–24.

67. Pavlish C, Hunt R. An exploratory study about meaningful work in acute care nursing. Nurs Forum 2012;47(2):113–22. Available at: http://onlinelibrary.wiley.com/doi/10.1111/j.1744-6198.2012.00261.x/abstract?deniedAccessCustomisedMessage=&userIsAuthenticated=false.

Aging Population

Deborah Ellison, PhD, RN*, Danielle White, RN, MSN,
Francisca Cisneros Farrar, EdD, MSN

KEYWORDS

- Older adult • Individualized aging • Complexity of care
- Physiologic changes with aging • ACES • Transitions • Pain management
- End of life

KEY POINTS

- Individualized aging is the process of aging from an individual perspective.
- It is important for frontline nurses to prevent hospital-acquired events by following best practice policies and providing evidence-based safe, quality, and accountable care to prevent complications during hospitalization.
- FANCAPES (fluids, nutrition, communication, activity, pain, elimination, mental status) is a comprehensive physical assessment tool to determine the basic needs and functional needs in an acutely ill, medically complex older adult.
- Frontline nurses need to focus on the assessment of function and how the chronic illness affects the quality of care for the older adult and the masking of acute illness.
- Individuals at high risk for vulnerability during transitions are older people with multiple conditions, depression, or other mental health disorders, isolated elders without family or friends, non–English-speaking individuals, immigrants, and low-income patients.
- Frontline nurses must be able to incorporate both the physiologic changes and the American Nurses Association's standards for the older adult into professional practice to provide quality, safe care.
- Frontline nurses are responsible for the assessment, treatment, and documentation of pain in all patients.
- Dying is an individual process. How one approaches the experience is a reflection of the way one has lived his or her life and responded to other losses, circumstances, and culture.
- There is a lack of discussion about palliative care and hospice.

INTRODUCTION

By 2050, 1 in 5 Americans will be more than 65 years of age, with those older than 85 years showing the greatest increase in numbers. The number of people living to

Disclosures: None.
School of Nursing, Austin Peay State University, PO Box 4658, Clarksville, TN 37044, USA
* Corresponding author.
E-mail address: ellisond@apsu.edu

100 years of age is projected to grow at more than 20 times the rate of the total population by 2050.[1] Frontline nurses are being called on to incorporate specific gerontological skills in order to meet the needs of the rapidly growing aging population (those aged 65 years and older). The aging population requires that nurses respond to the emerging issues in the health of older adults. These issues include coordination of care, helping older adults manage their own care, establishing quality measures, identifying minimum levels of training for people who care for older adults, and researching and analyzing appropriate training to equip providers with the tools they need to meet the needs of older adults.[2]

The current health care culture must change in order to respond to the aging population. Baby boomers in the United States may bring significant changes to how this country's health care system functions as a result of their past experiences. This generation of older adults is expected to have better health and, therefore, will live longer and be better educated, more connected to society, and more personally involved in health care decisions than any previous group.[3]

It is the responsibility of the nurse to assist the geriatric population to achieve the highest level of wellness in relation to whatever situation exits. Frontline nurses can, through knowledge and affirmation, empower, enhance, and support the person's movement to the highest level of wellness and quality of life possible.[1] The nurse can use several resources to assist in individualized care, the complexity of care for the elderly, and the issues of transitions of care. Healthy People 2020, Advancing Care Excellence for Seniors (ACES), and Clinical Preventive Services Guidelines are all excellent resources for frontline nurses.[4]

Healthy People 2020 has identified emerging issues in the health of older adults. The issues include

- Coordinate care
- Help older adults manage their own care
- Establish quality measures
- Identify minimum levels of training for people who care for older adults
- Research and analyze appropriate training to equip providers with the tools they need to meet the needs of older adults[2]

In 2007, the National League for Nursing in collaboration with the Community College of Philadelphia and funded by the Independence Foundation, the John A. Hartford Foundation, and Laerdal Medical embarked on efforts to improve on gerontological nursing education and research.[3] The project that emerged, ACES, is designed to enhance and improve gerontological nursing at the bedside. The ACES framework identifies 3 unique concepts integral to delivering high-quality care: individualized aging, complexity of care, and vulnerability during transitions.[3]

ESSENTIAL KNOWLEDGE DOMAINS
Individualized Aging

Individualized aging is the process of aging from an individual perspective.[3] The older adult has a unique background and health history. Frontline nurses need to recognize that stereotype characteristics do not apply to all older adults. For example, an 85 year old may have a biological age of 65 years because the older adult maintained a healthy lifestyle and remained active. Frontline nurses need to conduct a comprehensive assessment to determine the older adult's personal meaning of aging, their specific physiologic changes to aging, and how aging has impacted their activities of daily living.[1,3] Focused assessment to provide insight into individualized aging would include the following:

Cognitive abilities

Cognitive skills that decline with aging are verbal fluency, logical analysis, selective attention, object naming, and complex visuospatial skills.[3] Older adults are at risk for delirium secondary to acute infection, dementia, and depression. Assessment of cognition includes both biological and psychological factors. Frontline nurses need to assess the cognitive status of an older adult, including confusion, delusional ideation, paranoia, and hallucinations. Frontline nurses may need to make a recommendation for a neurologic assessment. If confusion is present, frontline nurses may need to recommend a sitter; implement an orientation program; and, as a last resort, use restraints per hospital policy. **Table 1** highlights the common examinations to assess individualized aging.

Table 1	
Individualized aging assessment tools	
Examination	**Description of Test**
MMSE	30-Item instrument to screen for cognitive difficulties Tests orientation, short-term memory and attention, calculation ability, language, and construction Score less than 24 shows impairment
Clock drawing test	Person draws a circle and the face of a clock for a designated time Requires some manual dexterity Scoring is based on position of numbers and hands on clock Used to measure severity of cognitive impairment
Mini-Cog	Combines short-term memory recall questions from the MMSE with the clock drawing test Can be administered quickly
Global deterioration scale	Seven-stage rating scale used to determine whether a person has cognitive impairment that is related to dementia reflected in deviation from skills, such as thinking, knowing, learning, and using judgment
Geriatric Depression Scale	Assesses mood, especially depression

Abbreviation: MMSE, Mini-Mental State Examination.
Data from ACES. Essential nursing actions. Available at: http://www.nln.org/facultyprograms/facultyresources/aces/pdf/essential_nursing_actions.pdf. Accessed July 1, 2014; and Eliopoulos C. Gerontological nursing. 7th edition. Philadelphia: Lippincott Williams & Wilkins; 2010.

Functional assessment

Activities of daily living and instrumental activities of daily living are measured by observation, self-report, or functional assessment. If the older adult is healthy and active, frontline nurses can document this finding. If potential problems exist, a functional assessment is needed. A recommendation for physical therapy, occupational therapy, and case management may be needed based on the assessment findings. Frontline nurses need to assess the gait, use of an assistive device, and history of any falls. Frontline nurses should implement fall and safety precautions for an older adult. **Table 2** overviews functional abilities that are evaluated in the functional assessment tools.

Table 2	
Functional assessment tools	
Assessment	**Measurement**
Activities of daily living	Eating, toileting, ambulation, bathing, dressing, and grooming
Instrumental activities of daily living	Cleaning, yard work, shopping, and money management
Focused questions	Identify deficit Identify changes from one period to another Determine specific services needed Determine if in unsafe living situation and needs higher level of care Referral to case management or social service

Data from Tagliareni E, Cline DD, Mengel A, et al. Quality care for older adults: advancing care excellence for seniors (ACES) project. Nurs Educ Perspect 2012;33(3):144–9.

Sensory assessment

Several changes occur in the sensory organs, especially in vision and hearing. Most older adults require reading glasses, and more than two-thirds of adults aged older than 65 years have a visual impairment. The leading causes of visual impairment in older adults are age-related macular degeneration, cataract, glaucoma, and diabetic retinopathy.[3] Frontline nurses need to respond to older adults' visual impairment by reading instructions, providing their eyeglasses, and recommending an ophthalmologist evaluation. Safety measures should be implemented to prevent falls and injuries.

Hearing assessment

Hearing loss in older adults is the third most common chronic condition. Age-related hearing loss is associated with miscommunication, depression, falls, loss of self-esteem, safety risks, and cognitive decline.[1] Frontline nurses need to assess hearing impairment and determine if the older adult has a hearing aid. The frontline nurses should request hearing aids be brought to and given to patients to wear, which will assist in decreasing safety issues such as falls and miscommunication.

Oral health assessment

Oral health is integral to general health. Dehydration, malnutrition, and systemic diseases, such as pneumonia, diabetes, and cardiac disease, are risk factors associated with poor oral health.[1,5] Older adults are prone to dental problems and may require dentures. Frontline nurses need to assess if a soft diet or pureed diet is needed because of oral health problems. Frontline nurses need to assess for dry mouth, dysgeusia (loss of taste), poor dentition, oral candidiasis, and mouth sores.[1] Frontline nurses need to make dentures available for meals and to allow older adult patients to communicate more clearly. A recommendation to an occupational therapist or a dentist may be needed for assistance in oral care.

Nutritional assessment

Generally, older adults need few calories because their metabolic rates slow down; it is recommended that they follow a heart-healthy diet of fruits, vegetables, whole grains, low-fat dairy products, poultry, and fish and restriction of salt intake.[1] Appetites and food consumption usually decline with age because of functional limitations, such as smell, taste, oral problems, decreased thirst sensation, and mood (touchy). Older adults are at risk for dehydration and malnutrition even though the prevalence of obesity, especially in the aging of the baby boomer generation, is increasing.[1,5] Dehydration is a risk factor for conditions such as delirium, infections, medication toxicity, electrolyte imbalance, and delayed wound healing.[1,4,5] Typical signs of dehydration are not always present in older adults because of the loss of subcutaneous tissue with aging. Dry mucous membranes in the mouth, orthostasis, speech incoherence, and a sunken eye may indicate dehydration. If dehydration is suspected in older adults, laboratory tests such be ordered. Frontline nurses need to assess intake and output, symptoms of dehydration, and assure that older adult patients receive adequate hydration unless fluid restriction is ordered. Frontline nurses need to assess the older adult for weight loss, conduct a diet history, assess appetite, and make a recommendation for a dietitian or nutritional consult if abnormalities are found. Nutritional supplements, such as protein or high-calorie drinks, may be ordered by the physician to supplement their diet and help restore nutritional needs.

Medication assessment

Adults older than 65 years are the largest consumers of prescriptions and over-the-counter medications, with 90% taking at least 5 prescriptions.[1] Polypharmacy can occur if more than 5 medications are taken. As the number of medications increase, the risk for ineffective and duplicate medications can occur. This situation can occur when new medications are prescribed or over-the-counter medications or supplements are added. Polypharmacy is usually accidental and puts the older adult at risk for drug interactions and an increased risk for adverse events that can result in hospitalization.[1] Polypharmacy can also put the older adult at risk for adverse drug withdrawal and therapeutic failures.[1] Misuse of medications can occur when multiple drugs are taken. Misuse may be accidental, such as misunderstanding, or deliberate, such as noncompliance of scheduled medication, insurance coverage problems, or intentional overdose of the medication.[1,3,5] Memory impairment, such as forgetting to take medications correctly, can be a causative factor of noncompliance. Visual impairment can cause problems with reading labels and instructions and requires an adjustment to large print. Health literacy and language need to be considered with medication teaching to the older adult or caregiver who will be administering the medication.[1,5] Frontline nurses need to conduct a comprehensive drug assessment and make sure correct medications are listed in the electronic medical record. Transition or discharge medications also need to be current and include over-the-counter medications along with supplements. Frontline nurses may need to recommend a clinical pharmacist consult and case manager if the older adult needs assistance with medication management.

Abuse and mistreatment assessment

Frontline nurses usually see families when an older adult is hospitalized. A family assessment needs to be conducted, including family history, family dynamics, and support systems. Frontline nurses need to be nonjudgmental and assess strengths to recognize the limitations in providing support and caregiving. A family member that is in the caregiver role experiences physical and emotional stressors.[1] Frontline nurses can decrease stress for the caregiver by recommending a referral for a social worker or case manager to help find respite services; recommending changing the situation, with the caregiver giving up the role and recommending assistive living or nursing home placement; and providing a list of support groups. Frontline nurses need to assess for potential abuse or mistreatment. If abuse is suspected, by law registered nurses are required to report suspicions of abuse to the state adult protective services. The facility policy should be followed. **Table 3** summarizes abuse and mistreatment that frontline nurses should assess.

Table 3 Elder abuse and neglect assessment		
Type	**Definition**	**Symptom Examples**
Physical abuse	Physical force that may result in bodily injury	Bruises, black eyes, lacerations, bone fractures, injuries in various stages of healing, slapped, kicked, visitors not allowed
Sexual abuse	Nonconsensual sexual contact of any kind without consent	Unexplained vaginal or anal bleeding, venereal disease, genital infections Bruises around genital area Elder report of rape
Emotional or psychological abuse	Infliction of anguish, pain, or distress through verbal or nonverbal acts	Being emotionally upset, withdrawn, uncommunicative
Neglect	Failure to fulfill any part of caregiving obligations	Unattended health problems, dehydration, malnutrition, untreated bedsores, poor personal hygiene, unclean living conditions
Abandonment	Desertion by caregiver	Desertion at hospital, nursing facility, public location

Data from Touhy T, Jett K. Ebersole and Hess' gerontological nursing & healthy aging. 4th edition. St. Louis (MO): Mosby; 2014; and Jarvis C. Physical examination and health assessment. 6th edition. Philadelphia: Saunders; 2011.

Atypical presentation assessment

Atypical presentation or a nonspecific presentation of illness can occur when an older adult has multiple chronic conditions. Symptoms of one condition can exacerbate or mask another condition causing overdiagnosis or underdiagnosis.[1,3,5] Atypical presentation can occur from physical or psychological conditions. Frontline nurses are challenged when completing a comprehensive assessment when atypical presentation occurs. Frontline nurses need to be aware of this issue and objectively document findings in their assessment for the correct diagnosis.

Learning assessment

Older adults may have learning barriers from hearing, vision, and cognitive impairment. Many older adults also have special learning needs because of their literacy level and cultural variations. These barriers and special learning needs may necessitate the need for teaching the caregiver. Frontline nurses need to assess the barriers and special needs to develop accommodations or alternative teaching to meet the health care learning needs. Instructions in the primary language and large print will facilitate learning and compliance. Older adults may need the instructions read to them along with written instructions for understanding (**Box 1**).

Box 1
Summary of individual aging focused assessment

- Cognitive abilities
- Functional assessment
- Sensory assessment
- Hearing assessment
- Oral health assessment
- Nutritional assessment
- Medication assessment
- Abuse and mistreatment assessment
- Atypical presentation assessment
- Learning assessment

Complexity of care

The care of older adults requires specialized knowledge in the art and science of both nursing and geriatrics to manage the interplay of factors that influence the quality of care. Older adults account for 46% of critical care patients and 60% of medical-surgical patients in the hospital setting.[1] These acutely ill patients are challenging to frontline nurses because they also frequently have multiple chronic conditions. Many older patients are at risk for functional decline and hospital-acquired events, such as catheter-associated urinary tract infections, pressure ulcers, and falls. Older patients are also at risk for geriatric syndromes, such as malnutrition, pneumonia, medication reactions, confusion, and falls.[1] It is important for frontline nurses to prevent hospital-acquired events by following best practice policies and providing evidence-based, safe, quality, and accountable care to prevent complications during hospitalization. Frontline nurses should screen for influenza and pneumonia vaccination on each patient. The FANCAPES (fluids, nutrition, communication, activity, pain, elimination, mental status) is a comprehensive physical assessment tool to determine the basic needs and functional needs in an acutely ill, medically complex older adult. Frontline nurses should obtain information in each area to determine a plan of care. **Table 4** overviews the FANCAPES acronym for the comprehensive assessment.

Table 4
FANCAPES assessment for complex older adult

Acronym	Assessment
Fluids (F)	State of hydrations
Nutrition (N)	Mechanical and psychological factors impacting nutrition
Communication (C)	Ability to communicate; form of communication
Activity (A)	Ability to participate in activities of daily living; assistance needed
Pain (P)	Assess physical, psychological, spiritual pain
Elimination (E)	Assess difficulty with bladder or bowel elimination
Mental status (M)	Assess mental status, cognitive ability, and mood

Data from Touhy T, Jett K. Ebersole and Hess' gerontological nursing & healthy aging. 4th edition. St. Louis (MO): Mosby; 2014.

In chronic illness, there is no cure. Frontline nurses need to focus on the assessment of function and how the chronic illness affects the quality of care for the older adult and masks the acute illness. **Table 5** summarizes the common chronic conditions that frontline nurses need to assess.

| Table 5 |
| Common older adult chronic conditions |

Chronic Condition	Complications
Rheumatoid arthritis	Chronic, systematic inflammatory disorder with progressive damage to joints Pain and swelling in multiple joints Weight loss common Impacts mobility
Diabetes	Complications develop more quickly and severely Control blood sugar and reduce risk of complications
Hearing loss	Third most prevalent chronic condition Risk for decreased function, miscommunication, depression, loss of self-esteem, safety risks, and cognitive decline
Macular degeneration	Progressive loss of vision and can lead to blindness Safety issues
Urinary incontinence	Involuntary loss of urine sufficient to be a problem Risk for urinary tract infection that if untreated can result in septicemia and delirium Can cause falls, skin irritations, pressure ulcers, and sleep disturbance
Constipation	Reflection of poor diet, activity, postponing passage of stool, and many chronic illnesses Can be signal to colonic dysfunction or colon cancer Can result in cognitive dysfunction, delirium, falls
Hypertension	Most common chronic cardiovascular disease Can result in stroke if not managed
Heart failure	Damage to heart from chronic heart disorder or myocardial infarction. No cure, just management of systems of edema, dyspnea, orthopnea, weight gain May seem confused and delirious with exacerbation
Chronic obstructive pulmonary disease	Chronic bronchitis, emphysema, or asthma Risk for pneumonia
Dementia	Need to differentiate between 3 Ds (dementia, depression, delirium) because of masking of symptoms; all 3 have behavior and cognitive changes *Dementia*: gradual onset and slow; steady decline in cognitive function without alterations in consciousness *Depression*: have inability to concentrate with memory impairment and other cognitive dysfunction; called pseudodementia *Delirium*: acute or subacute onset with symptoms developing over course of day; perceptual disturbances often accompanied by delusional thoughts, such as paranoia; caused by treatable conditions, such as infection

Data from Refs.[1,3,6]

The complexity of care challenges frontline nurse to differentiate between acute and chronic illnesses. They need to keep abreast of changes in health and cognitive status by conducting a comprehensive evaluation to differentiate symptoms that can be masked by underlying chronic illnesses (**Box 2**).

Box 2
Summary of complexity of care

- Many older patients are at risk for functional decline and hospital-acquired events, such as catheter-associated urinary tract infections, pressure ulcers, and falls.

- Older patients are also at risk for geriatric syndromes, such as malnutrition, pneumonia, medication reactions, confusion, and falls.

- The FANCAPES is a comprehensive physical assessment tool to determine the basic needs and functional needs in an acutely ill, medically complex older adult. Frontline nurses should obtain information in each area to determine a plan of care.

- Frontline nurses need to focus on the assessment of function and how the chronic illness affects the quality of care for the older adult and masks the acute illness.

Vulnerability during transitions

Although everyone has many transitions in life, the elderly may have to face major transitions, such as moving out of their homes to long-term care facilities or the death of a spouse or child. For the purpose of this article, transitions for the elderly population refer to the movement of patients from one health care provider or setting to another as their condition and care needs change.[1] Individuals at high risk for vulnerability during transitions are older people with multiple conditions, depression, or other mental health disorders; isolated elders without family or friends; non–English-speaking individuals; immigrants; and low-income patients.[7] Frontline nurses will see this process as patients are moved to either higher acuity levels that require specialty physicians or discharged to long-term care facilities. Often, patients will have new health care providers when they transition, as practitioners may not practice in multiple facilities. When new health care providers are introduced, there may be communication gaps that result in problems with care.

Many factors contribute to the gaps in care during transitions, including poor communication, incomplete transfer of information, inadequate education of older adults and their family members, medication errors, limited access to essential services, and the absence of a single point person to ensure continuity of care.[7,8] These areas are all areas that frontline nurses can impact, especially in the area of communication. Older patients often have complex problems that can be complicated when they experience transitions. Minimizing the number of transfers from unit to unit during a single hospitalization is associated with more consistent nursing care, fewer adverse incidents (eg, nosocomial infections, falls, delirium, and medication errors), shorter hospital stays, and lower overall costs.[9] Frontline nurses can minimize the number of complications associated from in-hospital transfers through understanding geriatric patients, interprofessional communication, and teamwork (**Box 3**).

Box 3
Summary of impacting transition of care for frontline nurses

- Using interprofessional educational concepts of teamwork and communication
- Using geriatric competencies
- Advocating for geriatric patients to minimize transfers
- Identifying high-risk patients

PHYSIOLOGIC CHANGES THAT ACCOMPANY AGING

Frontline nurses are responsible for accurate expert assessment skills. An accurate assessment is important for all patients but requires a few specific changes for geriatric patients. This section provides comprehensive physiologic changes for geriatric patients along with specific assessment, implications for care, and safety considerations. Frontline nurses must be able to incorporate both the physiologic changes and the American Nurses Association's (ANA) standards for geriatric patients into professional practice to provide quality, safe care.

The ANA has provided standards for gerontological nursing practice. They are as follows:

ANA (2010) standards of gerontological nursing practice are

- *Standard 1*: assessment
- *Standard 2*: diagnosis
- *Standard 3*: outcomes identification
- *Standard 4*: planning
- *Standard 5*: implementation
- *Standard 5A*: coordination of care
- *Standard 5B*: health teaching and health promotion
- *Standard 5C*: consultation
- *Standard 5D*: prescriptive authority and treatment
- *Standard 6*: evaluation[5,10]

The process of normal aging in the absence of disease is accompanied by a myriad of physiologic changes in the body systems.[11] The clinical presentation of these changes is of critical importance in the nursing assessment performed by frontline nurses. In order to differentiate from normal physiologic aging and changes associated with pathologic disease process, frontline nurses must be knowledgeable of the physiologic, psychosocial, and functional changes expected with the elderly population.[1]

According to Benner's novice to expert theory, assessment is a task for the expert. As all frontline nurses start as novices or advanced beginner nurses, it is imperative that the resources are available to assist in the health assessment. **Table 6** lists physiologic changes that are considered a normal part of aging with implications for nursing care. This type of resource will assist the nurse in transitioning from a novice to an expert in assessment of the aging population.

Table 6
Physiologic changes that accompany aging

Systems	Physiologic Changes	Implication for Elderly and Nursing Care	Assessment, Care, and Safety Precautions
Eyes	Eyebrows & eyelashes 1. Loss of pigment in hair Eyelids 1. Loss of orbital fat, ↓ muscle tone 2. Tissue atrophy, prolapse of fat into eyelid tissue Conjunctiva 1. Tissue damage related to chronic exposure to ultraviolet light or to other environment exposure Sclera 1. Lipid deposition Cornea 1. Cholesterol deposits in peripheral cornea 2. Tissue damage related to chronic exposure 3. ↓ In water content, atrophy of nerve fibers 4. Epithelial changes 5. Accumulation of lipid deposits Iris 1. ↑ Rigidity of iris 2. Dilator muscle atrophy or weakness 3. Loss of pigment 4. Ciliary muscle becoming smaller, stiffer Lens 1. Biochemical changes in lens proteins, oxidative damage, chronic exposure to ultraviolet light 2. ↑ Rigidity of lens	Eyebrows & eyelashes 1. Graying of eyebrows, eyelashes Eyelids 1. Entropion, ectropion, mild ptosis 2. Blepharodemachalasis (excessive upper lid skin) Conjunctiva 1. Pinuecula (small spot usually on medial aspect of conjunctiva) Sclera 1. Scleral color yellowish opposed to bluish Cornea 1. Arcus senilis (milky white-gray ring encircling periphery of cornea) 2. Pterygium (thickened, triangular bit of pale tissue that extends from inner canthus of eye to nasal border of cornea) 3. ↓ Corneal sensitivity and corneal reflex 4. Loss of corneal luster 5. Blurring of vision Iris 1. ↓ Pupil size 2. Slower recovery of pupil size after light stimulation 3. Change of iris color 4. ↓ In near vision and accommodation Lens 1. Cataracts 2. Presbyopia	Assess eyes every shift Monitor for dryness & irritation Assess history for wearing glasses/contacts Care & safety precautions Provide saline drops as needed Provide call bell within reach If patient has blurred vision, ↓ visual acuity, or changes in accommodation, provide safety protocols specific to facility Have patient's family provide glasses if not with patient Keep glasses within patient's reach Do not allow patient to get up without assistance; explain reasoning to patient and family

(continued on next page)

Table 6
(*continued*)

Systems	Physiologic Changes	Implication for Elderly and Nursing Care	Assessment, Care, and Safety Precautions
	3. Opacities in lens (may also be related to opacities in cornea and vitreous) 4. Accumulation of yellow substances Retina 1. Retinal vascular changes related to atherosclerosis and hypertension 2. ↓ In cones 3. Loss of photoreceptors cells, retinal pigment, epithelial cells, and melanin 4. Age-related macular degeneration as a result of vascular changes Lacrimal apparatus 1. ↓ Tear secretion 2. Malposition of eyelids resulting in tears overflowing lid margins instead of draining through puncta	3. Complaints of glare, night vision impaired 4. Yellow color of lens Retina 1. Narrowed, pale, straighter arterioles; acute branching 2. Changes in color perception, especially blue and violet 3. ↓ Visual acuity 4. Loss of central vision Lacrimal apparatus 1. Dryness 2. Tearing, irritated eyes	
Ear	External ear 1. ↑ Production of & drier cerumen 2. ↑ Hair growth 3. Loss of elasticity in cartilage Middle ear 1. Atrophic changes of tympanic membrane Inner ear 1. Hair cell degeneration, neuron degeneration in auditory nerve & central pathways, reduced blood supply to cochlea, calcification of ossicles 2. Less effective vestibular apparatus in semicircular canals	External ear 1. Impacted cerumen, potential hearing loss 2. Visible hair, especially in men 3. Collapsed ear canal Middle ear 1. Conductive hearing loss Inner ear 1. Presbycusis, diminished sensitivity to high-pitched sounds, impaired speech reception, tinnitus 2. Alteration in balance & body orientation	Assessment may be difficult because of hearing in a noisy environment, heightened sensitivity to loud sounds Speak in a normal voice, but may need to be closer to patient Assess if patient has hearing aid, if the batteries need to be changed, or if patient has hearing aid with them Care & safety precautions Aware that words may sound distorted Have family bring hearing aid if needed Implement safety protocols as needed specific to facility

Hair & nails	Hair 1. ↓ Melanin & melanocytes 2. ↓ Oil 3. ↓ Density of hair 4. Cumulative androgen effect; ↓ estrogen levels Nails 1. ↓ Peripheral blood supply 2. ↑ Keratin 3. ↓ Circulation	Hair 1. Gray or white hair 2. Dry, coarse hair, scaly scalp 3. Thinning and loss of hair; loss of hair in outer half or outer third of eyebrows & back of legs 4. Facial hirsutism, baldness Nails 1. Thick, brittle nails with diminished growth 2. Longitudinal ridging 3. Prolonged return of blood to nails on blanching	General assessment to include hair & nails every shift Assess circulation to extremities if nails are compromised because of the aging process
Integumentary	1. Epidermis thins, making blood vessels and bruises much more visible; T-cell function declines 2. Cell renewal time ↑ by up to one-third after 50 y of age; 30 or more days may be necessary for new epithelial replacement 3. Dermis loses about 20% of its thickness 4. ↓ Subcutaneous fat, collagen synthesis (stiffening)	1. May be a reactivation of latent conditions, such as herpes zoster (shingles) or herpes simplex, making a shingles immunization particularly important 2. Significantly affects wound healing 3. Thinness causes skin to look more transparent and fragile; dermal blood vessels reduced; cool skin temperature 4. Causes the skin to give less under stress and tear more easily; leads to loss of stretch (tenting) and resilience and sagging appearance (breasts)	Because of thinning of skin, tenting cannot be used as a measure of hydration status Skin breakdown happens quickly (can be within 2 h) Assessing skin can be done during bathing time Surgical wounds can be slow to heal Care & safety precautions Assess skin every shift Turn patients every 2 h & as needed Consult wound care specialist Special attention should be paid to prevent skin tears Avoid tape & friction tears

(continued on next page)

Table 6
(continued)

Systems	Physiologic Changes	Implication for Elderly and Nursing Care	Assessment, Care, and Safety Precautions
Cardiac system & blood vessels	1. Myocardial hypertrophy, ↑ collagen and scarring, ↓ elastin 2. Downward displacement 3. ↓ CO, HR, and SV in response to exercise or stress 4. Cellular aging and fibrosis of conduction system 5. Valvular rigidity from calcification, sclerosis, or fibrosis, impeding complete closure of valves 6. Arterial stiffening caused by loss of elastin in arterial walls, thickening of intima arteries, and progressive fibrosis of media 7. ↑ Venous tortuosity	1. ↓ Cardiac reserve, heart failure 2. Difficulty in isolating apical pulse 3. ↓ Response to exercise and stress; slowed recovery from activity 4. ↓ Amplitude of QRS complex and slight lengthening of PR, QRS, and QT intervals; irregular cardiac rhythms, ↓ maximal HR, and HR variability, ↓ 5. Systolic murmur (aortic or mitral) possible without an indication of cardiovascular disease 6. ↑ In systolic BP and possible ↑ or ↓ in diastolic BP; possible widened pulse pressure; pedal pulses diminished; ↑ in intermittent claudication 7. Inflamed, painful, or cordlike varicosities; dependent edema	Assess BP (lying, sitting, and standing) & pulse pressure Cardiac assessment: rate/rhythm/heart sounds; note altered landmarks, distant heart sounds, & extra heart sounds (Systolic grade 3 [S3] in CHF) Palpate carotid artery, peripheral pulses for symmetry Monitor heart rate and rhythm, note irregularity, ECG Assess for dyspnea with exertion, exercise intolerance Care & safety precautions For orthostatic hypertension: Have patient rise slowly from lying or sitting position Wait 1–2 min after position change to stand or transfer patient Monitor for overt signs of hypotension: changes in sensorium/mental status, dizziness, orthostasis,
Genitourinary system	1. ↓ Amount of renal tissue 2. ↓ Number of nephrons and renal blood vessels; thickened basement membrane of Bowman capsule and glomeruli 3. ↓ Function of loop of Henle and tubules 4. ↓ Elasticity and muscle tone 5. Weakening of urinary sphincter 6. ↓ Bladder capacity and sensory receptors 7. Estrogen deficiency leading to thin, dry vaginal tissue	1. Less palpable 2. ↓ Creatinine clearance, ↑ BUN level, ↑ serum creatinine 3. Alterations in drug excretion, nocturia, loss of normal diurnal excretory pattern because of ↓ ability to concentrate urine; less concentrated urine 4. Palpable bladder after urination because of retention	Assess renal function, particularly in acute/chronic illness Monitor BP (orthostatic) Assess for dehydration, volume overload, electrolyte imbalances, proteinuria Determine source of fluid/electrolyte imbalance, monitor laboratory data Assess choice/dose/need for nephrotoxic agents (eg, aminoglycoside antibiotics,

8. ↑ Prevalence of unstable bladder contractions
9. Prostate enlargement (men)

5. Stress incontinence (especially during Valsalva maneuver), dribbling of urine after urination
6. Frequency, urgency, nocturia, overflow incontinence
7. Stress or overactive bladder, dysuria
8. Overactive bladder
9. Hesitancy, frequency, urgency, nocturia, straining to urinate, retention, dribbling

radio contrast dye) and medications excreted through renals
Palpable bladder after voiding caused by retention
Assess for urinary incontinence, UTI
Assess for abnormal urine stream, urinary retention with BPH
Assess fall risk in nocturnal or urgent voiding
Care & safety precautions
• Maintain hydration, baseline fluid/electrolyte balance; prepare for fluid/electrolyte correction as indicated
• Monitor drug levels renally cleared medications
• Calculate creatinine clearance (see addendum)
• Monitor for normal renal function: constant serum creatinine level to baseline
• Safety precautions in nocturnal or urgent voiding & postural hypotension, institute fall prevention strategies

(continued on next page)

Table 6
(continued)

Systems	Physiologic Changes	Implication for Elderly and Nursing Care	Assessment, Care, and Safety Precautions
Respiratory system	Ventilatory capacity ○ ↓ Ventilatory capacity ○ Alveolar dilation ○ Larger air spaces ○ Loss of surface area ○ Diminished elastic recoil ○ ↓ Respiratory muscle strength ○ ↓ Chest wall compliance	• ↓ Cough, deep-clearance • Risk of infection & bronchospasm (airway obstruction) • Altered pulmonary function; lower maximal expiratory flow (FEV, FEV_1/FVC_1) ○ ↑ Residual volume ○ Reduced vital capacity ○ Unchanged total lung capacity • Dyspnea after exertion, ↓ exercise tolerance • ↓ Po_2, SpO_2; ↓ Capacity to maintain acid-base balance • Respiratory rate 12–24 (Breaths per minute)	Respirations: rate, pattern, breath sounds throughout lung fields Note thorax appearance, chest expansion Assess cough, deep breathing, exercise capacity Monitor arterial blood gases, pulse oximetry Monitor secretions, sedation, positioning, which can reduce ventilation/oxygenation Care & safety precautions Maintain patent airway through repositioning, suctioning, bronchodilators Prevention of respiratory infections with pulmonary Incentive spirometry as indicated, particularly if unable to ambulate or decline in function Education on cough enhancement, avoidance of environmental contaminants, smoking cessation Maintain hydration and mobility Provide oxygen as needed
Gastrointestinal system	Mouth 1. Gingival retraction 2. ↓ Taste buds, ↓ sense of smell 3. ↓ Volume of saliva 4. Atrophy of gingival tissue Esophagus	Mouth • Loss of teeth, dental implants, dentures, difficulty chewing • Diminshed sense of taste (especially salty and sweet) • Dry oral mucosa • Poor-fitting dentures	• Assess abdomen (note smaller liver), bowel sounds • Monitor weight, dietary intake, elimination patterns, fluid intake • Assess dentition, chewing, & swallowing abilities, eating habits/nutrition

1. Lower esophageal sphincter pressure ↓, motility ↓

Abdominal wall
1. Thinner and less taut
2. ↓ Number and sensitivity of sensory receptors

Stomach
1. Atrophy of gastric mucosa, ↓ blood flow

Small intestines
1. Slightly ↓ motility and secretion of most digestive enzymes

Liver
1. ↓ Size and lowered position
2. ↓ Protein synthesis, ability to regenerate ↓

Large intestine, anus, rectum
1. ↓ Anal sphincter tone and nerve supply to rectal area
2. ↓ Muscular tone, ↓ motility
3. ↑ Transit time, ↓ sensation to defecation

Pancreas
1. Pancreatic ducts distended, lipase production ↓, pancreatic reserve impaired

Esophagus
• Epigastric distress, dysphagia, potential for hiatal hernia and aspiration

Abdominal wall
• More visible peristalsis, easier palpation of organs
• Less sensitivity to surface pain

Stomach
• Food intolerances, signs of anemia as result of cobalamin malabsorption, slower gastric emptying

Small intestines
• Complaints of indigestion, slowed intestinal transit, delayed absorption of fat-soluble vitamins

Liver
• Easier palpation because of lower border extending past costal margin
• ↓ Drug & hormone metabolism

Large intestine, anus, rectum
• Fecal incontinence
• Flatulence, abdominal distention, relaxed perineal musculature
• Constipation, fecal impaction

Pancreas

• Assess lungs for basilar crackles, infection from aspiration
• Evaluate poor food intake

Care & safety precautions
• 3-d calorie count, consultation with dietician for poor intake/unplanned weight loss
• Monitor drug levels and liver function tests if on medications metabolized in liver; electrolytes, BUN/creatinine, albumin (nutritional indicator and if low effects drug levels like digoxin)
• Monitor for signs of dysphagia, coughing or choking with solids/liquids. Speech &/or swallowing evaluation as indicated
• Monitor for signs of aspiration particularly if decline in function/weakness; GERD
• Monitor nutrition/diet intake, fluid intake, elimination particularly if immobile. Maintain mobility.
• Provide laxatives if on constipating medications (eg, narcotics)

(continued on next page)

Table 6
(continued)

Systems	Physiologic Changes	Implication for Elderly and Nursing Care	Assessment, Care, and Safety Precautions
Musculoskeletal system	Muscle • ↓ Number and diameter of muscle cells; replacement of muscle cells by fibrous connective tissue • Loss of elasticity in ligaments, tendons, and cartilage • Reduced ability to store glycogen • ↓ Ability to release glycogen as quick energy during stress • ↓ Basal metabolic rate Joints • ↑ Risk for cartilage erosion that contributes to direct contact between bone ends and overgrowth of bone around joint margins • Loss of water from disks between vertebrae, ↓ height of intervertebral spaces Bone • ↓ Bone density and strength, brittleness • Slowed remodeling process	• Impaired fat absorption, ↓ glucose tolerance Muscle • ↓ Muscle strength and mass, abdominal protrusion, flabby muscles • ↑ Rigidity in neck, shoulders, back, hips, and knees • Fine-motor dexterity, ↓ agility • Slowed reaction times and reflexes as a result of slowing of impulse conduction along motor units; earlier fatigue with activity Joints • Joint stiffness, decreased mobility, limited ROM, possible crepitation on movement; pain with motion and/or weight bearing • Loss of height and shortening of trunk from disk compression; posture change Bone • Loss of height and deformity, such as dowager hump (kyphosis) from vertebral compression and degeneration • Back pain, stiffness • Bony prominences more pronounced • ↑ Risk of osteopenia and osteoporosis	• Assess functionality, mobility, symmetry and strength, fine & gross motor skills, ADLs • Ensure joint stabilization and slow movements in ROM examination to prevent injury • Conduct gentle passive ROM if active ROM is not possible; osteoarthritis is very common, and pain is often undertreated • Institute or implement facility policy for fall risk and mobility protocols Care & safety precautions • Maintain maximal function, encourage/provide active or passive ROM • Assess for pain and provide pain medication to enhance functionality • Demonstrate/encourage muscle strengthening exercises • Referrals to physical/occupational therapy • Fall risk interventions, avoid restraints
Nervous system & cognition	Brain 1. ↓ Cerebral blood flow and metabolism 2. ↓ Efficiency of temperature-regulating mechanism 3. ↓ Neurotransmitters, loss of neurons 4. ↓ O₂ supply	Brain 1. Alterations in mental functioning 2. Impaired ability to adapt to environmental temperature 3. Conduction of nerve impulses slowed, response time slowed	Assess baseline; periodic reassess of functional status during acute illness Assess gait and balance Assess muscle strength, which may be ↓ but should be equal on both sides

5. Cerebral tissue atrophy and ↑ size of ventricles	4. Changes in gait and ambulation; diminished kinesthetic	Assess baseline cognition and periodic reassessment
Peripheral nervous system: cranial & spinal nerves	5. Altered balance, vertigo, syncope, ↑ postural hypotension; proprioception diminished; ↓ sensory input	Monitor orthostatic BP
1. Loss of myelin and ↓ conduction time	Peripheral nervous system: cranial & spinal nerves	Care & safety precautions
2. Cellular degeneration, death of neurons	1. ↓ Reaction time in specific nerves	• Monitor for delirium during acute illness
Functional divisions: motor, sensory, & reflexes	2. ↓ Speed and intensity of neuronal reflexes	• Institute fall prevention strategies
1. ↓ Muscle bulk	Functional divisions: motor, sensory, & reflexes	• Rise slowly from lying, sitting positions; wait 1–2 min prior to transfer
2. ↓ Sensory receptors	1. Diminished strength and agility	
3. ↓ Electrical activity	2. Diminished sense of touch, pain, and temperature	
4. Atrophy of taste buds	3. Slowing of or alteration in sensory reception	
5. Degeneration of loss of fibers in olfactory	4. Signs of malnutrition, weight loss	
6. Degeneration changes in nerve cells in inner ear, cerebellum, and proprioceptive pathways	5. Diminished sense of smell	
7. ↓ Deep tendon reflexes	6. Poor ability to maintain balance, widened gait	
8. ↓ Sensory conduction velocity	7. Below-average reflex score	
Reticular formation: reticular activating system	8. Sluggish reflexes, slowing of reaction time	
1. Modification of hypothalamic function, ↓ stage IV sleep	Reticular formation: reticular activating system	
Autonomic nervous system: sympathetic nervous system & parasympathetic nervous system	1. Disturbances in sleep patterns	
1. Morphologic features of ganglia, slowing of autonomic nervous system responses	Autonomic nervous system: sympathetic nervous system & parasympathetic nervous system	
	1. Orthostatic hypotension, systolic hypertension	

Abbreviations: ADLS, activities of daily living; BP, blood pressure; BPH, benign prostatic hyperplasia; BUN, blood urea oxygen; CHF, congestive heart failure; CO, cardiac output; ECG, electrocardiogram; FVC, forced vital capacity; FEV, forced expiratory volume; FEV1, forced expiratory volume in 1 second; GERD, gastroesophageal reflux disease; HR, heart rate; O_2, oxygen; ROM, range of motion; SV, stroke volume; UTI, urinary tract infection.
Data from Refs[5,6,12]; Deborah Ellison, Critical Care work and educational experience, 1999–2014, unpublished.

ADVANCING CARE EXCELLENCE FOR SENIORS ESSENTIAL NURSING ACTIONS

The ACES project further identifies 4 essential actions to promote high-quality care for the elderly. These actions include assessing function and expectations, coordinating and managing care, using evolving knowledge, and making situational decisions.[4] **Table 7** gives the ACES explanation for each essential action.

Table 7 ACES essential nursing actions	
Assess function and expectations	• Assess, respond to, and respect an older adult's functional status and strengths, wishes, and expectations. • Determine the older adult's function and expectations, along with cognition, mood, culture, physiologic status, and comfort, to obtain a comprehensive assessment of the health care needs. • Use standardized assessment tools to assess the older adult's individual aging pattern.
Coordinate and manage care	• Manage chronic conditions, including atypical presentations, in daily life and during life transitions to maximize function and maintain independence. • Assist older adults and families/caregivers to access knowledge and evaluate resources. • Advocate during acute exacerbations of chronic conditions to prevent complications.
Use evolving knowledge	• Understand geriatric syndromes and unique presentations of common diseases in older adults. • Access and use emerging information and research evidence about the special care needs of older adults and appropriate treatment options. • Interpret findings and evaluate clinical situations in order to provide high-quality nursing care based on current knowledge and best practices.

Courtesy of the National League for Nursing, Washington, DC; with permission. Available at: http://www.nln.org/facultyprograms/facultyresources/aces/pdf/essential_nursing_actions.pdf.

PAIN MANAGEMENT

Frontline nurses are responsible for the assessment, treatment, and documentation of pain in all patients. The Joint Commission on Accreditation of Healthcare Organizations mandates health care workers must take a proactive persistent approach to the screening and assessment of pain, which is now considered the fifth vital sign. Although there are many ways that pain can be assess in patients, the gold standard for assessment and treatment is for the patient to self-report their pain. To further assist the frontline to accurately assess and treat pain, the PQRST should be used (**Box 4**).[11]

Box 4 PQRST method of pain assessment
P = Provokes the pain (what causes makes it better or makes it worse)
Q = Quality of the pain (sharp, dull, throbbing, stabbing, and/or crushing)
R = Radiation of the pain (does it move or stay in one place)
S = Severity of the pain (on a scale of 1 to 10)
T = Time (when did it start, how long did it last)

From Touhy T, Jett K. Ebersole and Hess' Gerontological nursing & healthy aging. 4th edition. Mosby; 2014; with permission.

Studies on pain in older adults show that pain is prevalent but often underreported.

- Fifty percent of adults aged 65 years and older report they experienced pain in the last 30 days.[13]
- One in 4 adults reported suffering daylong pain in the last month.[13]
- Up to 80% of nursing home residents experience pain regularly without treatment or relief of pain.[14]
- More than 80% of older adults have chronic medical conditions that are typically associated with pain, such as osteoarthritis and peripheral vascular disease.[15]
- Older adults often have multiple medical conditions, both chronic and/or acute, and may suffer from multiple types and sources of pain.[15]

It may be difficult for researchers to determine the accuracy of the reported prevalence of pain in older persons. The reasons for this difficulty are that pain may be overreported in order to seek attention from family and there may be a lack of reporting because of a fear of being labeled as complainer.

Pain Myths

Pain myths are barriers to seeking adequate pain management in the older adult. Frontline nurses need to educate patients and families about pain myths that could prevent treating the pain appropriately and prevent patients from reporting their pain.[16] **Box 5** summarizes these myths.

Box 5
Myths of pain in the geriatric population

Myth: Pain is a normal part of aging.

Fact: Pain is not normal with aging. The presence of pain in the elderly necessitates aggressive assessment, diagnosis, and management similar to younger individuals. The occurrence of pain increases with age and multiple disease processes.

Myth: Pain sensitivity and perception decrease with aging.

Fact: Research is conflicting regarding age-associated changes in pain perception, sensitivity, and tolerance. Chronic pain can cause a higher tolerance to pain, nevertheless the pain still exists and can be misleading to pain assessments and treatment.

Myth: If an elderly person does not complain of much pain, they must not be in pain.

Fact: Older individuals may not report pain for a variety of reasons. They may think pain is normal. Culturally they may think that the report of pain is inappropriate or that they are being a burden to nurses or family.

Myth: A person who seems to have no functional impairment and is occupied in activities of daily living must not have significant pain.

Fact: People have a variety of reactions to pain. Many individuals are stoic and refuse to give in to their pain. Over extended periods of time, the elderly may mask any outward signs of pain.

Myth: Narcotic medications are inappropriate for the elderly with chronic nonmalignant pain.

Fact: Opioid analgesics are often indicated in nonmalignant pain and are safe when pain is assessed and used appropriately. Although the elderly may be more sensitive to narcotics, this does not justify withholding narcotics and failing to relieve pain.

Data from Touhy T, Jett K. Ebersole and Hess' Gerontological nursing & healthy aging. 4th edition. St. Louis (MO): Mosby; 2014. p. 233–59; and Assessment and management of pain in the elderly: self-directed learning package for nurses in long-term care. Toronto: Registered Nurses' Association of Ontario; 2007. Available at: http://www.pulserx.ca/docs/Assessment_and_Management_of_Pain_in_the_Elderly.pdf.

Pain can be defined in many ways. It is a personal experience and integrates cultural and spiritual beliefs. Frontline nurses need to assess subjective pain data if possible because patients are the ones experiencing the pain. Objective data can be obtained if patients are unable to communicate and to validate the subjective data. Frontline nurses need to conduct a comprehensive pain assessment and review the physical history of patients to develop a pain management program.[5]

Subjective Pain Assessment

Frontline nurses need to ask patients specific questions to elicit the type of pain, level of pain, and duration of pain to develop an individualized pain program for patients. **Box 6** contains questions that frontline nurses can ask to collect subjective data.

Box 6
Subjective pain assessment

Sample self-report questions

Where is your pain?

How do you describe your pain? (sharp, dull, throbbing, pulling, constant, intermittent)

How often do you have the pain? (daily, all day, only when I walk, in the morning, and so forth)

How long does it last?

What makes your pain better? (heat, cold, walking, medicines)

What have you tried to relieve the pain?

What makes your pain worse? (weather, heat, cold, activity)

How does your pain affect your daily life? (sleep, attending activities, visiting with friends, appetite, and so forth)

What else do you want to tell me about your pain?

From National Institute of Nursing Research. Palliative Care. Available at http://cancer.ucsf.edu/_docs/sms/PalliativeCare.pdf.

Objective Pain Assessment

It is important for frontline nurses to assess objective data. These data can validate the pain experience of patients and let nurses know if the pain is being underreported. If patients are unable to communicate their pain, frontline nurses can assess the nonverbal expressions of pain, such as limiting movement, grimacing, swelling, rubbing a body part, limping, agitation, and/or discoloration. Also watch for changes in behavior from the patients' usual patterns.[15]

Another objective assessment tool is a numeric pain intensity scale. This tool asks patients to rate their pain by assigning a numerical value, with zero indicating no pain and 10 representing the worst pain imaginable. Although this may be valuable with some patients, the elderly may have trouble thinking in the abstract, making the tool unreliable. The verbal descriptor scale asks patients to describe their pain from *no pain* to *pain as bad as it could be*. Finally, the faces pain scale has been revised and validated for use with adults and the elderly. It can be accessed at www.iasp-pain.org/FPSR.[16,17]

Cognitive-Impaired Pain Patients

Older adults may have cognitive impairments, such as dementia, Alzheimer disease, or other illnesses that limit thinking. Patients who are not able to express themselves verbally usually receive less pain medicines. The nurse should try eliciting information from family members about patients' verbal and nonverbal/behavioral expressions of pain. Other signs of pain in those patients with dementia include increased agitation, aggression, increasing confusion, or passivity. If frontline nurses assess objective data for pain or patients have a condition that normally causes pain, nurses should assume they have pain and treat accordingly.[15]

Pain Management Modalities

An overall goal in pain relief might be that all older adults will either be pain free or their pain will be controlled to a level that is acceptable to patients and allows them to maintain the highest level of functioning possible. Specific goals in comfort care and pain relief might be the following: to report a reduced pain level to less than 5 in 5 days, patients will get at least 5 hours of uninterrupted sleep, and patients are able to perform activities of daily living without complaint. Goals for pain relief must be made mutually with the client. Treatment of pain in the elderly is diverse and includes pharmacologic and nonpharmacologic methods.

The World Health Organization has identified a pain ladder for pain relief. Begin with a nonopioid first plus ancillary activities. Acetaminophen is the most common, followed by nonsteroidal antiinflammatory drugs. Three basic principles for pain relief are to administer pain drugs on a regular basis to maintain therapeutic levels, use as-needed medications for breakthrough pain, and give pain medicine before starting an activity that causes pain. For mild to moderate or increasing pain that is not relieved with nonopioids, begin use of opioid analgesics. Begin with the lowest dose that relieves the pain, increasing as necessary. Nurses are traditionally afraid to give opioid medications to the elderly for fear of overdose or becoming addicted. When giving opioids to the elderly, nurses must watch closely for negative effects that may occur because of age and disease-related changes.[8,18]

Finally, there are nonpharmacologic pain reliefs that should be encouraged. These techniques must be tailored to the individual. Examples of these are relaxation therapy, distraction, heat, cold, transcutaneous electrical nerve stimulation units, tai chi, and yoga. It may be difficult to convince the elderly to try tai chi or yoga; research has shown that these activities improve movement, reduce pain and stiffness, enhance sleep, increase mental status, and perhaps increase immune response.[19,20]

END OF LIFE ISSUES

End-of-life issues are complicated at any time; but with the elderly, there are additional complexities. Two of these complexities are patients having comorbidities that are not related to the terminal illness and the attitudes of nurses about the elderly and death (you are old, so it is OK to die). Older Americans with chronic illness most often want their lives to end with a good death without persistent pain, uncomfortable symptoms, and additional technology.[21] A good death is one whereby the needs are met to the extent possible. The process of dying takes energy. The dying person, the caregivers, and the nurse all require extra energy to successfully work through the process. Helping those working through this process requires a specialized blend of sensitivity, insight, and knowledge to assess and plan effective interventions.[5] Dying is an individual process. How one approaches the experience is a reflection of the way one has lived their life and responded to other losses, the circumstances, and culture.

Death Theories

The most well-known theory related to the dying process is the work of Dr Elizabeth Kubler-Ross[22] from her 1969 book *On Death and Dying.* In this book, she developed the concept related to the coping mechanisms of the dying. The fluid stages of denial, anger, bargaining, depression, and acceptance serve as a framework to assist the nurse in supporting patients and families throughout the process. More about this theory can be found at http://psychcentral.com/lib/the-5-stages-of-loss-and-grief/000617. Another theory proposed by Pattison in 1977[23] refers to the living-dying interval. Phases are identified rather than stages. These phases are the acute, chronic, and terminal phase. The living-dying interval is accordionlike and may take weeks, months, or years to progress. No matter what theory is used, dying is a unique experience; theories of grief and bereavement can help to consolidate the many ideas about how people deal with the death of a loved one. Health care professionals need to ensure that they respect the individuality of the dying and the bereaved person and offer appropriate person-centered care and support.[5]

End-of-Life Fears and Wishes

Patients fear that their pain, symptoms, anxiety, emotional suffering, and family concerns will be ignored. Many fear that their wishes (advance directives) will be disregarded and that they will face death alone and in misery.[21] When seriously ill patients were asked to identify quality end-of-life care and measures to overcome their fears, several important themes emerged and are overviewed in **Table 8**.[5,24–26]

Table 8 End-of-life wishes	
Good Death Wishes	**Ways Nursing can Assist**
Freedom from pain and suffering	Offer palliative care early in treatment. Use opiate drugs as needed; addiction is not problem. Give emotional and spiritual support. Provide freedom from nausea, respiratory distress, constipation, and fatigue.
Being at peace with God or spiritually content	Remain sensitive to the preferences of patients. Ask the following questions: What gives you the strength to face life's challenges? Do you feel a connection with a higher being or spirit? What gives your live meaning?
Presence of family	Allow opportunities for reminiscing and talking with family. Assist patients to leave a legacy for family in the ways of letters, video, or tape. Encourage patients to express feelings: I love you, thank you, I forgive you, forgive me.
Being cognitively aware	Keep patients alert enough to say good-bye or to express feelings of peace and contentment.
Having treatment choices honored	Honor advance directives. Listened to patients when asked about removing tubes, not eating, or going home.
Having affairs in order	Facilitate communication regarding funeral plans. Facilitate discussion of wills or estate planning to complete.

Data from Refs.[5,24–26]

Obstacles to End-of-Life Experiences

Lack of communication between the stakeholders may be the largest obstacle to a good death. Communication is lacking in discussion of treatment options and advance directives. It is lacking in the area of palliative care and hospice. And there is a lack of knowledge by the health care providers on cultural and spiritual aspects of death.

Older adults want better discussions, information, and a chance to influence decisions about their care, whether to be at home or in the hospital. Having the talk about the end of life is difficult on both the patients' and the families' side. There is difficulty talking about dying and treatment options.[21] In an ideal world, the discussion about advance directives takes place when patients are healthy. Advance directives and health care surrogates are essential for the communication of a person's end-of-life wishes. Despite acceptance of advance care planning and advance directives in the care of older patients, less than 30% of Americans, including those with chronic disease, have advance directives. And of these 30%, only 15% have them noted in the chart or with family.[27] The nurse serves as an advocate for the client and must encourage discussions on end of life issues.[21] Once advance directives or health care surrogates are defined the information must be put in the chart and communicated to all persons involved in the care both in the hospital and at home.

There is a lack of discussion about palliative care and hospice. Many health care providers are not experts in symptom management. Palliative care is the standard for persistently ill or dying patients.[21,26] Additionally, many dying seniors are getting aggressive care spending time in intensive care units immediately before dying. Unless preferences are known, patients may undergo unwanted, distressing, and costly treatments that impair their quality of life, increase suffering, and distress loved ones. For many patients, palliative care and hospice are afterthoughts and are instituted at the last minute. Patients are unable to benefit from the psychosocial and physical support hospice offers. Nurses and health care providers need further education on the benefits of palliative care and hospice to dying patients. Additionally, patients and families need to talk to their health care providers early in their treatment about end-of-life care to avoid aggressive therapy.[28] Palliative care can be provided at any time and not just within the hospice benefit. **Box 7** summarizes palliative care.

Box 7
Palliative care

Palliative care strives to provide patients with

- Expert treatment of pain and other symptoms so patients can get the best relief possible
- Open discussion about treatment choices, including treatment of patients' disease and management of their symptoms
- Coordination of patients' care with all of their health care providers
- Emotional support for patients and their families
- Ensuring that care is more in line with patients' wishes
- Meeting emotional and spiritual needs of patients
- Comprehensive treatment of discomfort

Data from National Institute of Nursing Research. Palliative Care. Available at: http://cancer.ucsf.edu/_docs/sms/PalliativeCare.pdf. Accessed July 26, 2014.

Our knowledge of how culture influences choices about end of life is scant. The sociocultural values of many culturally diverse groups conflict with the values on which the use of advance directives is based. Clinicians may lack sensitivity to the sociocultural beliefs that influence decisions affecting end-of-life care and may not have the knowledge to increase flexibility in practices and standards in the application of advance directives.[21]

Caregiver Questions and Support

Nurses must be aware that the caregivers or families may travel through the emotional stages of dying at different times than the patients. Patients and their families have many questions and concerns about end-of-life care. **Table 9** summarizes possible questions a caregiver may present to the nurse.

Table 9 Caregiver questions	
Questions	**Possible Answers**
How long will they live?	• The time of death is unique for each individual. • Answer questions honestly as they arise. • Try not to instill false hope or destroy any hope.
When should the caregiver ask for professional help?	When patients • Are in unrelieved pain • Have trouble breathing and seem upset • Are unable to urinate or empty bowels • Have fallen • Seem depressed and talking about suicide • Have difficulty swallowing medicine or refuse to take medicine
How can I help? It is better not to ask the person "how can I help" but simply look for ways that will ease the time.	• Make a special meal or treat, take a drive, watch a movie, read to them. • Listen when your loved one wants to talk. They may not need advice but rather a sounding board for fears and concerns. • Allow them to reminisce about life. • Allow them to express fears and concerns about dying, and then assist them with actions or care. • Do not obsess about the illness and treatment unless they want to talk about it. • Help them maintain dignity and control by not treating them as invalids. Make them feel fears and concerns. Erm caremily planning. Go about your day as regular as possible. • Respect the need for privacy.
What are the signs of impending death?	• Drowsiness or increased sleeping • Confusion about time, place, and/or identity of loved ones • Visions of people and places that are not present (do not contradict or argue with what they see. These visions are normal). • Withdrawal from socialization (patients may be able to hear, so continue to talk with them). • Decreased need for food and fluids (allow patients to eat and drink what and when they want). • Loss of bladder or bowel control or darkened or decreasing urine • Skin cool to the touch; cover with blankets as needed • Rattling or gurgling sounds with breathing; raise head of bed with pillows to ease breathing

Data from Refs.[5,20]

Identifying the approach of death enables the family the chance to share the last minutes of the life with the loved one. The family or a pastor may be called in. It is especially important that during these last minutes patients are talked to and reassured. A simple holding of hands can be reassuring.

Finally, caring for dying patients and their families does not end with death. If families are in hospice, bereavement care is provided for family members for a minimum of 1 year following the death. This support includes visits, calls, and mailings from the social worker and chaplain. If not in hospice care, nurses assist families by providing support and helping them contact others who can assist in the process. Referral to a bereavement group, the funeral director, pastor, or a social worker can assist families through the many activities following death. There is no one way to grieve. Grief lasts as long as it takes to adjust to the changes in your life.[5,19]

There is one last word about the nursing staff. Caring for older adults at the end of life requires knowledge and skills related to the dying process and relief of symptoms. To be successful, it also requires that nurses have explored their own reactions to dying patients and have developed a personal philosophy related to life and death. It requires coping skills and a comfort with their own lives in order to work with the sadness and grief of others.[20]

SUMMARY

Our aging population is rapidly growing and accounts for 46% of critical care patients and 60% of medical-surgical patients in the hospital. These acutely ill patients are challenging to frontline nurses because they also frequently have multiple chronic conditions. Many older patients are at risk for functional decline and hospital-acquired events, such as catheter-associated urinary tract infections, pressure ulcers, and falls. Older patients are also at risk for geriatric syndromes, such as malnutrition, pneumonia, medication reactions, confusion, and falls. These vulnerable and complex older adults require the development of specific gerontological skills in order to meet their unique needs. Frontline nurses are charged with the ethical duty and responsibility to develop these skills. This article provides a tool kit of resources and clinical skills to develop safe, quality, and accountable care plans for positive patient outcomes. This article presents several resources to assist in individualized care, the complexity of care for the elderly, and the issues of transitions of care. **Table 6** presents comprehensive physiologic changes for geriatric patients along with specific assessment, implications for care, and safety considerations provides a framework for assessment skills to differentiate from normal physiologic aging and changes associated with pathologic disease process. Older adults may have cognitive impairments that limit their ability to participate in a pain management program. Aging adult pain tools and a tailored pain management program are presented as resources. End-of-life issues are complicated at any time; but with the elderly, there are additional complexities. An overview of end-of-life issues are discussed along with death theories, end-of-life fears and wishes, obstacles to the end of life, caregiver support, and the role of palliative care. This article empowers frontline nurses to develop gerontological skills and meet the unique needs of our aging population.

REFERENCES

1. Touhy T, Jett K. Ebersole and Hess' gerontological nursing & healthy aging. 4th edition. St. Louis (MO): Mosby; 2014.

2. U.S. Department of Health and Human Services. Healthy people 2020. Topics and objectives: older adults. 2012. Available at: http://www.healthypeople.gov/2020. Accessed July 1, 2014.

3. Tagliareni E, Cline DD, Mengel A, et al. Quality care for older adults: advancing care excellence for seniors (ACES) project. Nurs Educ Perspect 2012;33(3):144–9.

4. ACES. Essential nursing actions. Available at: http://www.nln.org/facultyprograms/facultyresources/aces/pdf/essential_nursing_actions.pdf. Accessed July 1, 2014.

5. Eliopoulos C. Gerontological nursing. 7th edition. Philadelphia: Lippincott Williams & Wilkins; 2010.

6. Jarvis C. Physical examination and health assessment. 6th edition. Philadelphia: Saunders; 2011.

7. Graham C, Ivey S, Neuhauser L. From hospital to home: assessing the transitional care needs of vulnerable seniors. Gerontologist 2009;49:23.

8. Naylor M, Keating S. Transitional care: moving patients from one care setting to another. Am J Nurs 2008;108(Suppl 9):58.

9. Kanak MF, Titler M, Shever L, et al. The effect of hospitalization on multiple units. Appl Nurs Res 2008;21(1):15–22.

10. The American Nurses Association. Geriatrics. Available at: http://www.nursingworld.org/MainMenuCategories/ThePracticeofProfessionalNursing/Improving-Your-Practice/Diversity-Awareness/Elderly. Accessed July 1, 2014.

11. Crozer Keystone Center for Nursing. Best practices: PQRST method facilitates accurate pain assessment. Available at: http://www.crozerkeystone.org/healthcare-professionals/nursing/crozer-keystone-nurses-in-the-news/eNewsletters/2010/february-march/best-practices-pqrst-method/. Accessed July 24, 2014.

12. Lewis S, Dirksen S, Heitkemper M, et al. Medical-surgical nursing: assessment and management of clinical problems. 9th edition. St. Louis (MO): Mosby; 2014.

13. National Center for Health Statistics. National Center for Health Statistics report: health, United States, 2006 special feature on pain. 2006. Available at: http://www.cdc.gov/nchs/pressroom/06facts/hus06.htm. Accessed September 27, 2014.

14. Zanocchi M, Maero B, Nicola E, et al. Chronic pain in a sample of nursing home residents: prevalence, characteristics, influence on quality of life (QoL). Arch Gerontol Geriatr 2008;47:121–8.

15. Horgas AL, Yoon SL. Pain: nursing standard of practice protocol pain management in older adults. Available at: http://consultgerirn.org/topics/pain/want_to_know_more. Accessed July 2, 2012.

16. Kapadia S, Rekai J, Rekai P. Assessment and management of pain in the elderly: self-directed learning package for nurses in long-term care. Toronto: Registered Nurses' Association of Ontario; 2007. Available at: http://www.pulserx.ca/docs/Assessment_and_Management_of_Pain_in_the_Elderly.pdf.

17. Flaherty E. Pain assessment for older adults from the Hartford Institute for Geriatric Nursing Care to older adults general assessment series, New York University, College of Nursing. Issue Number 7, revised 2012. Greenberg SA, PhD(c), MSN, GNP-BC, editor-in-chief. Available at: www.ConsultGeriRN.org. Accessed July 24, 2014.

18. World Health Organization. WHO's pain ladder. Available at: www.who.int/cancer/palliative/painladder/en. Accessed July 24, 2014.

19. National Hospice and Palliative Care Organization. Available at: http://www.nhpco.org/; http://cancer.ucsf.edu/_docs/sms/PalliativeCare.pdf. Accessed September 26, 2014.

20. Marlo S, contributing editor. 2014 Aging care. Available at: http://www.agingcare. com/Articles/end-of-life-care-for-dying-loved-one-123287.htm. Accessed July 3, 2014.
21. End-of-life care fact sheet. Prepared by Sharon Valente, RN, PhD, FAAN, in collaboration with the other members of the APA Ad Hoc Committee on End-of-Life Issues. APA 2014. Available at: http://www.apa.org/pi/aids/programs/eol/end-of-life-factsheet.aspx. Accessed July 24, 2014.
22. Kübler-Ross E. On Death and Dying [e-book]. London: Tavistock Publications; 1973.
23. Pattison EM. The experience of dying. In: Pattison EM, editor. The experience of dying. Englewood Cliffs (NJ): Prentice-Hall; 1977. p. 44–8.
24. Kuebler KK, Heidrich DE, Esper P. Palliative and end-of-life care. 2nd edition. St. Louis (MO): Mosby; 2007. p. 35.
25. Preparing for approaching death. Available at: https://www.hospicenet.org/html/preparing_for.html. Accessed July 26, 2014.
26. National Institute of Nursing Research. Palliative care. Available at: http://cancer. ucsf.edu/_docs/sms/PalliativeCare.pdf. Accessed July 26, 2014.
27. Yung VY, Walling AM, Min L. Elders' preferences for end-of-life care are not captured by documentation in their medical records: research activities, June 2011, vol. 370. Rockville (MD): Agency for Healthcare Research and Quality; 2011. Available at: http://archive.ahrq.gov/news/newsletters/research-activities/jun11/0611RA.pdf. Accessed July 1, 2014.
28. Nordqvist A. End-of-life care for elderly often too aggressive. MediLexicon, Intl. Medical News Today 2013;6. Web.

Index

Note: Page numbers of article titles are in **boldface** type.

A

ACTS. *See* Health literacy ACTS.

Advanced practice nurses, education for, Institute of Medicine's proposal for, 6

Advancing Care Excellence for Seniors (ACES), essential nursing actions in, 204

Advocacy strategies, transforming nursing care through health literacy ACTS, 92–95
  assess health materials and health environments, 92–94
  collaborate with patients and peers, 94
  survey evidence to maintain standards, 95
  train with peers to implement health literacy competencies, 94

Affordable Care Act (ACA), health care reform in, 10
  hospital readmission reduction program, 8–9

Agency for Healthcare Research and Quality, quality indicators from, 38

Aging population, transforming nursing care for, **185–213**
  Advanced Care Excellence for Seniors (ACES), essential nursing actions in, 204
  end-of-life issues, 207–211
  essential knowledge domains, 186–194
  pain management for, 204–207
  physiologic changes in, 194–204

Ambulatory care nursing, projected changes in, 11

American Association of Colleges of Nursing (AACN), integrating cultural diversity using tool kit from, 104–105

American Society for Quality, 37

Asthma, pediatric, case study of case management, 118–119

B

Balance, work-life, for a healthy practice environment, 176–179

Bariatric patients, ergonomics for safe patient handling and mobility in, 161–162

Best practices. *See* Evidence-based practice.

C

Cardiopulmonary resuscitation (CPR), family presence during, role of research in best practices for, 22, 24

Care coordination, projected changes in, 11–12

Case management, **109–121**
  characteristics, knowledge, and skill sets, 113–114
  current issues related to, 110–112
  definition, 110
  pediatric asthma case study, 118–119
  practice settings, 113
  process, 115

Nurs Clin N Am 50 (2015) 215–226
http://dx.doi.org/10.1016/S0029-6465(15)00011-0
0029-6465/15/$ – see front matter © 2015 Elsevier Inc. All rights reserved.

nursing.theclinics.com